Essential Procedures for Emergency, Urgent, and Primary Care Settings

Theresa M. Campo, DNP, APRN, FNP-C, ENP-BC, FAANP, received a doctor of nursing practice degree from Case Western Reserve University in Cleveland, Ohio, and a master's of science in nursing degree from Widener University in Chester, Pennsylvania. Theresa has over 23 years' experience in emergency medicine as a registered professional nurse and advanced practice nurse. She is board certified by the American Academy of Nurse Practitioners as a family nurse practitioner and the American Nurses Credentialing Center as an emergency nurse practitioner.

Dr. Campo is the co-director of the Family Nurse Practitioner track and associate clinical professor for the College of Nursing and Health Professions at Drexel University in Philadelphia, Pennsylvania. She works clinically as an emergency nurse practitioner in the emergency department at Atlanticare Regional Medical Center in Atlantic City, New Jersey, and is an adjunct professor at Case Western Reserve University. Dr. Campo has lectured nationally and internationally, as well as authored articles in peer-reviewed scholarly journals and is on the editorial board for the *Advanced Emergency Nursing Journal*.

Keith A. Lafferty, MD, FAAEM, received his BA in biology cum laude from Holy Family University in 1989 and his MD from the Medical College of Pennsylvania in 1994. At the completion of his training, his colleagues bestowed him with the "Senior Resident Teaching" award. Following his residency in emergency medicine and a fellowship in critical care, he spent 6 years in full academics as a medical student director and a critical care director. Dr. Lafferty currently is the emergency medicine director of education and process improvement at Gulf Coast Medical Center, adjunct assistant professor of emergency medicine at Temple University, director of emergency medical service education, and board member of the Holy Family University Pre-Medical Committee.

As a physician, Dr. Lafferty specializes in emergency medicine and practices in both Philadelphia and Florida. As an author, he has written numerous chapters and manuscripts, mostly having to do with critical care procedures of emergency medicine, with an emphasis on the airway. He has presented many of his research papers at the local and national levels.

Dr. Lafferty has traveled to Haiti, participating in mission expeditions after the devastating earthquake, and continues to work and educate Haitian physicians. Those experiences are reminiscent of his own humble beginnings, growing up with his mother and sister in a Philadelphia housing project. Providing medical care for the most indigent and teaching evidence-based medicine are the essence of his dedication to excellence in medicine.

Essential Procedures for Emergency, Urgent, and Primary Care Settings

A Clinical Companion

Second Edition

Theresa M. Campo, DNP, APRN, FNP-C,
ENP-BC, FAANP
Keith A. Lafferty, MD, FAAEM

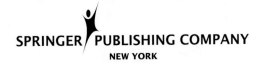

SPRINGER PUBLISHING COMPANY
NEW YORK

Springer Publishing Company, LLC
11 West 42nd Street
New York, NY 10036
www.springerpub.com

Acquisitions Editor: Margaret Zuccarini
Composition: diacriTech

Illustrations for this book were provided by Keisha Bonhomme, Bridgeport, Connecticut; Cathy Lafferty, Cape May, New Jersey; Joseph McDonough, Petersburg, New Jersey; Jodi Shoenfelt Glenn, Egg Harbour Township, New Jersey, with contributions from Graphic World.

ISBN: 978-0-8261-7176-4
e-book ISBN: 978-0-8261-7177-1

Videos can be found at springerpub.com/campo through the links provided in this text.

15 16 17 18 / 5 4 3 2 1

The author and the publisher of this Work have made every effort to use sources believed to be reliable to provide information that is accurate and compatible with the standards generally accepted at the time of publication. Because medical science is continually advancing, our knowledge base continues to expand. Therefore, as new information becomes available, changes in procedures become necessary. We recommend that the reader always consult current research and specific institutional policies before performing any clinical procedure or delivering any medication. The author and publisher shall not be liable for any special, consequential, or exemplary damages resulting, in whole or in part, from the readers' use of, or reliance on, the information contained in this book. The publisher has no responsibility for the persistence or accuracy of URLs for external or third-party Internet websites referred to in this publication and does not guarantee that any content on such websites is, or will remain, accurate or appropriate.

Library of Congress Cataloging-in-Publication Data
Campo, Theresa M.
  [Essential procedures for practitioners in emergency, urgent, and primary care settings]
  Essential procedures for emergency, urgent, and primary care settings : a clinical companion / Theresa M. Campo, DNP, APRN, FNP-C, ENP-BC, Keith A. Lafferty MD, FAAEM. —Second edition.
     pages cm
  Revision of: Essential procedures for practitioners in emergency, urgent, and primary care settings. 2011.
  ISBN 978-0-8261-7176-4
1. Nurse practitioners—Handbooks, manuals, etc. 2. Physicians' assistants—Handbooks, manuals, etc.
3. Medical protocols—Handbooks, manuals, etc. I. Lafferty, Keith A. II. Title.
  RT82.8.C36 2016
  610.73'72069—dc23
                        2015036223

Special discounts on bulk quantities of our books are available to corporations, professional associations, pharmaceutical companies, health care organizations, and other qualifying groups. If you are interested in a custom book, including chapters from more than one of our titles, we can provide that service as well.
For details, please contact:
Special Sales Department, Springer Publishing Company, LLC
11 West 42nd Street, 15th Floor, New York, NY 10036-8002
Phone: 877-687-7476 or 212-431-4370; Fax: 212-941-7842
E-mail: sales@springerpub.com

Printed in the United States of America by RR Donnelley.

This book evolved from the experiences and encounters I have had with mentors, students, colleagues, and patients, who have not only aided in the development of my career but have influenced my life. Clinical experiences alone do not make a person grow; the people along the journey do.

I am extremely lucky to have mentors that have not only had a positive effect on my life but a lasting effect on me as a person. Dr. Joyce Fitzpatrick, Dr. Elda Ramirez, and Dr. Sue Hoyt, I cannot thank you enough for believing in me and encouraging me to "step out of my comfort zone."

My family has helped to shape me into the person I am, and you mean more to me than words can express. Mom, you always said your children were the wind beneath your wings and now I am riding the wind of your angelic wings.

This book is dedicated to my husband, Jonathan Campo. You are my best friend and soul mate. Thank you for always standing by me with encouragement, pride and, most of all, love. You have put up with early mornings, late nights, and just plain long days while I was completing this book, yet you never complained. Your words are always of support and pride and I greatly appreciate them and you. You are the love of my life and you complete me. I truly would not be the person I am today without you. Everything I do is because of you. I love you more every day!

—**Theresa M. Campo**

At every one of my encounters with patients, I know my actions are guided by the thoughts, principles, and passion of my mentors, Dr. Lynda Micikas, Dr. Robert McNamara, and Dr. David Wagner. It is not only an honor to have been trained by the "best of the best," but even more so, to be a disciple of these pioneers and their relentless desire for perfection. I only hope the students I am privileged to teach are able to sense the illumination passed down to me, in order that they may also attempt to make this greatest of arts into the greatest of sciences.

The time, commitment, and dedication spent creating this manuscript are small in comparison to the sacrifice given by my beautiful family. Cathy, you are my love and my soul mate. I am truly a better person because of you, and I love you more every day. This text would not have come to fruition without your continued and relentless encouragement, support, and unselfishness. Karli, Koko, and Kory, Mom and Dad realize the sacrifice necessitated in inscribing such a document was very hard for you, especially in the last few months. "To win the respect of intelligent people and the affection of children . . . to know even one life has breathed easier because you have lived." —Ralph Waldo Emerson. *This is the true meaning of success. If you love what you do, it is not work! Daddy loves you so much and grows more proud of you every day. Always remember to equate success with the summation of one's virtuous acts.*

—**Keith A. Lafferty**

Contents

UNIT VII: PROCEDURES FOR THE MANAGEMENT OF NAIL AND NAIL BED INJURIES

UNIT VIII: INCISION AND DRAINAGE PROCEDURES

UNIT IX: PROCEDURES FOR EXAMINATION AND MANAGEMENT OF COMMON EYE INJURIES

UNIT X: PROCEDURES FOR MANAGING COMMON NASAL CONDITIONS

UNIT XIV: PROCEDURES FOR MANAGING COMMON GASTROINTESTINAL AND GENITOURINARY CONDITIONS

UNIT XV: MISCELLANEOUS PROCEDURES

Videos can be found at springerpub.com/campo through the links provided in this text.

Contributors

Lee Ann Boyd, MSN, ARNP-C, CUNP
Southwest Florida Urologic Associates
Cape Coral, Florida

Kathleen Bradbury-Golas, DNP, FNP-BC, ACNS-BC
Drexel University
College of Nursing and Health Professions
Philadelphia, Pennsylvania

Theresa M. Campo, DNP, APRN, FNP-C, ENP-BC, FAANP
Drexel University
College of Nursing and Health Professions
Philadelphia, Pennsylvania

Joseph Hong, MD
Jefferson Medical School
Atlantic Dermatology and Laser Center
Linwood, New Jersey

Larry Isaacs, MD, FACEP, FAAEM
Virtua Hospital, Voorhees Division
Voorhees, New Jersey

Keith A. Lafferty, MD, FAAEM
Atlanticare Regional Medical Center
Atlantic City, New Jersey

Christopher Lee Plaisted, MSN, FNP-C
Southwest Florida Emergency Physicians, PA
Fort Myers, Florida

M. Bess Raulerson, MMS, PA-C
Florida Urology Physicians
Fort Myers, Florida

Aubrey Rybyinski, BS, RDMS, RVT
Navix Diagnostix, Inc.
Taunton, Massachusetts

Reviewers

David Angelastro, MD, FACEP
Shore Memorial Hospital
Somers Point, New Jersey

Laurel Ballentine, MSN, FNP-C
Medford Family Practice
Medford, New Jersey

Omar Benitez, MD
Southwest Florida Urologic Associates
Cape Coral, Florida

Rachelle Beste, MD
Emergency Medicine Physicians, Supplemental Staff
Mayo Clinic
Rochester, Minnesota

Anne Marie Burkhardt, MSN, FNP-C
AtlantiCare Regional Medical Center
Atlantic City, New Jersey

Teresa Byrd, MSN, FNP-C
Ocean City Family Practice
Ocean City, New Jersey

James Cancilleri, DPM, FACFAS, FAPWCA
Private Podiatric Practice
Somers Point, New Jersey

Christopher Contino, MSN, FNP-C
Atlantic Emergency Associates
AtlantiCare Regional Medical Center
Atlantic City, New Jersey

Debra D. Fett Desmond, MD
Dermatology Solutions
Fort Myers, Florida

Valerie Dyke, MD
The Colorectal Institute
Fort Myers, Florida

Dian Dowling Evans, PhD
Emory University
Nell Hodgson Woodruff School of Nursing
Atlanta, Georgia

Darlene Ferrer, MSN, FNP-C
Atlantic Emergency Associates
AtlantiCare Regional Medical Center
Atlantic City, New Jersey

Victor Robert Frankel, MD
The Frankel Orthopedic and Sports Medicine Center, LLC
Linwood, New Jersey

Blanche Denise Hemby, MSN, FNP-C
Ocean City Family Medicine Practice
Ocean City, New Jersey

K. Sue Hoyt, PhD, FNP-BC
St. Mary Medical Center
Long Beach, California

Richard Juda, MD
Physician Regional Medical Center
Department of Critical Care
Naples, Florida

Todd Luyber, DO, FAAEM
Atlantic Emergency Associates
AtlantiCare Regional Medical Center
Atlantic City, New Jersey

Charles H. Nolte, DO
Virtua Health System
Voorhees, New Jersey

M. Bess Raulerson, PA-C
Naples, Florida

Janet E. Resop Reilly, DNP, APNP-BC
Professional Program in Nursing
Green Bay, Wisconsin

Mary Beth Saunders, DO
Gulf Coast Medical Center
Fort Myers, Florida

William Schumacher, DO, FACEP
Shore Memorial Hospital
Somers Point, New Jersey

Charles Springer, MD
Orthopedic Specialist of Southwest Florida
Fort Myers, Florida

Craig Stafford, DMD, PC
Private Practice—General Dentistry
Lancaster, Pennsylvania

Robert Turner, MD
Gulf Coast Medical Center
Fort Myers, Florida

Foreword

This distinctive book comprises procedures for practitioners for use in emergency, urgent, and primary care settings. *Essential Procedures for Emergency, Urgent, and Primary Care Settings, Second Edition* will assist providers in performing procedures commonly done in these settings. It is a friendly, procedurally focused resource that offers the necessary background information, illustrations, and step-by-step instructions for providing safe and efficient treatment to patients in these care settings, not only for the novice but for experts in emergent and urgent care. This new edition also offerd new chapters on ultrasound, in addition to videos. *Essential Procedures for Emergency, Urgent, and Primary Care Settings* furnishes today's providers with current information available in a concise and systematic framework. Procedures are those that providers perform on a daily basis.

Theresa Campo and Keith Lafferty, coauthors and coeditors, offer a wealth of information and knowledge combined with the expertise of Springer Publishing Company.

We know you will want to add this book not only to your medical library but more importantly so to your clinical setting as this book received the prestigious Doody's award the first year of its publication.

As practice evolves, new knowledge is acquired and procedures may change. In the meantime, we know you will enjoy utilizing *Essential Procedures for Emergency, Urgent, and Primary Care Settings, Second Edition.*

K. Sue Hoyt, PhD, RN, FNP-BC, CEN, FAEN, FAANP, FAAN
Emergency Nurse Practitioner, St. Mary Medical Center
Long Beach, California
Co-owner, EmergeED, Education and Consultation
San Diego, California

Elda G. Ramirez, PhD, RN, FNP-BC, FAANP
Associate Professor of Clinical Nursing
Director of Simulation and Clinical Performance Lab
and Emergency Concentration
University of Texas Health Science Center at Houston
Houston, Texas

Preface

Welcome to the only book of procedures for practitioners in emergency, urgent, and office settings. The intention of this book is to aid the practitioner (advanced practice nurse, physician assistant, and other specialty health care professionals) and students alike in performing common and not so common procedures in these settings. It is meant to be a clinical companion that is easy to understand and follow.

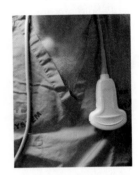

CLINICAL EXPERTS

This book has been prepared by clinical experts with numerous years of experience in both the academic and clinical arenas of their respective fields. Utilizing the most up-to-date literature as well as experience-based pearls of practice, we have organized this book to be user friendly and broad-based. As busy clinicians, we all understand time constraints and the need for a well-organized and simplified procedural book.

NEW TO THE SECOND EDITION

The addition of chapters on ultrasonography as a modality to assist in many of the previous and newly added procedures is an important plus. It is the only resource to include two chapters completely devoted to bedside ultrasonography and how it is used as a tool to enhance the accuracy of numerous bedside procedures. Grounded in fundamental sonography principles, these chapters provide readers with a clear and fundamental understanding of ultrasound guidance, when applicable, which can be followed with confidence and ease. Also, the book has been expanded to include many other clinical techniques, including more advanced procedures.

ORGANIZATION

The book is divided into 15 units covering the spectrum of common procedures performed by practitioners in emergency, urgent, and office settings. This collection of thoroughly described procedures is intended for use as a clinical companion and is an easy-to-use reference when performing such techniques. Current evidence-based literature has been utilized during the writing of this book. For ease of reading, all resources will be noted at the end of each chapter.

Chapters are organized in a format describing the background of the procedure, including pathophysiology of particular disorders requiring the procedure about to be performed. Current treatments along with the actual procedures are outlined in each chapter. It is the intent of the authors to purposely describe in some detail the disease process for a better understanding of the indication and performance of the procedure. **Videos have been prepared by the authors to support the understanding and accuracy of a procedure when performed in a clinical setting. The link to the videos is found in the text (springerpub.com/campo).**

PREPARATION

The authors recommend classroom didactics accompanied with hands-on experience before performing any procedure. Practitioners should always work within the scope of practice designated by their regulating agencies in their respective states and institutions. The authors and contributors are not responsible for any actions resulting from the use of this text.

People are entitled to their own opinions but not to their own facts. The authors of this textbook strongly believe that evidence-based practice is the only way to effectively treat patients.

Theresa M. Campo
Keith A. Lafferty

UNIT I

Introduction

CHAPTER 1

The Basics of Patient Procedures: Standard Precautions, Infection Control, Patient Preparation, and Education

Theresa M. Campo

Standard precautions and infection control are key to minimizing the spread of infection to health care workers, patients, and family members. In our age of resistance, it is becoming more challenging to effectively treat bacterial infections. Consistent practices of hand hygiene and universal precautions can be the best defense against infections, either community or hospital acquired.

Proper patient preparation and education are methods of ensuring time efficiency when performing procedures and of increasing a patient's level of satisfaction with the health care system. This book illustrates how to effectively prepare for each procedure in a confident, organized, and time-efficient manner. It also covers important educational points to share with patients to ensure a rapid and complete recovery.

STANDARD PRECAUTIONS

Standard precautions, previously termed "universal precautions," have been practiced since the late 1980s when the Centers for Disease Control and Prevention (CDC) published guidelines recommended for use by all health care workers to protect themselves from contamination from bodily fluids. Universal precautions are defined as "An approach to infection control in which all human blood, tissue, and certain fluids are treated as if known to be infectious for human immunodeficiency virus (HIV), hepatitis B virus (HBV), and other blood-borne pathogens" (OSHA, n.d.). The CDC recommendations should be followed when the risk of contact with any body fluids and/or secretions is present and suspected. These precautions replaced the traditional isolation category of blood and body fluids precautions.

Standard precautions apply not only to visible blood and body fluids, but also to nonvisible semen, vaginal fluids, tissue, and other fluids (e.g., amniotic, cerebrospinal, pleural, peritoneal). Other bodily excretions and secretions do not require universal

3

precautions unless blood is visualized or suspected. Examples include feces, nasal secretions, sputum, sweat, tears, urine, and vomitus.

Implementation of standard precautions includes using barriers to protect the health care worker from contamination. Examples of these protective barriers include gloves, masks, goggles, and gowns. Additional precautions must be taken to protect health care workers from needle puncture by using needleless systems and needle-free products, and the use of vacutainers when possible. The required degree of protection depends on the potential threat to the health care worker for exposure to infected bodily fluids.

Gloves should be worn whenever the potential for contact with blood or body fluids arises. They should also be worn if handling contaminated items such as sheets, absorbent pads, bedside tables, and other equipment. Gloves should be changed if their integrity is compromised (ripped, punctured, or torn) after patient contact and if grossly contaminated. Handwashing should always be performed before and after wearing gloves.

Masks, protective eyewear, and gowns should be used during any patient contact or procedure when the risk of contact with fluids and/or tissue is present. These barrier methods are best worn if splashing of the fluid is a potential threat, for example, droplets of blood or fluids, mucous membrane droplets (sneezing, coughing, etc.), or splashing of blood or body fluids during a procedure (active bleeding from a vein or artery, fluid under extreme pressure such as the contents of an abscess). Protective gear can also protect the patient, especially the immunocompromised, from the provider and assistants.

INFECTION CONTROL

Infection control procedures are important in protecting both the health care worker and the patient. In addition to using the standard precautions, basic handwashing is key in preventing the spread of infection to the health care worker as well as to other patients. Handwashing before and after any patient contact, with or without gloves, should be part of everyday practice. Handwashing has reduced the rate of community- and hospital-acquired infections and methicillin resistant *Staphylococcus aureus* (MRSA) transmission. Creamer et al. (2010) demonstrated that MRSA was present on the fingertips of health care workers ($n = 523$) even after hand hygiene practices were performed with either 4% alcohol, chlorhexidine, or soap and water. They also found MRSA present on the fingertips of health care workers who had contact with the patient, the patient's environment, and even with no specific contact. Handwashing should be done for a minimum of 15 seconds to be effective.

Debate continues as to whether handwashing is the sole method of cleansing the hands. Alcohol-based hand sanitizers are an alternative and accepted method of proper hand cleansing. The current recommendations state that hand rubbing with an approved sanitizer can be more effective than handwashing with soap and water. Kocak Tufan et al. (2012) found that alcohol-based hand rub was the most effective method for reducing MRSA colonization and soap alone was least effective. This method is best used when cleansing between patients, with handwashing with soap and water being the best method for gross contamination.

Good handwashing techniques and universal precautions are to be implemented before and after all procedures presented in this book. Gloves, gowns, and protective eye wear should be worn whenever there is potential exposure to blood or body fluids.

Use of needleless or needle-free products is encouraged but is dependent on what equipment your institution provides.

PATIENT PREPARATION

Preparing the patient, mentally and physically, for a procedure is as important as performing the procedure. All procedures, whether seemingly basic and trivial or obviously more advanced and emergent, are invasive to the patient and should be discussed with the patient in as much detail as the situation allows. Discussions should include the potential risks and benefits of performing the procedure versus not performing the procedure and should include the required follow-up and care. Care should be taken to include options if various techniques are available for the particular situation at hand (i.e., suture closure versus skin adhesive) and the risks and benefits of each method.

Continued reassurance should be given not only to the patient but also to the family member(s). Communicating confidence to the patient and family member(s) during the initial discussion makes a difference in the course of the procedure. When speaking to a patient, remember to keep your voice low and slow, and to pause at regular intervals to provide the patient the opportunity to ask questions. Always speak directly to the patient, even if the patient is a young child. You may need to first calm and reassure the parent before you can explain a procedure to the pediatric patient. On completion of the discussion, allow ample time for questions and further discussions. After explaining the intended procedure, consent must be obtained before initiating the procedure. Confidence and trust go a long way. Remember, anxiety spreads faster than fire.

Every effort should be made to make the patient and family member comfortable for the procedure. Place the patient in a comfortable position, especially if the procedure will be lengthy. Have the family member sit in a secure chair on the opposite side of the stretcher or examination table, so he or she is not only out of the way but in case the family member becomes "squeamish." Have your assistant also stand on the opposite side so that he or she cannot only assist you but also ensure the visitor remains safe during the procedure.

In this book, the required equipment is listed in the "Procedural Preparation" section of the chapters. All efforts to list what will be needed as well as alternative equipment have been made. Developing a checklist of equipment is helpful for the provider and his or her assistant to ensure everything that is needed will be at the bedside. Exiting to obtain necessary equipment during the procedure is time consuming and may have a negative effect on the patient's confidence.

Once the equipment is at the bedside and consent has been obtained, continued reassurance should be given to the patient and any family members present. Parents and family members should be allowed at the bedside when appropriate; this should be up to the provider's discretion. Universal precautions should be strictly followed for procedures involving or potentially involving blood and body fluid. When performing the procedure, every effort should be made for the provider to be in a comfortable position. Body mechanics are key for the provider as well as the assistants. Some procedures can be lengthy and stress the neck and back. Simple measures to ensure proper body mechanics and comfortable positioning are sitting in a chair, adjusting the height of the stretcher/examination table, having the patient positioned close to you to avoid reaching, and maintaining proper lighting.

PATIENT EDUCATION

Taking the time to properly educate the patient on follow-up, medications, wound care, and any other pertinent wound-related information can save time and frustration to the patient and provider. Verbal instructions followed by written instructions are ideal. Taking the time to review the procedure that was performed, proper care and management at home, and follow-up are key components of any discharge instructions. Always allow time for questions and further discussion to ensure the patient and family members have a good understanding. Once the information has been presented to the patient and family members, simply ask the patient and/or family member to repeat what you have discussed to ensure understanding.

Patient's anxiety levels, medications, and even simply the trauma of experiencing a procedure can affect what information the patient actually absorbs. Providing written instructions assists the patient and guides his or her follow-up. Written instructions can be obtained through software companies specializing in patient instructions or via the Internet. Always fully review the instructions before distributing them to patients. Instructions that are consistently updated based on current evidence-based practice are best. Review and update of the instructions for accuracy and current measures should be done on a daily basis.

Whenever instructions are given to a patient, ample time should again be given for review and questions. It can be frustrating for a patient with questions to be rushed out of the examination area. The patient either returns upset and angry or continuously calls to clarify the instructions. Such patients may never return for follow-up or continued care.

Documentation of verbal and written instruction is extremely important. Be sure to document what was discussed and provided to the patient, the place and time for follow-up (i.e., primary care physician [PCP], emergency department [ED], urgent care, or specialist), and whether the patient and/or family member verbalized understanding of the instructions and specific questions that were addressed. Detail is key.

SUMMARY

Take a time-out break before starting any procedure. Review the particular procedure in this book, the video when provided, and then review it once again in your head. Plan how to proceed and envision the parameters of the procedures before you begin. Take a deep breath. Doing this will help to ensure that you place yourself in a comfortable position and state of mind, which will sustain you throughout the procedure. There is nothing worse than bending over too far or standing during a time-consuming procedure and suffering a resultant stiff back or sore legs. When possible, sit on an adjustable chair or stool while performing a procedure. Adjustments can be made during the procedure, if necessary, to avoid bending over for prolonged periods of time, causing posture strain that can lead to provider discomfort, pain, sloppiness, and inferior results. Be sure to take care of yourself before taking care of others.

Universal precautions and patient preparation and education are key elements to any procedure performed in the emergency, urgent, or primary care setting. Providers need to deliver high-quality, efficient care while keeping the patient comfortable and calm. Achieving these goals requires taking extra steps to prepare properly for the procedure, to educate your patient and his or her family, and to be compassionate during every patient encounter. It is always important to treat your patients as if they were your family or close friend.

RESOURCES

Barnes, T. A., & Jinks, A. (2009). Methicillin resistant *Staphylococcus aureus*: The modern-day challenge. *British Journal of Nursing, 27,* 14–18.

Clock S, A., Cohen, B., Behta, M., Ross, B., & Larson, E. L. (2010). Contact precautions for multidrug-resistant organisms: Current recommendations and actual practice. *American Journal of Infection Control, 38,* 105–111.

Creamer, E., Dorrian, S., Dolan, A., Sherlock, O., Fitzgerald-Hughes, D., Thomas, T., . . . Humphreys, H. (2010). When are the hands of health care workers positive for methicillin resistant *Staphylococcus aureus*? *Journal of Hospital Infection, 75*(2), 107–111.

Croft, A. C., & Woods, G. L. (2011). Specimen collection and handling for diagnosis of infectious disease. In R. A. McPherson & M. R. Pincus (Eds.), *Henry's clinical diagnosis and management by laboratory methods* (22nd ed.). New York, NY: Elsevier.

di Martion, P., Ban, K. M., Bartonloni, A., Fowler, K. E., & Mannelli, F. (2011). Assessing the sustainability of hand hygiene adherence prior to patient contact in the emergency department: A 1-year postintervention evaluation. *American Journal of Infection Control, 39,* 14–18.

Del Rio, C. (2008). Prevention of human immunodeficiency virus infection. In L. Goldman & D. A. Ausiello (Eds.), *Cecil's medicine* (23rd ed.). New York, NY: Elsevier/Saunders. Retrieved from http://www.mdconsult.com/das/book/body/187068169-3/962478166/1492/1372.html#4-u1.0-B978-1-4160-2805-5..50416-X–cesec15_17320

Haas, J. P., & Larson, E. L. (2008). Impact of wearable alcohol gel dispensers on hand hygiene in an emergency department. *Academy Emergency Medicine, 15,* 393–396.

Henderson, D. K. (2010). Immunodeficiency virus in health care settings. In G. L. Mandell, J. E. Bennett, & R. Dolin (Eds.), *Principles and practice of infectious diseases* (7th ed.). Philadelphia, PA: Churchill Livingston/Elsevier. Retrieved From http://www.mdconsult.com/book/player/book.do?meod=display&type=bookPage&decorator=header&eid=4-u1.0-B978-0-443-06839-3..00306-4-s0080&displayedEid=4-u1.0-B978-0-443-06839-3..00306-4-s0085&uniq=187068169&isbn=978-0-443-06839-3&sid=962478166

Hughes, C., Tunney, M., & Bradley, M.C. (2013). Infection control strategies for preventing the transmission of methicillin-resistant *Staphylococcus aureus* (MRSA) in nursing homes for older people. *Cochrane Database Systematic Review, 11,* CD006354. Retrieved from https://www.clinicalkey.com/#!/ContentPlayerCtrl/doPlayContent/2-s2.0-24254890/{"scope":"all","query":"infection control"}

Jabbar, U., Leischerner, J., Kasper, D., Gerber, R., Sambol, S. P., Parada, J. P., . . . Gerding, D. N. (2010). Effectiveness of alcohol-based hand rubs for removal of *Clostridium difficile* spores from hands. *Infection Control Hospital Epidemiology, 31,* 565–570.

Kimlin, L. M., Mittleman, M. A., Harris, A. D., Rubin, M. A., & Fishman, D. N. (2010). Use of gloves and reduction of risk of injury caused by needles or sharp medical devices in healthcare workers: results from a case-crossover study. *Infection Control of Hospital Epidemiology, 31,* 908–917.

Kocak Tufan, Z., Irmak, H., Bulut, C., Cesur, S., Kinikli, S., & Demiroz, A. P. (2012). The effectiveness of hand hygiene products on MRSA colonization of health care workers by using CHROMager MRSA. *Mikrobiyoloji Bulteni Impact Factor, 46*(2), 236–246.

Lafferty, K. (2006). Femoral phlebotomy: The vacuum tube method is preferable over needle syringe. *Journal of Emergency Medicine, 31*(1), 83–85.

Lederer, J. W. (2009). A comprehensive handwashing approach to reducing MRSA health care associated infections. *Joint Commission Journal of Quality and Patient Safety, 35*(4), 180–185.

Messina, M. J., Brodell, L. A., & Brodell, R. T. (2008). Hand hygiene in the dermatologist office: To wash or to rub? *Journal of the American Academy of Dermatology, 59*(6), 1043–1049.

Nicholau, D., & Arnold, W. P. (2010). Environmental safety including chemical dependency. In R. D. Miller (Ed.), *Miller's anesthesia* (7th ed.). Philadelphia, PA: Churchill Livingston/ Elsevier. Retrieved from http://www.mdconsult.com/das/book/body/187068169-3/ 962478166/2053/104.html#4-u1.0-B978-0-443-06959-8..00101-1-s0210_6196

Occupational Safety & Health Administration (OSHA). (n.d.). Retrieved from https:// www.osha.gov/pls/oshaweb/owadisp.show_document?p_table=STANDARDS& p_id=10051#1910.1030(b)

Parmeggiani, C., Abbate, R., Marinelli, P., & Angelillo., I. F. (2010). Healthcare workers and health care-associated infections: Knowledge, attitudes, and behavior in emergency departments in Italy. *BMC Infection Disease, 23,* 35.

Stedman. (2008). *Stedman's concise medical dictionary for the health professions and nursing* (6th ed.). Philadelphia, PA: Wolters Kluwer Health.

WHO (2009). *WHO guidelines on hand hygiene in health care* (pp. 1–262). Retrieved from http:// www.who.int/gpsc/5may/tools/9789241597906/en/index.html

CHAPTER **2**

Consent, Documentation, and Reimbursement

Theresa M. Campo and Kathleen Bradbury-Golas

The legal aspects of medicine and nursing are often overlooked, yet, they are very important. Obtaining the proper consent, becoming familiar with the ethics of good practice, documenting thoroughly and accurately, and learning about insurance reimbursement and the Patient Protection and Affordable Care Act (PPACA) and its impact on American health care are integral aspects of practicing medicine and performing procedures. Having even a basic understanding can aid the provider in making good, sound decisions for the patient, health care team, and self.

CONSENT

Consent can be defined as "to give approval, assent, or permission. A person must be of sufficient mental capacity and of the age at which he or she is legally recognized as competent to give consent (age of consent)" (http://medical-dictionary. thefreedictionary.com/consent). *Informed consent* is the patient's right to be presented with sufficient information about a recommended procedure by the provider or a representative for the purpose of enabling the patient to make an informed decision. Patients or their representatives have the right to fully participate in this decision. As the health care professional recommending the procedure, the senior health care provider must participate in the process of explaining the procedure or treatment being offered to the patient, including the risks, benefits, and alternatives. In certain situations, a student can explain the procedure to the patient, along with the relevant benefits and risks, as long as the student is accompanied by the health care professional who is responsible for the patient. The essential elements that must be presented to the patient include diagnosis, the purpose of the treatment or procedure, what the procedure entails, the possible risks/benefits, the alternative risks of not receiving the treatment or procedure, prognosis, and consequences if the treatment is not provided at all. Patients must be deemed competent in order to sign or verbalize consent.

Informed or *"understood" consent* is necessary for any patient who is physically touched and for any invasive procedure. Not obtaining this beforehand can lead to communication discrepancies. Informed consent can be divided into two areas: expressed consent and implied consent. All forms of consent have become more important as a result of the increasing amount of litigation in the health care field.

Expressed consent is where the patient consents to treatment or procedures through direct words. This can be written or oral. *Written consent* requirements are stipulated by individual hospitals and mandated by the Joint Commission. Written consent is used as a method of proof that the information was explained to the patient/patient representative and is valid for 30 days. Oral consent can be obtained and then documented on the chart, but requires two witnesses to verify the consent. *Implied consent* can be obtained through the patient's behavior. One example of implied consent is when patients wait for hours to get the H1N1 influenza vaccine.

Emergency consent can be obtained when there is risk to the patient's life or if serious impairment to life or limb can occur with no intervention. The provider may act with responsibility to avert loss of limb or life. Examples of this include cardiac arrest, trauma, and significant fracture with neurovascular compromise. However, a patient's relatives or members of the health care team cannot give consent on behalf of patients who are incompetent or unconscious in a nonemergency situation unless they possess power-of-attorney status (S. A. Jawaid & Jawaid, 2006).

Consent for minors must be obtained from either a parent or legal guardian. A family representative can give consent for treatment as long as it is in writing from the parent or guardian. Minors may be treated as adults if they are emancipated (legally free of parental control). Emancipation can occur by being a mature minor, married, being parents themselves, or being in active military service. In some states a 14- or 15-year-old may be considered a mature minor and, therefore, may give consent for his or her own care. Reference your individual state laws regarding minors as they vary for each state. However, although the child cannot give consent for the procedure, the procedure should be explained in terms that the child will understand.

Anyone who is competent, autonomous, and not experiencing central nervous system dysfunction (i.e., alcohol, drugs, ischemia, or metabolic derangement) has the right to refuse treatment even if the provider feels it is necessary. Make sure that the patient is aware of any risks of not having the procedure or treatment. Always refer to your institution's policy and procedures with regard to consent as they differ from institution to institution, and state to state.

Prior to beginning any procedure discussed in this book, discuss the procedure, potential complications, risks, benefits, and alternatives with the patient. In addition, discuss the importance of follow-up and the expected time to return to the treatment area or primary care provider for reevaluation. Consent should be obtained based on your institution's policies and procedures.

OTHER LEGAL CONSIDERATIONS

Malpractice is a concern for providers with regard to health care delivery, especially when performing procedures. *Malpractice* is defined as the provider deviating from the standard of practice through an act or omission that can result in injury or complication to the patient. Providers must be cognizant of the most current guidelines and standards of practice. Care must be taken to "first do no harm," which can be accomplished by regular review of the current literature, regulations, and practice guidelines.

Ethical issues can also lead to legal ramifications. Cultural, ethnic, and religious beliefs can place the provider in a difficult situation. What is standard care for the majority of the patient population may not be acceptable to the patient based on one or several of these factors. Receiving blood products or certain medications and treatments may be thought to be detrimental or unacceptable by a particular religious group, culture, or ethnic group. When the provider faces this situation, he or she should always consult the ethics committee of the institution immediately, regardless of whether the outcome of altered or no treatment can be potentially life threatening. It is often very difficult for providers to "sit and wait" for an acceptable conclusion.

Respecting the patient's beliefs and practices can be frustrating and difficult. However, it may be a priority of the patient, not necessarily the provider. Always engage a collaborative approach with the patient, family, community, and health care team.

Medical liability and resulting litigation are a great concern for every provider. Medical malpractice reform, tort reform, and capitation are methods used to better regulate this rapidly growing problem. The medical record has become more of a weapon in the provider's defense of lawsuits and litigation. Proper and thorough documentation are essential not only for preventing litigation, but also positively effecting reimbursement from third-party payers.

DOCUMENTATION AND REIMBURSEMENT

Reimbursement for services rendered is even more essential in the present economic times. *Reimbursement in health care* is defined as the payment for health care services (Castro & Layman, 2006). As many societies attempt to stop soaring health care costs, it is important for the health care provider to document accurately and completely, thereby maximizing potential reimbursement. With the Affordable Care Act (2010) mandate for the electronic health record (EHR), a system in which the patient has access to view his or her record and results, the U.S. health care payment becomes integrated into one universal information source. As more and more individuals are required to have some form of reimbursement, health care providers must become more knowledgeable on how to determine what procedures are reimbursable and which ones are not.

Coding of disorders and causes of death can be traced to the 17th century. The *International Classification of Diseases (ICD)* was started in the 1900s in France. It originates from the international classification of causes of death, which was developed during a conference on the revision of the Bertillon system. It listed 179 groups of causes of death and an abridged classification of 35 groups. In 1946, the responsibility for the *ICD* was transferred to the WHO, which continually reviews and revises this classification system. Currently the *ICD-10* is in use.

In order to determine reimbursement, health care providers should research what the Centers for Medicare & Medicaid Services (CMS) and private insurance agencies have designated as reimbursable procedures, what technology assessment recommendations are required, and what the assigned Current Procedural Terminology (CPT) codes are for each procedure (BioDesign, n.d.). EHRs should be set up to include all of the essential elements necessary for adequate reimbursement.

CPT codes use a universal system of numbers (five) and descriptors that identify medical services that involve payment. These codes were designed and are updated yearly by the American Medical Association (AMA). The system assists in streamlining reporting of services and increases accuracy of documentation providing for a more efficient means of communicating medical services provided. If a procedure does not have a code, it may not be reimbursable or is too new to have one designated to it. An example of this is new technology. Coverage for new technology may be integrated directly into the diagnosis coding for the patient condition and not as a separate procedure (Princeton Reimbursement Group, n.d.).

The EHR must reflect the pertinent information with regard to history, physical examination findings, plan of care (episodic and/or continual), and diagnosis. Communication paired with thorough documentation can promote realistic expectations for the patient and help protect the provider against malpractice allegations. Documentation needs to be complete and legible for claims review, quality management, and peer review. The use of electronic records has provided greater capability for chart and claims reviews, along with a faster billing mechanism.

The CMS published evaluation and management (E&M) guidelines in 1995 and 1997 that are still used today. There are three key components in this process. These three components include the history, physical examination, and medical decision making (MDM).

The history is the subjective narrative that provides information on the current problem and/or symptomatology for the encounter. It is composed of (a) the chief complaint, (b) history of the present illness (HPI), (c) review of systems (ROS), and (d) past medical/family/social history. The E&M guidelines also note that the history increases in complexity and detail. There are seven characteristics of an HPI, which include location, quality, severity, duration, timing, context, modifying factors (relieving and aggravating), and associated signs and symptoms. Therefore, the history can be one of four levels, which include (1) problem focused, (2) expanded problem focused, (3) detailed, and (4) comprehensive. Table 2.1 outlines the criteria for these four levels of history. No matter what, all levels of history require the chief complaint and some form of an HPI.

TABLE 2.1 Criteria Required for History Levels

Level of History	HPI Elements	ROS	Medical/Family/ Social History
Problem focused	1–3	None	None
Expanded problem focused	4 HPI or status of 3 or more chronic conditions	1 system	None
Detailed	4 HPI or status of 3 or more chronic conditions	2–9 systems	Pertinent elements
Comprehensive	4 HPI or status of 3 or more chronic conditions	10 systems	Complete

HPI, history of present illness; ROS, review of systems.

The physical examination is the second component of E&M documentation. It also has four levels of detail. These levels are (1) problem focused, (2) expanded problem focused, (3) detailed, and (4) comprehensive. The details for the physical examination must follow the criteria designated in the 1997 E&M guidelines, not the 1995 ones.

The 1997 guidelines rely on more than documentation in organ systems but also include specific bullet points as well. There are a total of 10 systems but only nine are required. For a comprehensive examination, two bullet points per each of nine systems are required. Therefore, there must be a minimum of 18 bullet statements listed for a comprehensive physical examination to occur; though if all 10 systems are addressed there may be 20 bulleted statements documented. Documentation of vital signs counts as one bullet (Table 2.2).

TABLE 2.2 Physical-Examination Level Criteria

Level of Physical Examination	Number of Systems and Bullets	Total Number of Bullets Required
Problem focused	1–5 bullets from 1 *or* more organ systems	1 but 4 or more is better
Expanded focused	At least 6 from any organ systems	Minimum of 6
Detailed	At least 2 bullets from 6 organ systems *or* 12 bullets from 2 or more organ systems	Minimum of 12
Comprehensive	2 bullets for each of 9 organ systems	Minimum of 18 but 20 is better

MDM is the most important of the three components. It involves many steps to determine the level. There are four levels of MDM, which increase based on complexity. These levels are (1) straightforward, (2) low complexity, (3) moderate complexity, and (4) high complexity. Please note that not all states quantify as does the CMS, therefore, it is necessary for providers to check for specific state deviations.

The first determinant of MDM is determining risk. Risk is based on the number of diagnoses or management options; the amount or complexity of data reviewed and the potential risk of complications and/or morbidity/mortality. The highest in any of those three areas determines risk. However, this method has been found to be very subjective and CMS has now developed a "point" system in order to audit charts accordingly. Though this point system is not part of the E&M guidelines, and was voluntarily recommended for all Medicare carriers to use, it is what is used in all chart audits that the CMS conducts.

The "point" system makes risk and MDM more objective by assigning a numerical scale to describe each problem(s), then gives points to discuss how much information the health care provider needs to process. As an example, for a self-limiting or minor problem (up to two), a provider would receive one point. For a new high-risk problem with the need for additional studies, the provider would receive four points. Data points are then added to each encounter/diagnosis. Data points are determined by the diagnostic studies that are either reviewed or ordered for the encounter. An example of this is if a provider reviews blood work, the audit would show one point. Likewise if a provider orders blood work, the audit would show one point. However, a provider cannot get two points for reviewing current blood work and ordering future blood work.

Only one point would be allowed. Lastly, management options that are recommended or ordered are determined. All three of these factors add up to complexity of MDM. All three areas have "points" determined thereby allowing the provider to actually see the complexity level (Table 2.3).

TABLE 2.3 Summary of Medical Decision Making

Complexity of Medical Decision Making	Problem Points	Data Points (Diagnostics)	Risk Level
Straightforward	1	1	Minimal: 1 self-limited or minor problem
Low complexity	2	2	Low: 2 self-limited or minor problem *or* 1 stable chronic *or* 1 acute stable condition
Moderate complexity	3	3 (complex, often invasive)	Moderate: 1 or more chronic illnesses with exacerbation; 2 or more stable chronic conditions; acute illness with systemic symptoms; *or* acute complicated injury
High complexity	4	4 (often invasive)	High: 1 or more chronic illnesses with exacerbation or progression; acute or chronic illness that poses a threat to life *or* body function; *or* abrupt change in neurological status

Some providers have chosen to work diligently to understand and master the complexity of the E&M guideline system with the intention of avoiding fraud. Davidson (2007) created a tool to assist providers in the primary care setting to audit and review charts in order to accurately determine proper billing.

The combination of *ICD-10* and CPT codes yields the billable medical service. However, documentation must support the CPT code. Should the documentation not meet the required elements for billing, the health care provider can be charged with fraud. The Office of the Inspector General of the Department of Health and Human Services is responsible for prosecuting Medicare fraud. The EHR is an efficient, time-reducing, and cost-containing method of documenting patient encounters. It allows for more readily available medical information and sharing, resulting in more thorough care of the patient, reducing duplication of services. In some programs, E&M codes can be activated to ensure that the proper billable documentation has been achieved. However, the provider must still enter the MDM complexity, which institutions and primary care providers can share via satellite sites and vice versa. This is essential as in the past pertinent patient information would have been delayed or unobtainable.

THE PPACA AND ITS IMPACT ON AMERICAN HEALTH CARE

Though the United States spends the most money per capita (approximately $8,900 in 2012), Americans have lower life expectancy and higher rates of infant mortality, low birth weight, injuries/homicides, adolescent pregnancy and sexually transmitted infections, obesity, diabetes, heart disease, chronic lung disease and disability, drug-related deaths, and HIV/AIDS than people in other industrialized countries (Bradley, Taylor, & Finebert, 2013; CMS, Health Expenditures, 2012). Yet, before implementation of the PPACA there were an estimated 50 million people without health insurance living in the United States. That does not include the 25 million undocumented immigrants living within the country.

Every president since Teddy Roosevelt in 1912 has tried to reform American health care. However, none was ever able to get legislation through the U.S. bureaucratic system. Lyndon B. Johnson accomplished the most in 1965 with the implementation of Medicare and Medicaid. However, since 1970 health care costs have risen about 1,600%, which hampers the U.S. ability to compete internationally in manufacturing and trade.

The PPACA is a compromise solution that is making incremental changes to the existing convoluted health care system. The law maintains a mixture of public/government health insurance, veterans/military care, federal employees' health care, and private/commercial insurance. It strives to "fix" areas so that the government is no longer paying for iatrogenic-caused complications and to slow down health care costs to a sustainable level.

The PPACA has several themes through which it will impact care and costs. Those themes are access, cost control, quality improvement, prevention, workforce, revenue, and other. Each of these themes will be discussed in more detail (Emmanuel, 2014). All insurance policies within the United States were expected to adopt 10 elements thereby guaranteeing all Americans have minimum essential coverage (MEC). These benefits (see Table 2.4) include ambulatory patient services, emergency services, hospitalization, maternity and newborn care, mental health/substance use disorder services, prescription drugs, rehabilitative/habilitative services and devices, laboratory services, preventative/well services and chronic disease management, and pediatric services, which include oral and vision care (Folger, 2014).

TABLE 2.4 Essential Health Benefits Under the Affordable Care Act

Ambulatory Patient Services	Emergency Services
Hospitalization	Maternity and Newborn Care
Mental Health and Substance Use Disorder Services	Prescription Medications
Rehabilitative and Habilitative Devices	Laboratory Services
Preventative/Wellness Services and Disease Management	Pediatric Services, Including Oral and Vision Care

Access to care is defined as a person's ability to obtain health insurance. The PPACA improves this through the expansion of Medicaid and the health care exchanges. Beginning in 2010, temporary exchanges were created to sell policies to people with preexisting conditions (many of whom could not get insurance previously); private insurers were not permitted to turn away children with preexisting medical conditions and lifetime limits started to be eliminated. The government offered the opportunity to expand Medicaid to all people/families (not just children) who lived below the federal poverty level. The federal government agreed to pay 100% of the costs for the new beneficiaries from 2014 to 2016. After that, the states would have to pay up to 10% of funding from 2020 thereafter. Although the federal government attempted to "force" the states to do this, the Supreme Court found that part of the law unconstitutional. Therefore, the states could refuse to implement this part of the law. Several states, many with the poorest health care outcomes in the country, refused to accept the expansion. This pushes more people into the exchange system who normally did not belong there or who would again be uninsured (Medicaid, n.d.).

The goal of the act was to have companies who have more than 50 employees provide health insurance. These employees were considered eligible for these benefits if they worked greater than or equal to 30 hours per week. For those businesses with fewer than 50 employees, the individual could either apply for Medicaid or purchase health benefits through the health care exchange system. However, it was expected that employers provide health benefits; this is known as the employer mandate. This mandate was expected to take effect in 2014 but its implementation was postponed to January 2015.

The health care exchange system created a "marketplace"-like environment in which individuals could go online to sign up and buy health care coverage during an open enrollment period. This went into effect on October 1, 2013, with disastrous results from the poor technology used and a "nonbusiness" person running the entire system. Since then, the website has been fixed and a new leader has been hired, and only time will tell if its functionality is improved. Although expansion to small-group/business coverage is expected, it may actually be too difficult to create a website for groups to use. Under the exchange system, a person can choose a plan based on level of coverage. Much of the difference in levels is based on the amount of the deductible. Those levels of coverage are listed in Table 2.5. Depending on income, a person/family may receive a subsidy from the federal government to help in covering the cost of health care.

For those people/families with health care insurance from their employers, children up to the age of 26 years can remain on their parents' insurance. This was expanded so that the older child could remain on the family insurance even if she or he had health care benefits offered by employment.

Cost control attempts to slow health care cost growth or to decrease the amount of what is being spent to pay for health care. Cost-control initiatives include the creation

TABLE 2.5 Levels of Coverage

Payment Responsibilities	Bronze Plan	Silver Plan	Gold Plan	Platinum Plan
What Patient Pays	40%	30%	20%	10%
What Insurance Pays	60%	70%	80%	90%

of accountable care organizations (ACOs), elimination of fee for service, bundled payments, CMS technology innovation, Cadillac tax, and the Independent Payment Advisory Board (IAPB). ACOs are really part of Medicare's Shared Savings Program, in which a medical organization focuses more on patients than on procedures. These organizations are composed of providers and suppliers who will use evidence-based practice plans to improve patient outcomes for a specific patient population (must care for 5,000 patients to be eligible). Patients enroll in an ACO and receive their care from ACO providers. At the present time, health care payment follows the traditional "fee for service" model, however, eventually this will move to a "prepayment method." Health care providers will be paid a set fee for each patient; if the ACO provides services that cost less than revenues, it will keep the difference. This requires ACOs to put quality over quantity (CMS, Shared Savings, n.d.).

One of the major CMS technology requirements is the meaningful use of an EHR by 2015. If acute care facilities and providers have not implemented electronic medical records by January 1, 2015, the CMS will penalize them. As providers join together in an ACO, they are able to share the cost of the EHR, develop protocols for various patient populations, and hire a professional manager, who then reviews all the data on patient outcomes and quality indicators. All of this leads to improved quality care, lower costs, and potentially improved patient outcomes.

The Cadillac tax will be implemented by 2018. This 40% tax on all health care insurance plans that are over the accepted standard limits will produce revenue as well as set control-cost standards on "top of the line" plans. The limits that have presently been set specify that any plan costing more than $10,200 and $27,500 for individual and family plans, respectively, will cost employers 40% more (Parks, 2012).

The IAPB is to be a 15-member federal agency that would review the calculated Medicare growth rate on a yearly basis. If the growth rate is higher than what was targeted, the team would develop a proposal on how to reduce the rate. The board is prohibited from rationing care, raising premiums, increasing cost sharing, restricting benefits, or modifying eligibility. In addition, Congress must approve of this plan. If Congress does not approve of the IAPBs plan, then Congress must come up with its own plan to meet the target rate. No matter which plan is chosen, all the decisions must be made on sound research and evidence. At this time there are no members on the IAPB since the target rate for health care costs have been less than predicted.

Quality-improvement initiatives are a significant part of the Patient Protection section of the National Strategy for Quality Improvement in Healthcare. These initiatives were meant to reduce hospital-acquired infections, reduce hospital readmission rates, encourage use of EHRs, and Patient-Centered Outcomes Research Institute. It is estimated that between 44,000 and 98,000 patents die annually in U.S. hospitals due to medical errors. Beginning in 2011, CMS began to track hospital-acquired conditions. If there are better patient outcomes (fewer errors), the hospital will get better payments. Medicare will no longer pay for the care of hospital-acquired conditions, which leaves the burden of longer length of stay and treatment modalities on the hospital. The cutting of payments began in 2014. In addition, error track records are published for every hospital so the public can view the quality of care the hospital provides. The Patient-Centered Outcomes Research Institute recommends the most effective treatment modalities (Emmanuel, 2014).

CMS has begun posting 30-day readmission rates for all hospitals. In an effort to decrease the readmission rates (within 30 days) of the top five disease processes, Medicare began implementing penalties as of 2012. These disease processes include congestive heart failure, diabetes mellitus, chronic obstructive pulmonary disease, hypertension, and coronary artery disease. Hospital payments are now readjusted according to the readmission rate, and for lower readmission rates, incentives have been offered. The goal of combining quality-improvement initiatives and ACOs is for interprofessional coordination of care with effective communication, with providers working as a team for improved patient outcomes (Emmanuel, 2014).

Disease prevention and public awareness are integral parts of the PPACA. First, it provides no-cost preventive services to all individuals. There are no longer copayments for well child, women's health, and adult physical examinations. The law infused money into public awareness through the National Public Health Improvement Initiative, the National Prevention Council, National Prevention Strategy, and Community Transformation Grants. The PPACA requires nonprofit hospitals to engage in community health needs assessments (CHNAs). These CHNAs are to be conducted once every 3 years and the hospital is to adopt an implantation strategy to meet the community health needs. The hospital must file a report, and any hospital that does not meet the CHNA requirements can be fined yearly. Through the National Prevention Strategy, the National Prevention Council engages states, communities, and public partners to create a blueprint for creating a healthier America at every stage of life. This is the first mandatory funding that has been given to public health (Parks, 2012).

Other key public health initiatives have been public education campaigns for tobacco-free lifestyle choices, active living and healthy eating, chronic disease awareness, and workplace wellness programs. Menu labeling for all restaurants with more than 20 locations is now on the horizon. These restaurants are now required to post a list of calories of the food on their menus. In addition, the PPACA has more than 40 provisions to support, increase, and encourage innovation in the health care workforce. The National Health Service Corps offers scholarship and loan repayment money for those health care providers who are willing to work in underserved communities. In addition, there are innovation awards and grants encouraging the development of community health centers and school-based health centers to care for low-income Americans with little or no insurance.

The revenue piece of PPACA includes new fees on pharmaceutical companies that manufacture, sell, or import drugs in the United States; a 3.2% excise tax on the sale of human medical devices, such as pacemakers and MRIs; limits contributions to health flex accounts to only $2,500 instead of $5,000; raises the Medicare threshold from 7.5% to 10% of adjusted gross income; and institues a 10% tax on tanning salons (Parks, 2012).

The final theme covers those areas that made financial information more public. Financial disclosures regarding the relationship between pharmaceutical companies and health care providers were required to be transparent. The medical loss ratio rules were implemented, limiting the amount that insurance companies can spend on administrative salaries and fees. Beginning in 2010, insurance companies must spend specific portions of premium dollars for actual medical care of its policyholders, limiting their profits. Medicare spends over 90% on care, but many private insurance companies were spending as little as 70% on care. Presently, insurance companies are required to spend 80% for individuals and small businesses and 82% for larger employer plans. Although medical loss ratio rules were included in the PPACA, several states have chosen to waive the implementation of this rule.

In summary, the PPACA offers many changes to the American health care system. It increases reimbursement to primary care providers, supports graduate and medical school funding (especially primary care programs), alters practice toward evidence-based care with a change from treatment to prevention, and expands the development of community health and school-based health centers to provide health promotion and screening/preventive services to move America's health care toward a wellness model of service provision (Davidson, 2013).

SUMMARY

Communication between health care providers and patients, obtaining consent, and accurate documentation provide the foundation for competent and thorough care. Providers should always take the time to listen and communicate with their patients. Discussion and education with patients provide a basis for realistic expectations and outcomes. Thorough and accurate documentation lead to decreased liability and fraud, resulting in accurate reimbursement: If it was not documented, it was not done.

Keeping patients informed throughout their care and thorough documentation make sense legally and ethically.

RESOURCES

American Medical Association. (n.d.) *Patient physician relationship topics. Informed consent.* American Medical Association. Retrieved January 9, 2012 from http://www.ama-assn .org/ama/pub/physician-resources/legal-topics/patient-physician-relationship-topics/ informed-consent.shtml

BioDesign. (n.d.). *Reimbursement basics.* Retrieved from http://web.stanford.edu/group/ biodesign/cgi-bin/ebiodesign/index.php/concept-selection/reimbursement-basics-menu

Bitterman, R. A. (2010). Medicolegal issues and risk management. In J. A. Marx, R. S. Hockenberger, R. M. Walls, J. G. Adams, W. G. Barsan, M. H. Biros, et al. (Eds.), *Rosen's emergency medicine* (7th ed.). Philadelphia, PA: Elsevier. Retrieved from http:// www.mdconsult.com/book/player/book.do?method=display&type=bookPage&decor ator=header&eid=4-u1.0-B978-0-323-05472-0..00202-4-s0200&displayedEid=4-u1. 0-B978-0-323-05472-0..00202-4-s0205&uniq=187068169&isbn=978-0-323-05472-0& sid=962492495

Bradley, E., Taylor, L., & Fineberg, H. (2013). *The American health care paradox: Why spending more is getting us less.* Public Affairs.

Castro, A., & Layman, E. (2006). *Principles of healthcare reimbursement.* Chicago, IL: American Health Information Management Association.

Centers for Medicare & Medicaid. (1997). *CMS 1997 documentation guidelines for evaluation and management services.* Retrieved from https://www.cms.gov/Outreach-and-Education/ Medicare-Learning-Network-MLN/MLNEdWebGuide/Downloads/97Docguidelines.pdf

Centers for Medicare & Medicaid. (2009). Medicare physician guide. A resource for residents, practicing physicians, and other health care professionals. *Department of Health and Senior Services.* Retrieved from http://gme.sites.medinfo.ufl.edu/files/2010/03/Physician-Guide- to-Medicare-Services.pdf

Centers for Medicare & Medicaid Services (CMS). (2012). National Health Expenditures 2012 Highlights. Retrieved from http://www.cms.gov/Research-Statistics-Data-and-Systems/ Statistics-Trends-and-Reports/NationalHealthExpendData/downloads/highlights.pdf

Centers for Medicare & Medicaid Services. (n.d.). Medicare Shared Savings Program. Retrieved from https://www.cms.gov/Medicare/Medicare-Fee-for-Service-Payment/sharedsavings program/index.html?redirect=/sharedsavingsprogram

CMS tightens documentation and signature requirements. Retrieved from http://www .healthcarefinancenews.com/blog/cms-tightens-documentation-and-signature-requirements

Davidson, J. (2007). A simple system for coding E&M services. *AAOS Now*. Retrieved from http://www.aaos.org/news/bulletin/may07/managing7.asp

Davidson, S. (2013). *The new era in U.S. healthcare: Critical next dteps under the Affordable Care Act* (Sanford Briefs). Palo Alto, CA: Sanford University Press.

E/M University. (2003–2015). *Medical decision making*. Retrieved from http://emuniversity.com/ MedicalDecision-Making.html

Emmanuel, E. (2014). *Reinventing American health care: How the Affordable Care Act will improve our terribly complex, blatantly unjust, outrageously expensive, grossly inefficient, error prone system*. Public Affairs.

Folger, J. (2014). Essential health benefits under the Affordable Care Act. Retrieved from http:// www.investopedia.com/articles/personal-finance/100913/essential-health-benefits-under-affordable-care-act.asp

International statistical classification of diseases and related health problems. *Encyclopedia of public health*. Retrieved from http://www.answers.com/topic/icd

Jawaid, S. A., & Jawaid, M. (2006). Patient's rights and the practice of obtaining informed consent: The need for some corrective measures. *Pakistan Journal of Medical Science, 22*(1), 7–9.

Loughlin, K. R. (2008). Medical malpractice: The good, the bad, and the ugly. *Urology Clinics of America, 36*, 101–110.

Medicaid. (n.d.). Affordable Care Act. Retrieved from http://www.medicaid.gov/ affordablecareact/affordable-care-act.html

Medical documentation requirements. Retrieved from http://www.usbr.gov/mp/mp500/leave_ share/medical_documentation_requirements.pdf

Medical liability reform. Retrieved from http://www.ama-assn.org/ama/pub/advocacy/current-topics-advocacy/practice-management/medical-liability-reform.shtml

Medical templates: Demystifying medical documentation. Retrieved from http://www.scribd .com/doc/7540597/Demystifying-Medical-Documentation

Parks, D. (2012). *Health care reform simplified* (2nd ed.). New York, NY: Apress/Springer Verlag.

Princeton Reimbursement Group. (n.d.). *Key elements of reimbursement*. Retrieved from http:// www.prgweb.com/resources/key_elements_of_reimbursement.php

Snyder, K. E., West, R. W., Lai, W. S., & Gay, S. B. (n.d.). Elements of informed consent. *University of Virginia Health Sciences Center Department of Radiology*. Retrieved from http:// www.med-ed.virginia.edu/courses/rad/consent

Stern, T. A., Rosenbaum, J. F., Fava, M., Biederman, J., & Rauch, S. L. (2008). Informed consent, competency, treatment refusal, and civil commitment. *Massachusetts General Hospital Comprehensive Clinical Psychiatry*. Retrieved from http://www.mdconsult.com/das/ book/body/187068169-6/962489283/1657/774.html#4-u1.0-B978-0-323–04743-2.. 50086-X–cesec4_2389

Teichman, P. G. (2000). Documentation tips for reducing malpractice. *Family Practice Medicine*. Retrieved from http://www.aafp.org/fpm/20000300/29docu.html

U.S. Department of Health and Human Services. (n.d.). Affordable Care Act. Retrieved from http://www.hhs.gov/healthcare/rights

UNIT II

Introduction to Sonography

CHAPTER **3**

Overview of Sonography

Aubrey Rybyinski

Ultrasound is a safe and effective form of imaging that has been used by physicians for more than half a century to aid in diagnosis and guide procedures. The growth of point-of-care ultrasound and its application has exponentially increased over the last decade as more compact, higher quality, and less expensive equipment has become more available. Furthermore, there is a good deal of literature demonstrating its ability, in the trained hands of clinicians making real-time decisions, to significantly decrease morbidity and mortality, eliminating previous diagnostic delays, and increasing procedural precision. Because of this, the technology is now ubiquitous in many acute care clinical settings. Sonography is a highly user-dependent technology, and as its clinical usage grows, there is a need to ensure education as well as limit unnecessary imaging and its consequences. While it is not the intent for the practitioner to become a certified sonographer, the use of this bedside tool in a focused manner will greatly enhance the ability to diagnose, resuscitate, monitor, guide, and treat acute medical conditions. Education in emergency or point-of-care ultrasound is currently an essential part of emergency training programs. Comprehensive training guidelines are published to ensure proficiency in ultrasound education and are currently the standard of care in modern-day emergency departments. The days of indirectly ascertaining pathology via auscultation and palpation have now been augmented by real-time bedside imaging thanks to current mobile sonography.

PRINCIPLES

Ultrasound is defined as a frequency above that which humans can hear, more than 20,000 Hertz (Hz). The frequency of diagnostic ultrasound is in the millions of Hertz (MHz). Ultrasound uses a quartz or composite piezoelectric material that generates a sound wave when an electric current is applied. When the sound wave returns, the material in turn generates a current. The crystal that lies in the probe itself, thus both transmits and receives the sound.

The standard screen image that machines display is known as B-mode (also called two dimensional or gray scale), and is created by an array of crystals (often 128 or more) across the face of the transducer. Each crystal produces a scan line that is used to create an image or frame, which is refreshed many times per second to produce a moving image on the screen.

TRANSDUCERS

Ultrasound transducers come in many various sizes, shapes, and frequencies, as they have to be used on different body areas. Lower frequency ultrasound has better penetration, but at lower resolution. Higher frequency ultrasound provides better images, but it does not visualize deep structures well. The face of the transducer, or footprint, is where the sound waves are transmitted. Convex transducers are curved and ideal for abdominal imaging or in areas where rocking the transducer will improve visualization. Linear transducers are flat and generally offer higher frequencies and are used for imaging small parts (testicles, breast, thyroid, superficial imaging, etc.). Appropriate transducer selection is based on the depth of the area of interest and anatomical region (Figure 3.1).

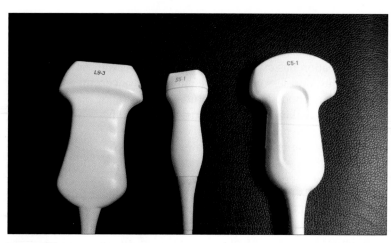

FIGURE 3.1 Transducers are constructed with different frequencies and footprints because selection is based on body region and depth to the area of interest. Linear transducers are more suitable for superficial imaging (far left). Curved transducers (far right) are more suitable imaging the abdomen since the transducer can be rocked. Cardiac probes have a small footprint in order to be used in intercostal acoustic windows (middle).

Equipment Maintenance

Ultrasound transducers must be cleaned with an appropriate disinfectant after each use. Using an autoclave, gas, or other methods may damage your transducer. When using ultrasound for needle guidance do not allow sharp objects, such as scalpels and cauterizing knives, to touch transducers or cables. Transducers have crystals so it is important not to bump them on hard surfaces. Be sure to follow the manufacturer's instructions when using disinfectants; if you are unsure call the equipment manufacturer.

IMAGING

Sonography offers the ability to image dynamically and in multiple patient positions. Patients can be evaluated in the supine, prone, left or right lateral decubitus, erect, or oblique positions. Two-dimensional ultrasound is used to visualize a plane that is then shown on the screen. An indicator or "notch" on the probe is used to orient the user to the orientation of the plane on the screen. This is displayed on the screen as a manufacturer's emblem or a symbol. The imaging plane may be directed by the user in any anatomical plane on the patient or area of interest: sagittal, coronal, transverse, or a combination (oblique).

Sagittal (Longitudinal)

The transducer orientation for a sagittal longitudinal plane has the indicator in the 12 o'clock position in relation to the organ or area of interest. The sound waves are transmitted from either a usual anterior or posterior approach. The superior aspect of the region is displayed on the left side and inferior aspect on the right side of the sonographic image. The sagittal (longitudinal) plane does not demonstrate the organ in a lateral dimension (Figure 3.2).

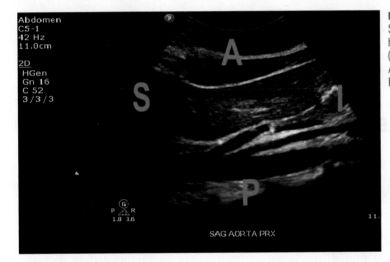

FIGURE 3.2
S superior (patient's head), I inferior (patient's feet), A anterior, and P posterior.

Coronal

The transducer orientation for a coronal plane has the indicator in the 12 o'clock position in relation to the organ or area of interest. The sound waves are transmitted from a right or left surface (e.g., the flank/kidney). The superior aspect of the region is displayed on the left side of the image and inferior aspect on the right side. This plane does not demonstrate the organ in an anterior or posterior dimension (Figure 3.3).

Transverse (Anterior or Posterior Surface)

The transducer orientation for the transverse plane has the indicator in the 9 o'clock position in relation to the organ or area of interest. The sound waves are transmitted from either anterior (usual) or posterior dimension. From the typical anterior view, the patient's right side is displayed on the left of the screen and patient's left side on the right side of the screen when sound waves are transmitted from an anterior approach (similar to

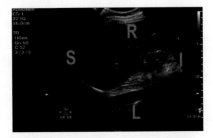

FIGURE 3.3 S superior (patient's head), I inferior (patient's feet), R right, and L left. Right is at the top of the image because the patient is in a left lateral decubitis position and the transducer is on the patients right side.

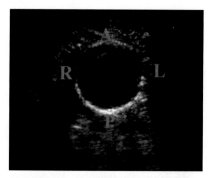

FIGURE 3.4 R patient's right, L patient's left, A anterior, and P posterior. Note this picture represents an abdominal aortic aneurysm and, as stated in the text, think of viewing in the transverse plane as if you were standing at the patient's feet looking toward his or her head, analogous to studying a CT scan.

viewing CT scans) (Figure 3.4). From a posterior view, the patient's left is seen to the left of the screen and patient's right on the right side of the screen.

Transverse (Right or Left Surface)

The transducer orientation for the transverse plane has the indicator in the 9 o'clock position in relation to the organ or area of interest. The sound waves are transmitted from either the right or left surface (e.g., the flank/kidney). The area anterior to the patient is displayed on the right side of the screen and the posterior on the left side of the screen when sound waves are transmitted from the right surface. From a left-surface view, the patient's anterior is seen to the left of the screen and posterior on the right side of the screen. This plane does not demonstrate superior or inferior.

DEFINITIONS OF SONOGRAPHIC CHARACTERISTIC

Because of the nature of how the ultrasound image is created, descriptive terms are used based on the echogenicity or strength of the sound wave reflected back to the transducer. Echogenicity is not something that can be measured like mass or length. In order to effectively communicate sonographic findings, the use of specific terms is required. Normal tissues and organ structures have a characteristic appearance *relative to surrounding structures*. A normal relationship in this inherent sonographically detected echogenicity of various organs means that there is no apparent pathology, though subtle pathology may not be appreciated. In diseased states, this organ-specific and characteristic echogenicity is abnormal. This underlies the importance in using correct nomenclature in describing findings for a precise diagnosis. Common ultrasound terms are defined in the chart (Table 3.1, Figures 3.5 and 3.6).

TABLE 3.1 Echogenicity

Term	Definition	Example
Hypoechoic	Not as bright as surrounding tissues	Muscle is less bright than fat
Hyperechoic	Brighter echoes than surrounding tissues	Bone, renal stone (Figure 3.5)
Isoechoic	Same intensity as surrounding tissues	The liver and right kidney cortex may appear isoechoic in normal patients.
Anechoic	Echo free	Simple cyst, urinary bladder, blood (within vessel), free fluid (Figure 3.6)
Homogenous	Imaged echoes of equal intensity	Normal liver or spleen
Heterogenous	Structures having varied echo characteristics	Normal kidney exhibits different echotextures (cortex, medulla, and sinus)

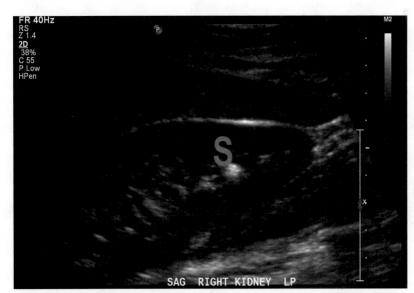

FIGURE 3.5
Arrow indicates a renal stone. The stone (labeled as "S") has an increased (brighter) echogenicity than the kidney.

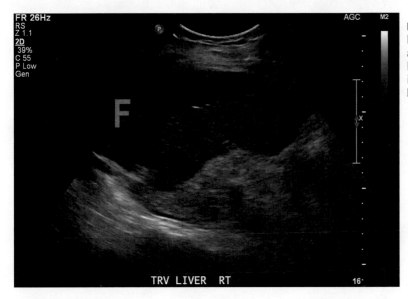

FIGURE 3.6
F Free fluid around the liver. Note the fluid is anechoic and homogeneous.

RESOURCES

Dean, A. J., Lafferty, K., & Villanueva, T. C. (2003). Emergency medicine bedside ultrasound diagnosis of intussusception in a patient with chronic abdominal pain and unrecognized Peutz-Jeghers syndrome. *Journal of Emergency Medicine, 24*(2), 203–210.

Edelman, S. (2012). *Understanding ultrasound physics* (4th ed.). Houston, TX: ESP.

Kawamura, D. (2012). *Diagnostic medical sonography* (3rd ed.). Philadelphia, PA: Wolters Kluwer Health/ Lippincott Williams & Wilkins.

National Center for Biotechnology Information. (2009). Retrieved from http://www.ncbi.nlm.nih.gov/pmc/ articles/PMC2967679

PHILIPS Healthcare. (2010, July 14). *Transducer cleaning, disinfecting, and sterilizing.* Retrieved from http://www.healthcare.philips.com/main/products/ultrasound/transducers/transducer

CHAPTER 4

Ultrasonography: Physics, Equipment, and Clinical Uses

Aubrey Rybyinski

PHYSICS

Ultrasound physics can be an obstacle for many individuals. The information provided in this chapter serves as an introduction, and foundation to utilize, ultrasound for diagnostic, procedural, and therapeutic interventions.

The speed of ultrasound does not depend on its frequency but rather the medium or tissue it is traveling in. Generated sound waves travel faster in dense materials and slower in compressible materials. In soft tissue sound travels at about 1,500 m/sec, in bone about 3,400 m/sec, and in air 330 m/sec. Acoustic gel is used as a coupling medium because air is an impenetrable barrier to ultrasound, and fluid offers the least resistance.

When ultrasound waves interact with the tissue medium attenuation occurs. Attenuation is the loss of the sound wave caused by the absorption of ultrasound energy by conversion to heat. Reflection, refraction, and scattering also result in reduced beam penetration. Attenuation is increased when the sound waves distance from the transducer increases, higher frequency transducers are used and when there are mismatches in acoustic impedance.

Acoustic impedance is a measure of how ultrasound traverses a tissue; it depends on the density of the medium and the relative propagation velocity of the sound wave traveling through the medium. In essence, it is the resistance for propagation of ultrasound waves. This varies according to the density of the material in which the ultrasound waves pass through. When the material is more solid, than the particles are denser and more sonographic waves will reflect back to the crystals within the probe and less will penetrate this medium. Fluid transmits more sound waves than solid material (less dense) so less ultrasound waves will reflect back from fluids and more can go through this medium, thereby producing an echogenic "black" image. Bones reflect more sound waves than fluid and produce a bright "white" image; therefore a black acoustic shadow (void of waves) will be present behind it. Air is a strong ultrasound beam reflector making it difficult to visualize structures behind it. A large difference in acoustic impedance is referred to as acoustic impedance mismatch. The greater the acoustic mismatch, the greater the percentage of ultrasound reflected and the less transmitted. An example of a large acoustic impedance mismatch is soft tissue bone interface and soft tissue air interface.

RESOLUTION

Resolution refers to the ability to identify two or more objects or points as separate entities within a special plane. It is measured in units of distance such as millimeters. The higher the resolution, the smaller the distance that can be differentiated. There are three types of resolution that pertain to ultrasound imaging: axial, lateral, and temporal. Axial (or longitudinal) resolution is the ability to recognize two different objects at slightly different depths from the transducer along the longitudinal axis of the ultrasound beam. The resolution at any point along the beam is the same. Axial resolution is improved with the use of higher frequency transducers, but comes at the expense of penetration. Higher frequencies, therefore, are used to image structures close to the transducer.

Lateral resolution is the ability to distinguish objects that are side by side or 2 points in the direction perpendicular to the direction of the sound waves. Lateral resolution is generally poorer than axial resolution and is dependent on beam width. The ultrasound machine assumes that any object visualized originates from the center of the beam, so two objects side by side cannot be distinguished if they are separated by less than the beam width. Lateral resolution is improved with optimal focal zone placement.

Temporal resolution is the ability to detect that an object has moved over time and is dependent on frame rate. Temporal resolution is improved by minimizing depth and narrowing the sector (sector angle) to the area of interest.

ARTIFACTS

Artifacts can be defined as any structure in the ultrasound image that does not have a corresponding anatomic tissue structure. They are a common occurrence in an ultrasound image since they are often the sequelae of the physical properties of ultrasound itself. All ultrasound machines make various assumptions in generating an image. These assumptions include the following: the ultrasound beam only travels in a straight line with a constant rate of attenuation, the depth of a reflector is accurately determined by the time taken for sound to travel from the transducer to the reflector and return, and the speed of sound in all tissues is 1,540 m/sec. In order to provide technically accurate images, the operator needs to have a basic knowledge of artifacts and how to reduce or eliminate them. The following artifacts are the most commonly encountered during routine sonographic exams.

Reverberation artifact occurs when the ultrasound wave is repeatedly reflected between two highly reflective surfaces. For example, if the transducer acts as another reflective surface to a returning echo, this echo will then be re-reflected and retrace itself, resulting in an artifactual image identical to the real image, but at twice the distance from the transducer. Due to the process of attenuation, each subsequent echo is weaker than the first. To avoid this, move the transducer to a slightly different location and avoid the strong reflecting surface.

Mirror-image artifact is a type of reverberation artifact that occurs in highly reflective air with fluid interfaces such as the lung/diaphragm. The first image is displayed in the correct position, whereas a false image is produced on the other side of the reflector due to its "mirror"-like effect.

Posterior enhancement artifact occurs when the area behind an echo-weak or echo-free structure appears brighter (more echogenic) than its surrounding structures. This occurs because neighboring signals had to pass through more attenuating structures and return with fainter echoes. This explains why cysts or fluid collections demonstrate a brighter echo deep to the fluid as the sound wave is traveling faster through it. To avoid this move the transducer to a slightly different position (Figure 4.1).

An acoustic shadow results when the sound beam is unable to pass through an area posterior, or beyond, a strongly reflecting or attenuating structure. It is seen, for example, deep to areas of calcification such as stones or bones. Tissue dropout occurs due to poor beam penetration and the shadow obscures the area (Figure 4.2).

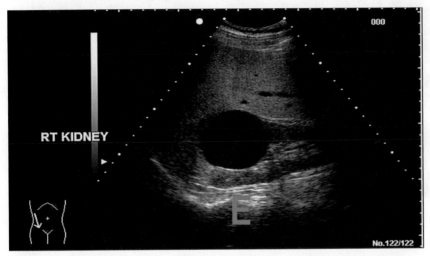

FIGURE 4.1 Arrow indicates a simple renal cyst. Note the enhancement (E) of the sound beam posterior to the cyst. The speed of sound is faster in the cyst (simple fluid) than the organs (liver and kidney).

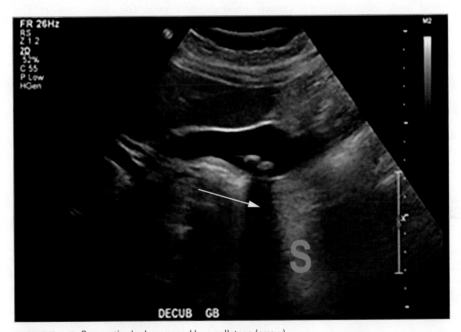

FIGURE 4.2 S acoustic shadow caused by a gallstone (arrow).

Image is overgained (bright from too much overall gain), which can create or obscure information. This is of great importance when attempting to evaluate for renal stones (Figure 4.3).

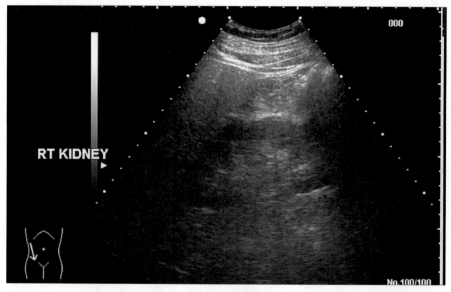

FIGURE 4.3 Image is overgained (bright from too much overall gain), which makes it difficult to assess renal anatomy.

CLINICAL USES OF ULTRASOUND

Advancements in technology have fueled the clinical application for the use of ultrasound and, as such, have grown exponentially over the past decade. The increased use of medical ultrasound can also be attributed to rising demand for point-of-care testing and the increasing number of diagnostic procedures. The expediency of bedside and real-time diagnosis of various pathologies, including life-threatening ones, precision enhancement for many procedures, avoidance of transportation delays, evasion of radiation, and potential aversion of costly additional imaging modalities are some major factors in the emergence and continued growth in clinical sonography. The clinical usefulness of ultrasound is only limited by the operator's imagination. Throughout this text the usefulness of sonography is described in order to heighten the clinician's practice reminiscent to what the stethoscope did upon its discovery in 1816 by René Laennec in 1816.

RESOURCES

Abu-Ziden, F. M., Hefny, A. F., and corr, P. (2011). Clinical ultrasound physics. *Journal of Emergencies, Trauma, and Shock, 4*(4), 501–503.

Edelman, S. (2012). *Understanding ultrasound physics* (4th ed.). Houston, TX: ESP.

Kawamura, D. (2012). *Diagnostic medical sonography* (3rd ed.). Philadelphia, PA: Wolters Kluwer Health/Lippincott Williams & Wilkins.

Medical ultrasound equipment market analysis and global forecast to 2020: Size, share, trends and growth. (2014, November 10). Retrieved from http://www.releasewire.com/press-releases/medical-ultrasound-equipment-market-analysis-and-global-forecast-to-2020-size-share-trends-and-growth-560306.htm

Tayal, V.S. (2014). Emergency ultrasound. In J. A. Marx, R. S. Hockberger, and R. M. Walls (Eds.), *Rosen's emergency medicine* (8th ed., pp. 2492–2504). Philadelphia, PA: Elsevier/Saunders.

UNIT III

Procedures for Airway Management

CHAPTER 5

Procedures for Basic Airway Management and Foreign-Body Removal

Keith A. Lafferty

BACKGROUND

Although advanced airway management skills may be beyond the scope of many practitioners, it behooves any provider who is performing minor surgical procedures using sedatives and potentially large doses of local anesthetics to have a fundamental understanding of basic airway maneuvers. Indeed, it is paramount for the provider to recognize potential airway compromise and to act on it early, before its sequelae of hypoxemia, acidosis, and obstruction may ensue.

Knowledge of the airway anatomy is mandatory. An appreciation of the importance of proper airway tone in maintaining airflow is crucial. Any decrease in consciousness, whether it is via trauma or iatrogenic medications, may allow the tongue to fall against the posterior pharyngeal wall, as well as induce a decrease in tone of the pharyngeal soft tissue. This causes a collapse of the hypopharynx and may induce a partial and/or full airway occlusion.

PATIENT PRESENTATION

Signs of partial or complete airway obstruction include the following:

- Decrease in mentation
- Pooling of oral secretions
- Stridor
- Difficulty in phonation
- Hypoxemia may be a late sign
- Cyanosis may be a late sign

TREATMENT

Often, partial or complete airway obstruction can be overcome by simple techniques, such as the chin lift or jaw thrust, which overcomes lax musculature and tongue occlusion of the posterior pharynx, especially in the patient with a decreased level of consciousness.

A chin lift or jaw thrust should be performed on every unconscious patient. This maneuver pulls the hyoid bone anteriorly, which in turn pulls the epiglottis and posterior tongue superiorly and anteriorly away from the posterior pharyngeal wall (Figure 5.1). Note that a child's airway demands greater attentiveness as children have a relatively larger tongue and a smaller luminal airway diameter relative to adults.

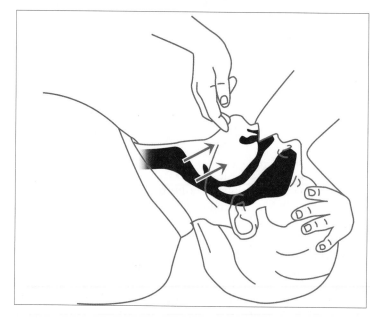

FIGURE 5.1 Sagittal view of chin lift with airway anatomy.

SUPPLEMENTAL OXYGEN

Besides proper head positioning, supplemental oxygenation (O_2) may be all that is required for patients in respiratory compromise. The signs of hypoxemia include agitation, cyanosis, and change in heart rate. A pulse oximeter should be used in all cases of conscious sedation. Furthermore, all patients with an altered mentation should be assumed to be hyopglycemic or hypoxic until proven otherwise. Physiologically, it is key to keep a patient's oxygen saturation near 100% because when it gets down to 90%, the corresponding PaO_2 is 60 mmHg, which is on the descending segment on the oxyhemoglobin dissociation curve. A further decrease will drop a patient's oxygenation rapidly and exponentially, potentially causing dysarrhythmia and/or death.

Nasal Cannula

- Generally is better tolerated than a mask
- Cannot deliver O_2 in excess of 3 L/min reliably under normal circumstances
- Not a closed system, so the FiO_2 gain may be only modest unless utilized in rapid sequence intubation (see Chapter 6)

- Further increases in flow cause nasal irritation and are not well tolerated by the patients

Simple O$_2$ Mask

- Delivers oxygen more readily than a nasal cannula
- Not as tolerable
- A minimum O$_2$ flow rate of 6 L/min must be maintained
- Note that room air is allowed to enter the mask through exhalation ports; for this reason a FiO$_2$ of 35% to 60% is all that is delivered

Nonrebreather Mask

- Contains one-way valves over the exhalation port, which allow egress of exhaled air while preventing the introduction of room air into the mask during inhalation
- There is a one-way valve between the reservoir bag and the mask
- Flow should be 10 to 12 L/min and a FiO$_2$ of 95% can be maintained

Bag-Valve Mask

- Must be utilized when all other methods fail
- Experience lends a hand here as a tight seal is a must
- Often used in conjunction with proper head positioning
- May require an oral or nasopharyngeal airway
- Tight seal is mandatory to prevent loss of air volume during ventilation
- Problems encountered include inadequate tidal volume and gastric distention
- An FiO$_2$ of 100% can be achieved with a proper seal

SUCTIONING

Occasionally, patient positioning and supplemental oxygen may be inadequate to achieve airway patency. Blood, vomitus, and secretions may require devices connected to tubing; wall suctioning may be used to clear and maintain airway passage.

A soft catheter tip suction device may be used for gentle suction of the nasopharynx, especially for infants younger than 6 months of age, as they are obligate nasal breathers. This can also be used to clear tracheostomy cannulas. They are not designed for suctioning thick secretions and/or particulate matter as the lumen can easily become occluded by such material.

The Yankauer or tonsil-tip suction device is used to clear upper airway hemorrhage and secretions. A dental tip suction device may also be used and may offer a greater ability to remove particulate matter because its tip is not rounded like the Yankauer, although it may cause more pharyngeal trauma. Oral and pharyngeal suctioning should be performed at intervals no longer than 15 seconds to prevent further hypoxemia.

Complications of suctioning include the following:

- Induction of vomiting
- Possibility of creating a complete airway obstruction from a partial obstruction if material cannot be suctioned and becomes lodged
- Bleeding
- Pharyngeal wall injury
- Brady dysrhythmias

ARTIFICIAL AIRWAYS

Artificial airways must be used when basic head positions do not alleviate tongue/pharyngeal obstruction. These devices will bypass obstructive tissue, allowing for smooth nonturbulent airflow.

Oropharyngeal Airway

The oropharyngeal airway is limited to use in the unconscious patient as it causes pharyngeal irritation that can induce vomiting in the awake patient. It is composed of a piece of hard plastic with a central air channel and a flanged end that rests on the lips (Figure 5.2).

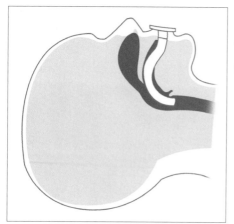

FIGURE 5.2 Oropharyngeal airway in its correct placement.

Nasopharyngeal Airway

The nasopharyngeal airway is among the simplest of artificial airways and its use is highly effective in preventing the tongue from falling back against the posterior pharyngeal wall and obstructing the airway. This device is less noxious than the oropharyngeal airway in stimulating the gag reflex. It is made of a soft rubber material. Its size can be estimated by placing the flange end from the naris to the lobule of the ear. At this length, it will rest just above the epiglottis (Figure 5.3).

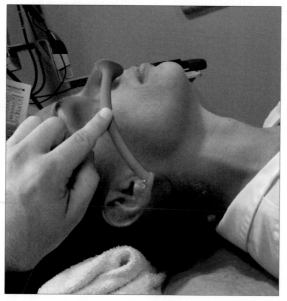

FIGURE 5.3 Nasopharyngeal airway measurement.

PROCEDURE

Chin Lift

- Place the tips of the fingers beneath the patient's chin.
- Lift the mandible forward.

Bag-Valve Mask

- Rescuers' hands must be large enough to apply pressure anteriorly by while simultaneously lifting the jaw forward.
- The thumb and index finger provide anterior pressure while the fourth and fifth fingers lift the jaw, placing pressure on the mandible, not the soft tissue.
- Complete compression of the bag must occur in order to give enough tidal volume for adequate ventilation (Figure 5.4).
- An assistant should apply firm posterior pressure on the cricoid ring in order to alleviate gastric inflation, although recent literature disputes this clinical dogma.

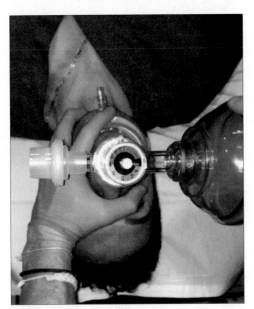

- Dentures should be left in place to help ensure a better seal with the mask.
- Attach tubing to supplemental oxygen with a flow rate of 15 L/min in order to prevent hypoxemia.

Bag-valve mask complications lead to inadequate ventilation and result from:

- A poor mask seal
- Failure to achieve proper airway patency
- Insufficient tidal volume
- Gastric distention can result from poor airway patency as air is insufflated in the esophagus and stomach, with an inherent risk of regurgitation and aspiration.

FIGURE 5.4 Bag-valve mask ventilation technique.

OROPHARYNGEAL AIRWAY

- Contraindicated in the awake patient.
- Estimate proper size by placing it adjacent to the patient's face with the flange at the level of the anterior teeth and the distal component at the angle of the mandible.
- Patient should be in supine position.
- Tongue is depressed inferiorly with a tongue depressor.
- Place the concave side inferiorly until the distal part rests in the posterior hypopharynx.
- An alternative method would be to insert the device into the oral cavity in an inverted manner, then rotate it 180 degrees and advance until its distal end is pointed caudal in the hypopharynx.

- This device essentially molds to the posterior tongue.
- It separates the tongue from the posterior pharyngeal wall and pushes the epiglottis forward.

Complications

- Vomiting
- If device is too small, it can push the epiglottis inferiorly, occluding the glottic opening.
- If the device is too big, it can impinge and displace the tongue posteriorly and occlude the hypopharynx (Figure 5.5).

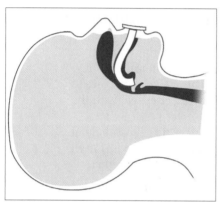

FIGURE 5.5
Incorrect size of oropharyngeal airway.

NASOPHARYNGEAL AIRWAY

- Contraindicated in facial trauma
- Lubricate the device
- Place in the nostril of least resistance.
- Insert posteriorly and toward the nasal septum.
- May have to rotate upon placement.
- If there is too much resistance, use other nostril.

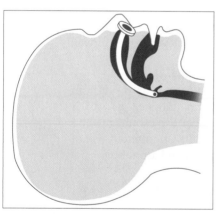

FIGURE 5.6
Incorrect size of a nasopharyngeal airway.

Complications

- Epistaxis
- Injury to nasal mucosa in adenoid tissue
- Sinusitis
- If device is too long, it can push epiglottis inferiority, occluding the glottic opening (Figure 5.6).
- In the presence of a basilar skull fracture, it may be inadvertently placed through the cribriform plate into the anterior cranial fossa.

PEARLS

- Always use supplemental oxygen when administering sedatives or large amounts of local anesthetics.
- The chin-lift maneuver by itself commonly alleviates partial airway obstruction.
- Routinely check resuscitation equipment and have it nearby for procedures involving sedatives or large doses of local anesthetics.
- In almost all instances except teeth clenching, the nasopharyngeal airway is superior to the oropharyngeal airway.

BACKGROUND

Airway foreign bodies can be divided into upper (main bronchi and proximal) and lower (distal to main bronchi) impactions. More than 3,000 deaths occur annually secondary to foreign-body aspirations; delayed presentation is common, outside of acute asphyxiation. Lower airway tract foreign bodies are a diagnostic challenge because of the following: 80% occur in children younger than 3 years of age; the event is usually not witnessed and most foreign bodies are radiolucent such as peanuts, hot dogs, grapes, and so on. Because of this, one must maintain a high index of suspicion. In general, lower airway foreign bodies are not amenable to removal in the office or acute care setting. Note that, even though many signs are nonspecific at the initial presentation, 90% of children who have aspirated will have a history of choking, coughing, wheezing, or stridor. No doubt, recurrent croup, pneumonia, atelectasis, new-onset asthma, pneumothorax, and pneumomediastinum should alert the clinician to arrange for a bronchoscopy, as this modality has decreased mortality from 50% to less than 1%. Even when the physical examination is unremarkable, if the history is possibly consistent with an acute aspiration (sudden symptoms or an object in the mouth that is suddenly missing) one must pursue this diagnosis.

Because more than two thirds of aspirated foreign bodies are radiolucent, x-rays may show indirect evidence of their presence, such as air trapping, mediastinal shift with expiration, atelectasis, pneumothorax, and pneumomediastinum. If the object is radiopaque, it may be seen oriented in the sagittal plane on the posteroanterior (PA) x-ray, as the cartilaginous tracheal rings are not fused posteriorly.

The sudden and acute asphyxiation induced by a lodged upper airway foreign body (oropharynx, hypopharynx, supraglottic, subglottic, or trachea) is a medical emergency. Any patient presenting with an acute upper airway aspiration who is not coughing, speaking, or displaying respiratory distress, needs to be treated immediately. The cough reflex is the body's primary means of expelling a foreign body. This occurs via deep inspiration followed by a forced expiration against a closed glottis, which suddenly opens after high pressure forces it to do so. All immediate emergent treatments (Heimlich, back blow, and chest thrust maneuvers) essentially mimic this protective reflex. Patients presenting in this way should be treated as a 9-1-1 emergency, and standard basic life support/advanced life support (BLS/ALS) algorithms should be followed.

Further discussion pertains to patients who present with a fish/chicken bone or pill foreign-body sensation in the throat (Figure 5.7). As a rule, these patients are stable, give a clear history, and do not display any signs or symptoms of asphyxiation. They usually present immediately and can localize by pointing to the neck, where the foreign-body sensation is felt. Indeed, most of these patients have a minor mucosal defect, which appears as a foreign-body sensation. These usually heal within 24 hours.

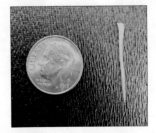

FIGURE 5.7 Fish bone. Note the size in relation to a dime.

Although most of the foreign bodies are in the hypopharynx, occasionally, with careful inspection with a tongue blade and light, some can be found in the oral pharynx (tonsils and base of the tongue). Clinically, the challenge is determining whether this is a foreign body or, more commonly, an abrasion. Adding to this diagnostic challenge is the following:

- Plain x-rays are less than 50% sensitive, as not all fish or chicken bones are radiopaque secondary to their high cartilaginous content (Figure 5.8).
- Less than 25% of patients who complain of a foreign body actually have it found endoscopically.

The sensitivity of CT scans is more than 95% and they are widely available. Also, as a complementary modality, the nasopharyngeal laryngoscope (NPL) provides direct and complete visualization and is easy to use. Combining these two modalities essentially rules out the possibility of this diagnosis (Figure 5.9).

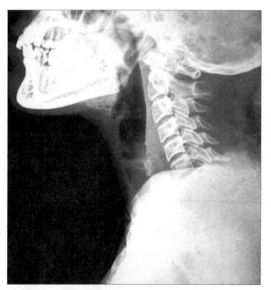

FIGURE 5.8 Lateral neck x-ray. Note that the fish bone is not seen.

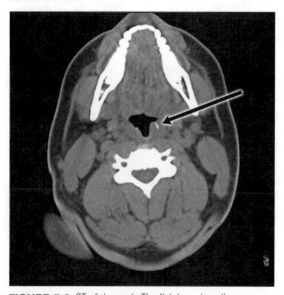

FIGURE 5.9 CT of the neck. The fish bone is radiopaque.

PATIENT PRESENTATION

- Patients usually present a few hours after the initial event.
- They sit upright and often point with a finger to the area of the throat where the foreign body is felt.
- They may experience odynophagia if the foreign body is placing pressure on the esophagus.

TREATMENT

Treatment differs depending on the clinical setting and one's familiarization with fiberoptic equipment and/or the use of a laryngoscope. Patients are initially evaluated with a careful oropharyngeal inspection. If the foreign body can be identified at this point and removed with forceps, the patient can be discharged. If further inspection is required, it usually includes the following modalities:

- Indirect laryngoscopy
- Direct laryngoscopy
- NPL
- CT scan

Fiberoptic visualization instruments, specifically the NPL, are being used with much more frequency in recent years (Figure 5.10). With a basic understanding of the upper airway anatomy, NPL use is easily mastered with minimal practice. It is attached to a light source and inserted through the nares, through the nasopharynx, and into the hypopharynx. Its distal end moves superior and inferior with the control of a dial using the dominant hand. Its lateral movement is controlled with the nondominant hand holding the end just outside the patient's naris (Figure 5.11).

In recent years, because of much-increased sensitivity, CT scans have replaced plain x-rays and the NPL has replaced indirect laryngoscopy.

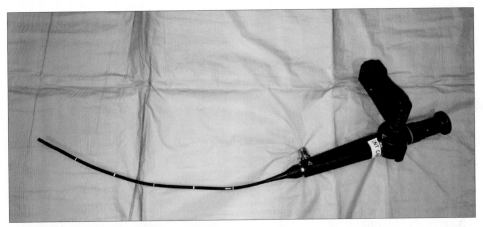

FIGURE 5.10 Naspharyngeal laryngoscope.

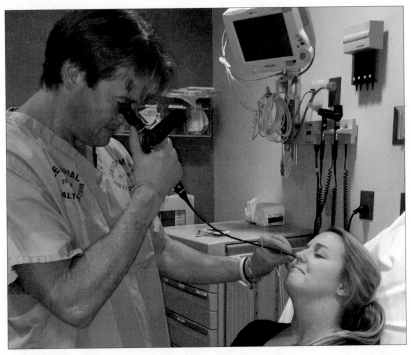

FIGURE 5.11 Naspharyngeal laryngoscope technique.

CONTRAINDICATIONS

Unfamiliarity with the use of:

- NPL
- Laryngoscope

PROCEDURE PREPARATION

Nasopharyngeal Laryngoscopy

- NPL
- Light source
- Benzocaine spray
- Water-based lubricant

Direct Laryngoscopy

- Laryngoscope and blade
- Benzocaine spray
- Viscous lidocaine
- Yankauer wall suction
- McGill forceps

Indirect Laryngoscopy

- Laryngeal (dental) mirror
- Head lamp
- Gauze
- Benzocaine spray

PROCEDURE

Nasopharyngeal Laryngoscopy

- Patient should sit in an upright position leaning slightly forward (sniffing position) with the head leaning back on a fixed surface to prevent head movement.
- Apply lubricant to the distal end of the NPL excluding the tip.
- Spray the posterior pharynx with benzocaine.
- Insert the NPL through the most patent naris (have the patient exhale through each naris separately while compressing the other).
- Insert the NPL posteriorly past the turbinates and visualize the posterior pharynx, hypopharynx, and supraglottic and glottic structures (Figure 5.12).
- If fogging occurs, move the distal end to rub against the mucosa.
- Have the patient say "e e e e," as this moves the vocal cords together and moves the glottis away from the larynx, providing a better view.
- If a foreign body is seen, proceed to direct laryngoscopy.

Direct Laryngoscopy

- After spraying the posterior pharynx with benzocaine, have the patient gargle for 1 minute three times with viscous lidocaine.
- Patient should be lying on a stretcher in the supine position.
- Provider should be standing at the head of the bed.
- Check the light on the laryngoscope blade.
- Using the left hand, place the laryngoscope blade along the floor of the mouth and gently lift up at a 45-degree angle.
- Identify the foreign body and grasp with forceps.

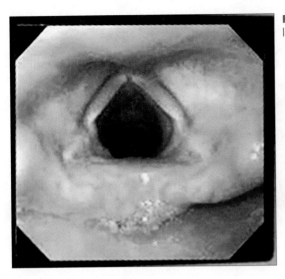

FIGURE 5.12 Naspharyngeal laryngoscope visualization.

Indirect Laryngoscopy

- Patient should sit in an upright position leaning slightly forward (sniffing position) with the head leaning back on a fixed surface to prevent head movement.
- Spray the posterior pharynx with benzocaine.
- Place the dental mirror in warm water to prevent condensation.
- Wrap the tongue in gauze and grab it with the nondominant hand.
- Place the mirror upside down in the posterior oropharynx and visualize the hypopharyngeal/supraglottic structures.

COMPLICATIONS

Retained Foreign Body

- Infection (retropharyngeal abscess)
- Asphyxiation

Nasopharyngeal Laryngoscopy

- Bleeding
- Abrasions
- Cough
- Vomiting

Direct Laryngoscopy

- Vomiting
- Bleeding
- Teeth trauma

Indirect Laryngoscopy (Dental Mirror)

- Cough
- Vomiting

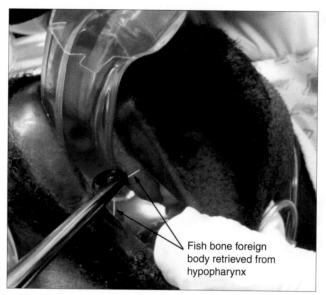

FIGURE 5.13 Retrieval of upper airway foreign body via video-assisted laryngoscopy. Note fish bone retrieval with forceps.

Fish bone foreign body retrieved from hypopharynx

PEARLS

- Because of the low sensitivity of plain x-rays, x-rays can be eliminated in practices with access to an NPL and CT.
- CT scans have a sensitivity of more than 95% in identifying fish/chicken bones.
- If symptoms persist more than 24 hours, fiberoptic identification and extraction are indicated, as these usually will not dislodge and secondary bacterial infection will ensue (Figure 5.13).

RESOURCES

Bingham, R. M., & Proctor, L. T. (2008). Airway management. *Pediatric Clinics of North America, 55,* 873–886.

Bosson, N., & Gordon, P. E. (2009, March 6). *Bag-valve-mask ventilation.* Retrieved from http://emedicine.medscape.com/article/80184-overview

Clinton, J. E., & McGill, J. W. (2004). Basic airway management and decision-making. In J. Roberts & J. Hedges (Eds.), *Clinical procedures in emergency medicine* (pp. 53–68). Philadelphia, PA: Saunders, Elsevier.

Cordle, R. (2004). Upper respiratory emergencies. In J. Tintinalli & G. Kelen (Eds.), *Emergency medicine: A comprehensive study guide* (pp. 848–858). New York, NY: McGraw-Hill.

Digoy, G. P. (2008). Diagnosis and management of upper aerodigestive tract foreign bodies. *Otolaryngology Clinics of North America, 41*(3), 485–496.

Lafferty, K. A., & Kulkarni, R. (2010, June 10). *Tracheal intubation, rapid sequence intubation.* Retrieved from http://emedicine.medscape.com/article/80222-overview

Munter, D. W., & Heffner, A. C. (2004). Esophageal foreign bodies. In J. Roberts & J. Hedges (Eds.), *Clinical procedures in emergency medicine* (pp. 775–793). Philadelphia, PA: Saunders, Elsevier.

Riviello, R. J. (2004). Otolaryngologic procedures. In J. Roberts & J. Hedges (Eds.), *Clinical procedures in emergency medicine* (pp. 1280–1316). Philadelphia, PA: Saunders, Elsevier.

Santillanes, G., & Gausche-Hill, M. (2008). Pediatric airway management. *Emergency Medicine Clinics of North America, 24*(4), 961–975.

Scarfone, R. J. (2008). Oxygen delivery, suctioning, and airway adjuncts. In C. King & F. Henretig (Eds.), *Textbook of pediatric emergency procedures* (pp. 93–108). Philadelphia, PA: Lippincott Williams & Wilkins.

Takada, M. (2000). 3D-CT diagnosis for ingested foreign bodies. *American Journal of Emergency Medicine, 18*(2), 192–193.

Thomas, S. H., & Brown, D. F. (2006). Foreign bodies. In J. Marx, R. Hockberger, & R. Walls (Eds.), *Rosen's emergency medicine concepts and clinical practice* (pp. 859–881). Philadelphia, PA: Mosby, Elsevier.

CHAPTER 6

Advanced Airway Management

Keith A. Lafferty

BACKGROUND

Few procedures have the same capacity to affect patient outcome as advanced airway management. Specifically, an appreciation of airway anatomy and oxygen physiology, coupled with the skills required for proper bag-valve-mask (BVM) ventilation and endotracheal tube intubation (ETTI) are vital to one's competency and proficiency. No doubt, this knowledge is fundamental and the cornerstone of caring for the critically ill patient. When basic airway skills are inadequate in terms of oxygenation and ventilation, competency and dexterity in such techniques are a must. For the most part, these treatment modalities trump all other actions and, as such, are the focus of this chapter.

In general, patients may be divided into those who need an immediate airway (crash airway) and those who can be managed in an orchestrated, stepwise, and escalating manner, potentially avoiding ETTI. The focus of this chapter is on rapid sequence intubation (RSI) via video-assisted laryngoscopy (VAL) in favor of direct laryngoscopy (DL). The reason behind this can also be found in the chapter describing central venous catheter (CVC) placement using ultrasound guidance rather than the landmark technique; namely the (VAL) equipment is ubiquitous and the literature supports its ease of use, superior success rate, and retention.

ETTI is still the preferred technique used to secure the airway and apply mechanical ventilation when advanced airway management is required. VAL offers the advantage of abandoning the need for alignment of the optical axes in the mouth, pharynx, and larynx in order to visualize the entrance of the glottis and therefore is more effective. Unfortunately, standard ETTI via DL, performed by untrained medical personnel and those who perform it only occasionally, carries a high risk of failure. In several studies looking at the success rate of ETTI via DL performed by medical support staff, medical students, and novice anesthesia residents, the initial success rate varied between 35% and 65%. Mulcaster et al. (2003) and Konrad, Schüpfer, Wietlisbach, and Gerber (1998) have shown that in order to improve the success rate of DL to over 90%, one would require about 47 to 56 intubations. In stark contrast, VAL has been shown to be easily learned and highly successful with minimal training necessary.

In a prospective trial, Howard-Quijano, Huang, Matevosian, Kaplan, and Steadman (2008) compared 37 novice residents in VAL versus DL and found that the former yielded a 14% higher success rate and 14% fewer esophageal intubations. Nouruzi-Sedeh, Schumann, and Growben (2009) evaluated medical personnel with no prior experience in ETTI (paramedic students, nurses, and medical students) and after a brief didactic/manikin session compared their laryngoscopy skills in the operating room (OR) between VAL and DL. As in many other similar studies, they showed that VAL led to a significantly higher success rate (93%) as compared with DL (51%) *in nonphysicians with no prior laryngoscopy experience.* Subjects were also noted to have a dramatic improvement after only five ETTIs; they neared a 100% success rate using VAL. In a meta-analysis, Griesdale et al. looked at VAL compared with DL in 17 trials with 1,998 patients. The pooled relative risk for nondifficult intubations was 1.5 and for difficult intubations was 3.5; the authors concluded that VAL improves glottic visualization, particularly in patients with potentially difficult airways.

We briefly touch on other advanced airway modalities, which may at times alleviate patient symptoms and progression to further airway modalities.

- Noninvasive positive-pressure ventilation (NIPPV)
  - Bilevel positive airway pressure (BIPAP)
  - BVM
- Laryngeal mask airway (LMA)

ANATOMY
Upper Airway

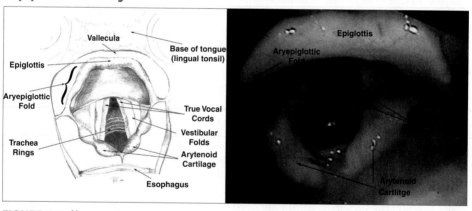

FIGURE 6.1 Airway anatomy.

Pertinent upper airway anatomical structures/divisions can be divided into the following regions (Figure 6.1):

Nasal cavity—conduit for air entry into the pulmonary system. It is the primary pathway for normal breathing.

Oral cavity—consists of the upper and lower teeth, the tongue and floor of the mouth, and the hard palate.

Oropharynx/Oral airway—begins at the soft palate and continues to the level of the hyoid bone. The tongue is the principal source of obstruction when its tone is diminished (sedatives and or cerebral insult) as it falls posteriorly against the pharyngeal wall in a supine patient. It arises from the hyoid bone and all basic airway maneuvers (chin lift, jaw thrust) elevate the hyoid bone and therefore bring the tongue anteriorly, lifting it off the pharyngeal wall.

Nasopharynx/Nasal airway extends from the back of the internal nasal cavity to the soft palate.

Laryngopharynx/Oral airway begins at the level of the hyoid bone and extends downward, where it branches into two passages: the anterior larynx and the posterior esophagus.

Larynx is the major cartilaginous skeleton of the larynx is formed by the thyroid cartilage anteriorly, the cricoid cartilage circumferentially, and the cartilaginous arytenoids posteriorly, where the true vocal cords attach. Also contains the epiglottis superiorly, which varies in size and acts as a cape superiorly draping the anterior lateral surfaces of the vocal cords. The triangular opening between the vocal cords is called the glottic opening and is the entry point to the larynx. In the adult, the glottis is the narrowest point, whereas in small children the subglottic area is narrowest. Patency of the glottic opening is dependent upon muscle tone.

- During difficult laryngoscopy, the posterior arytenoids may be the only structure visualized and one can guide the (endotracheal tube) ETT into the glottic opening by anteriorly placing its tip, knowing that these structures form the base of the triangle formed by the attaching vocal cords.

Trachea is 12 cm in length from the glottic opening to carina. The carina normally lies at the T4 to T5 interspace, so the ETT tip needs to be at least 5 cm above this to allow for ±2-cm movement that occurs with head and neck movement.

- 10% of ETTs migrate and can lead to serious complications.

Pediatric Airway Anatomy

There are some fundamental differences between the pediatric and adult airway.

- Occiput is proportionally larger
    - Causes neck to already be in slight flexion when supine
    - No need for cushion under head
    - Only slight head extension may be needed
- Obligate nasal breathers until 3 months of age
- Mouths are proportionally smaller
- Tongue is proportionally larger
- Epiglottis covers more of the glottis
    - Hypoepiglottic ligament is more lax; therefore, it creates a more floppy epiglottis
        - Reasoning behind recommended straight blade use in DL is that it lifts the epiglottis up
- Glottis is more cephalad
    - Located at the C3 to C4 level (C4–C5 in adults)
    - More anterior, causing it to be at a more acute angle in relation to the oral airway
- Narrowest segment is at the cricoid cartilage until the age of 10
- Trachea
    - 4 to 5 cm in newborns

- 7 cm in children 18 months of age
- 12 cm in adults
  - Because of the smaller trachea size, a 1- to 2-cm difference in ETT depth or height may result in an endobronchial intubation or supraglottic position.

Pediatric partial/full airway obstruction is more likely to occur than in the adult because:

- Laryngeal cartilage is more compliant than in the adult and partial airway obstruction via dynamic collapse secondary to negative intraluminal pressure is more likely to occur in the pediatric airway.
- A small change in the pediatric airway size (edema, inflammation) causes a greater increase in air resistance than a similar change in the corresponding adult airway.
  - Poiseuille's law states that the resistance to a gas (air) flowing through a tube (airway) is inversely proportional to the fourth power of the radius of the tube (airway) (Table 6.1).

TABLE 6.1 Poiseuille's Law Demonstrating the Effect of Decreasing Airway Diameter in Pediatric Versus Adult Patients

Airway	Adult	Pediatric
Decreasing by 1 cm	8 → 7 cm	4 → 3 cm
Resistance	↑ 3 x	↑ 16 x
Cross-sectional area	↓ 44%	↓ 75%

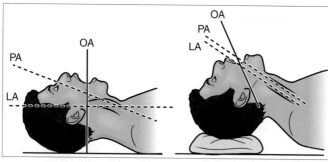
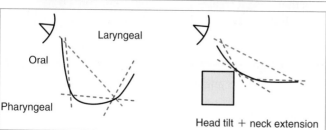

FIGURE 6.2 Oral axis, pharyngeal axis, and the laryngeal axis. Note that the oropharyngeal curve in comparison to the pharyngeotracheal curve is much more angled.

Positioning

Optimal head positioning not only creates the least obstructive anatomical alignment of the upper airway for ease of the patient's breathing but also dictates the initial straightforwardness on the application of any advanced airway in any patient in respiratory distress. The fundamental principles are:

- Separation of the tongue from the posterior pharyngeal wall
  - Alignment of the three upper airway axes to the most similar angles possible (Figure 6.2)
    - Oral axis (OA)
    - Pharyngeal axis (PA)
    - Laryngeal axis (LA)

As stated previously, the most common cause of upper airway obstruction is posterior displacement of the tongue against the pharyngeal wall, usually secondary to loss of tone and partial collapse of the pharyngeal soft tissue (history of snoring/sleep apnea are risk factors).

- Chin lift
- Jaw thrust
    - Both elevate the mandible and hyoid bone and therefore move the tongue anteriorly, lifting it off the pharyngeal wall.
    - Both cause some movement to the atlanto-occipital joint (other cervical vertebrae do not/minimally move).

In the neutral position, the OA forms roughly a 90-degree axis in relation to the LA and inherently creates a technical challenge in terms of glottic visualization. In order to decrease these three angles and subsequently decrease airway resistance, the patient should be placed supine in the "sniffing" position. Any maneuvering position that decreases airway resistance also provides better glottic visualization via laryngoscopy.

The sniffing position describes the anatomic position of slight neck flexion, head elevation (cushion of 6–7 cm), and extension. However, recent debate questions the relevance of this maneuver. Adnet et al. (2001) found no difference in glottic visualization by DL between simple head extension versus classic sniffing position and, in fact, glottic visualization was reduced with the latter in 11% of the patients. Subgroup analysis did show that patients who most benefitted from the sniffing position were the obese and those with limited neck mobility. Nur et al., in a prospective randomized trial of 378 patients undergoing elective surgery, compared the sniffing position to simple head extension (head flat) and noted that in terms of the Cormack and Lehan laryngeal view scores:

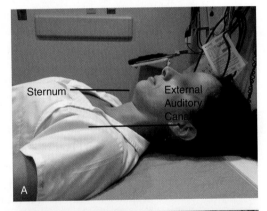

- Sniffing
    - 58% improvement
    - 40% no change
    - 5% worse

Recent meta-analysis of 2,759 adult patients compared the sniffing position with other head positions and failed to show an improvement in glottic visualization, success rate of first intubation, or intubation time.

Studies are less indicative of the sniffing position but rather reinforce the importance of head extension in all patients (providing no cervical injury).

- The external auditory meatus should be aligned with the sternum ("ear to sternum") as seen in Figure 6.3A. Note the positioning in Figure 6.3B is the incorrect positioning.

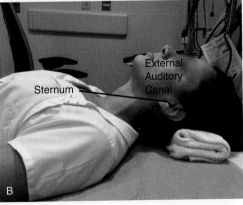

FIGURE 6.3A and 6.3B External auditory canal aligned with sternum. Note that in Figure 6.3A the external auditory canal is aligned with the sternal line; therefore correct. Figure 6.3B shows an incorrect alignment.

Head/torso elevation prevents the posterior lung from atelectasis. Lane et al. (2005) compared preoxygenation in patients undergoing RSI with head/torso raised 20 degrees compared with those in the supine position and noticed it took 1 minute and 43 seconds longer to go from an oxygen saturation (O_2 sat) of 100% to 95% in those with the head/torso up position.

- 20 degrees increases the functional residual capacity (FRC) by 20% (not in suspected C-spine injury).
- 30 degrees reverse the Trendelenburg position.

PATIENT PRESENTATION

Any patient presenting in respiratory distress or with an altered mental status is a potential candidate. Specifically, patients may be categorized into the following:

- Respiratory failure
  - Hypoxic
  - Hypercapnic
- Altered mentation (protective airway reflexes diminished)
- Partial/complete airway obstruction

NOTE *Impending respiratory failure is primarily a clinical diagnosis superseding blood gas analysis.*

- pH < 7.35
- $PaCO_2$ > 45 mmHg
- PaO_2: FiO_2 < 200 mmHg

TREATMENT

Preoxygenation

Initial goals are to bring the patient's O_2 sat as close to 100% as possible by means of displacing the alveoli/airway's 78% nitrogen storage with that of O_2. In essence, we wish to replace the ambient alveoli air with a high concentration of O_2 and in doing so create an O_2 bank.

Though the anesthesia literature states that having a patient take eight tidal volume (TV) breaths utilizing an FiO_2 of 1.0 can provide safe apnea time of over 3 minutes, this does not apply to emergent respiratory distressed patients with limited pulmonary reserve.

The nonrebreather mask (NRB) does not fully denitrogenate the alveoli, as its FiO_2 is 0.7 at 15 L/min flow. However, by opening the flow valve on the wall completely (calibration stops at 15), one can obtain a flow rate of 30 L/min, thereby increasing the FiO_2 to 0.9. Note the calibration on the wall stops at 15, but by opening the flow valve it can be significantly increased. This will in turn more fully denitrogenate and create the desired O_2 bank, which will be needed for ETTI during the safe apnea period (> 90% O_2 sat) of the procedure.

Patients who cannot maintain their O_2 sat ≥ 95% by preoxygenation for 3 minutes by means of the NRB are displaying physiologic shunting and require NIPPV with positive end-expiratory pressure (PEEP). Physiologic shunting is basically mimicking anatomical shunting in that venous blood is being redistributed back into the arterial circulation without being fully oxygenated. This is because the alveoli are not allowing O_2 to diffuse across the alveolar epithelium/pulmonary capillary endothelium (Hgb is leaving "empty handed") secondary to them being diseased with (Figure 6.4):

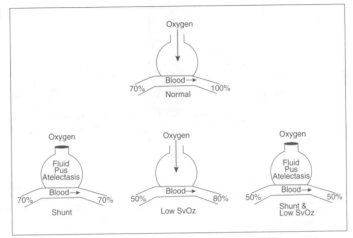

FIGURE 6.4 Physiological pulmonary shunt. Note that the pulmonary blood flow is leaving the alveoli without being adequately oxygenated.

- Congestive heart failure (CHF)—water
- Pneumonia—pus
- Pulmonary contusion—blood
- Atelectasis

Besides physiologic shunting, another reason patients may not be able to increase their O_2 sat greater than 95% after adequate NRB preoxygenation is if their VO_2 (venous O_2) sat is lower than the normal 65% to 70%. This can occur in shock states in which the tissue is attempting to compensate for a decrease in cardiac output by extracting more O_2 than normal from Hgb, thereby causing a lower VO_2 sat on entry into the pulmonary capillary bed. The answer to this is volume resuscitation. Though this seems somewhat unrelated, increasing one's cardiac output can dramatically benefit one's O_2 sat.

In order for patients to tolerate safe apnea after RSI medications are given, they must have a sufficient O_2 bank to tolerate possible minutes without ventilation. This only can occur if their O_2 sat is as close to 100% as possible in order for them to be as far away as possible from the steep part of the O_2 sat curve.

It takes some time, especially with a proper O_2 reserve, for one to go from an O_2 sat of 100% to an O_2 sat of 90%, but a rapid and precipitous time to go from an O_2 sat of 90% to an O_2 sat of 70% (Figure 6.5).

Desaturations less than 70% (danger zone) impose a high risk of:

- Dysrhythmias
- Vascular collapse
- Hypoxic brain injury
- Death

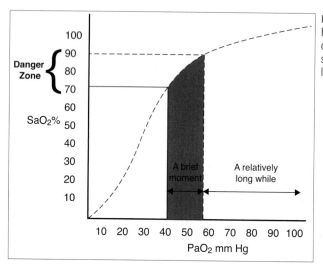

FIGURE 6.5 Oxygen hemoglobin dissociation curve. Note that the O_2 sat does not decline in a linear manner over time.

NIPPV with PEEP is the only method to address patients with physiologic shunting who are in need of preoxygenation above an O_2 sat of 95%. This is because PEEP, via increasing the mean airway pressure, induces (Table 6.2):

- Hydrostatic movement of fluid from the alveoli into the interstitium
- Distention of damaged/atelectatic alveoli
  - Because nitrogen has alveoli distention qualities, preoxygenation/denitrogenation can lead to absorption atelectasis.
- Recruits alveoli

TABLE 6.2 Examined Hypoxic Critically Ill Patients Requiring Displaying Physiologic Shunting and Compared Preoxygenation With PPV and Without

Oxygen Saturation	PPV Group	Non-PPV Group
Preoxygenation O_2 sat	98%	93%
O_2 sat during apneic time/ETT placement	93%	81%

EET, endotracheal tube; PPV, positive-pressure ventilation.

Adapted from Baillard et al. (2006)

Mort et al. evaluated patients with physiologic shunting before and after 4 minutes of preoxygenation using a BVM without PEEP and noticed a mean arterial PaO_2 of 67/104 mmHg before/after and concluded BVM without PEEP increases the PaO_2 only negligibly in these patients.

From an operation point of view, it is difficult to set up BIPAP for a few minutes in order to preoxygenate the patient then disassemble the equipment for ETTI and switch ventilators. For this reason and to aid simplicity, one can still provide PPV with PEEP using the standard BVM by means of adding a PEEP valve to the exhalation port (Figure 6.6).

Because the one-way valve in the BVM between the mask and bag opens mainly by squeezing the bag or by negative pressure induced by a patient's spontaneous inspiration, applying a constant stream of air via an attached nasal cannula (NC) at a flow rate of 15 L/min satisfies the pressure needed between ventilations to maintain PEEP.

Apneic Oxygenation

Because pulmonary blood flow is still occurring during the apneic period of ETT placement, O_2 is continually being diffused out of the alveoli epithelium at 250 mL/min and into the capillary endothelium, attaching itself to circulating Hgb. This creates an O_2 concentration gradient from the alveoli to the pulmonary capillary bed and, in doing so, likewise between the more proximal airways and the alveoli. Despite no ventilations (RSI dictates this, assuming the patient has a full stomach unless O_2 sat is low) after the patient is paralyzed, there is actual flow and movement of O_2 down these concentration gradients, as the alveoli are somewhat subatmospheric and a mass flow of gas (O_2) flows from the airways into the alveoli. By applying an NC at 15 L/min (noxious and otherwise not tolerable in the awake patient), proximal airways can come close to an FiO_2 of 1.0 and serve to replace the alveoli O_2.

Taha et al. (2006) have shown that apneic oxygenation via an NC during RSI in comparison to those without apneic oxygenation desaturated in 6 minutes rather than 3.65 minutes.

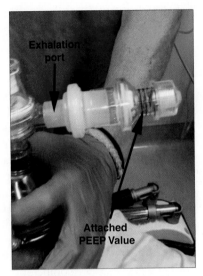

FIGURE 6.6 Bag-valve mask with positive end-expiratory-pressure valve. Note that this simple device attaches to the exhalation port and can be dialed from 5 to 20 mmHg.

Rapid Sequence Intubation

The ultimate goal is to place the ETT quickly into the trachea, alleviating the patient's respiratory distress and not inducing any iatrogenic hypoxia. Emergent patients usually have nonfasting stomachs, which poses an aspiration risk. These patients are inherently different than those prepared for the OR who have fasted for a minimum of 8 hours and therefore have a negligible risk for aspiration. Also, unlike the elective OR patients, emergent dyspnea patients by definition have limited pulmonary reserve secondary to acute and/or chronic pulmonary pathology. Because of this, immediate and simultaneous rapid-acting sedative and paralytic medications after adequate preoxygenation has been developed. Coupled with this swift transformation from the conscious to the unconscious state is the need to keep positive pressure ventilation to a minimum as any gastric insufflation coexisting with a potentially full stomach is a precursor to gastric regurgitation and possible pulmonary aspiration. For this reason, RSI has been the mainstay of emergent ETTI for decades and continues to be the standard of care.

- Preoxygenate for 3 minutes in order to establish and maintain an O_2 sat of $\geq 95\%$
  - NRB at 30 L/min to establish an FiO_2 of 0.9
  - Head/torso up, position 45 degrees (20 degrees upon laryngoscopy)
  - Do not administer PPVs throughout procedure, even when the patients has apnea.
  - NC under mask using separate O_2 source (turn on at 15 L/min after NRB removed on ETT placement)
- If unable to increase the O_2 sat $\geq 95\%$ with these steps, do the following
  - BVM at 15 L/min to establish an FiO_2 of 0.9 with a PEEP valve attached (5–15 mmHg) and NCO_2 at 15 L/min
  - Proper airway positioning, including:
    - Nasopharyngeal airway (NPA)
    - Head up 20 degrees or reverse Trendelenburg at 30 degrees
  - Continue bagging after RSI meds are given during the apnea period as shunting is still present and will still need PEEP
    - Use manometer to ensure airway pressure ≤ 20 mmHg (lower esophageal sphincter opens at 25 mmHg)
    - PEEP valve dialed to 5 to 15 mmHg

  Steps include:

- Give RSI meds
  - Sedative—etomidate or ketamine
  - Paralytic—succinylcholine or rocuronium
- NCO_2 at a flow rate of 15 L/min to ensure apneic oxygenation
- VAL

  Medications used in RSI:

- Essentially is a two-drug procedure
  - Induction agent (Table 6.3)
  - Paralytic agent (Table 6.4)
- Because of the expediency needed to make an awake patient unconscious and paralyzed, and for because in the advent of a failed airway it behooves the clinician to have the patient rapidly awake (pharyngeal tone and protective reflexes), the medications must possess the following properties:
  - Rapid onset
  - Rapid offset
  - High potency

Bilevel Positive Airway Pressure

Initially developed for patients with sleep apnea (continuous positive airway pressure [CPAP]) and those with neuromuscular disorders, this respiratory modality has become first line for many patients with acute respiratory distress. Keenan, Sinuff, Cook, and Hill (2003) have shown that in the acute chronic obstructive pulmonary disease (COPD) patient, BIPAP has decreased ETTI by 28% (other studies have shown higher rates) and hospitalization length of stay by 4.57 days. Other studies have shown a decrease in nosocomial pneumonia from 22% to 8%, with also a decrease in mortality campared to patients treated with ETTI.

TABLE 6.3 RSI Induction Medications

Induction Agent	Dose	Onset	Duration	Advantages	Cautions
Etomidate	0.3 mg/kg IV (intravenous) push (normal adult dose about 20 mg)	45 sec	7–10 min	Does not alter hemodynamics or intracranial pressure (ICP); no histamine release; does not induce apnea; useful for patients with multiple trauma and hypotension (does not alter systemic BP)	Myoclonus; adrenal suppression (clinical significance with one bolus is in dispute at this time); vomiting; lowers seizure threshold; does not provide analgesia
Ketamine	1.5–2.0 mg/kg IV push (not to exceed 0.5 mg/kg/min)	1 min	10 min	Bronchodilatory effects advantageous if hypotension or lung disease present (leaves airway and other protective reflexes intact); may possess neuroprotective effects as it increase CPP (cerebral perfusion pressure) without increasing the ICP	Has recently been shown not to increase ICP and may in fact be neuroprotective; hallucinations; increases sympathetic tone (good in shock patients); potent cerebral vasodilation, mild cardiovascular stimulation; emergence delirium more of a concern when used for conscious sedation

TABLE 6.4 RSI Paralytic Medications

Paralytic Agent	Dose	Onset	Duration	Advantages	Cautions
Succinylcholine	1.5 mg/kg	45 sec	7–10 min	Depolarizing neruomuscular block (NMB); drug of choice for emergency pediatric intubation; rapid onset (45 sec) and brief duration of action	Increases serum potassium; muscle fasciculation; malignant hyperthermia; cardiac arrest in children with muscular dystrophy; dysrhythmia with multiple doses
Rocuronium	1.0–1.5 mg/kg IV push	1 min	45 min	Nondepolarizing NMB; minimal effect on hemodynamics; low incidence of histamine release (0.8%)	Duration prolonged with hepatic impairment

In general, when one describes NIPPV, he or she is describing this airway modality. BIPAP offers the benefit of mechanical ventilation without the risk associated with ETTI. The main reason for BIPAP is to assist in patient's ventilation (IPAP [inspiratory positive airway pressure]) and to improve oxygenation by means of keeping alveoli extended, recruitment of other aveoli, and to force fluid from the alveoli into the interstitium.

Besides for the acute respiratory distress patient, this airway adjunct can be used in chronic conditions as well. Also, BIPAP is becoming used more often as a transition from invasive mechanical ventilation to spontaneous breathing. It behooves the clinician to be familiar with appropriate patient-selecting criteria as well as basic ventilator settings. One can think of BIPAP as a more precise, controlled, and cycled form of BVM in which the exact TVs and respiratory rate are set with a peak valve in place and a perfect seal.

BIPAP is composed of two ventilatory cycles/pressures; the difference between these two settings is representative of the given pressure support or TV.

- IPAP
  - Always the higher pressure number
- EPAP (expiratory positive airway pressure)
  - Always the lower pressure number
  - Analogous to PEEP

Studies have shown that BIPAP improves the outcome in acute respiratory distress patients:

- COPD exacerbation secondary to acute hypercapnia.
- In a meta-analysis, Ram et al. reviewed 14 studies evaluating the effect of BIPAP in acute COPD versus standard medical therapy and showed a decrease in:
  - Mortality (RR [respiratory rate] 0.52)
  - Need for intubation (RR 0.41)
  - Treatment failure (RR 0.48)
- CHF in the absence of shock or ischemia.
  - Recent literature shows no difference in clinical outcome between BIPAP and CPAP.

There is no evidence that BIPAP improves the outcome in patients with:

- Pneumonia
- Asthma
- Adult respiratory distress syndrome (ARDS)

Contraindications

- Cardiac arrest
- Respiratory arrest
- Vomiting
- Large amount of secretions
- Upper gastrointestinal (GI) bleed
- Status epilepticus
- Partial/full airway obstruction

Relative Contraindications

- Mask discomfort that cannot be relieved with adjustments and sedatives
- Patients at risk for aspiration, including but not limited to those with an altered mental status unless secondary to hypercapnia

- Limit use in patients who have had recent gastric surgery to avoid inadvertent gastric distention and possible intra-abdominal anastomosis dehiscence

Special Consideration

- Often eliminates the need for ETTI

Procedure Preparation

- Respiratory therapy should be at the patient bedside assisting in ventilatory settings and assuring proper mask size.
- There are various types of masks but the oral–nasal mask is the most common (Figure 6.7).
  - The silicon cushion forms a seal around the nose and the mouth.
    - Typically, the smallest mask providing a proper fit is the most effective.
    - Though the nasal-only mask induces less claustrophobia, the seal is often lost as patients may have difficulty keeping the mouth closed.

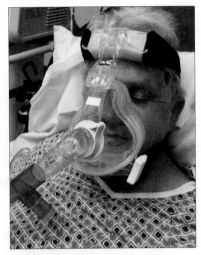

FIGURE 6.7 BIPAP oral–nasal mask.

- Patient may require a small dose of a sedative to ensure mask comfort as the mask often induces some anxiety/claustrophobia.
- Ventilatory settings include but are not limited to
  - IPAP/EPAP (TV)
  - RR
    - Besides the set rate, a patient's spontaneous negative inspiratory pressure will activate a full preset TV.
  - FiO_2
  - PIP (peak inspiratory pressure)
  - Detection of air leak

Procedure

- Apply mask and straps.
  - Should be able to place two fingers easily between the straps and the patient's head.
  - The mask should not extend over the chin.
  - If the mask continues to be uncomfortable or there are large air leaks, replace the mask with a different size.
- Initial settings are generally that of an IPAP of 10 and an EPAP of 5.

Post-Procedure Considerations

- If patient continues to have persistent hypercapnia
  - Increase the IPAP number to increase the TV
    - Typically increase by increments of two
- If patient has persistent hypoxia
  - Increase the FiO_2
  - Increase the EPAP number
    - If this is done one may have to increase the IPAP as well, in order to maintain a constant TV (pressure support).

- In general, trials of 1 to 2 hours are useful to determine if the patient is improving or needs more advanced intervention (i.e., ETTI); predictions of success include:
  - Clinical improvement in respiratory status
  - Decrease in $PaCO_2 > 8$ mmHg
  - Improvement of pH > 0.06

Complications

- Skin pressure injuries from masks that are too tight
- Anxiety/claustrophobia
- Gastric distention
  - Generally avoided with IPAP < 20

BAG-VALVE MASK

These skills are imperative to anyone working with potentially ill patients. These self-inflating bags have a one-way valve between the reservoir and the bag on the distal end and a similar valve in the proximal end between the bag and the mask (with a manometer), which only opens via (Figure 6.8):

- Squeezing the bag
- Negative inspiratory breath of the patient providing a mask seal

Can assist a patient's spontaneous ventilatory efforts ("bagging with the patient") or may need to solely ventilate the apneic patient ("bagging the patient").

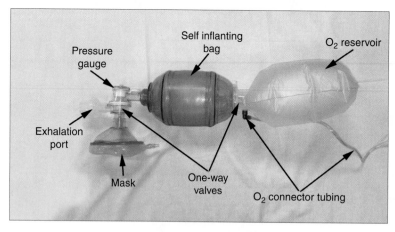

FIGURE 6.8 Anatomy of bag-valve mask.

Absolute Contraindication

- Inability to form and or maintain a mask/face seal

Relative Contraindications

- Beards (use lube)
- Facial trauma
- Micrognathia

Studies have also shown the following subset of patients to propose potential difficulty:

- Obesity
- Edentulous
- Age older than 57
- History of sleep apnea
- High Mallampati score

Special Considerations

- Use of an airway conduit is highly recommended (see Chapter 5).
  - Authors strongly recommend the use of an NPA over that of an oropharyngeal airway (OPA) because the former:
    - Induces no gagging
    - Easier to place
    - Leaves the oral cavity unoccupied
    - Can be left in place during ETI
- Have a Yankauer suction catheter at arm's reach.
- Use a roll or ramp under the shoulders of obese patients.
- Pull the mandible upward rather than pushing the mask down.

Procedure Preparation

- Proper patient positioning (as described previously)
- NPA
- PEEP valve (patients with a physiologic shunt)
- Ensure a tight mask seal
- Gather adequate personnel
- Assemble necessary equipment (Figure 6.9)

Procedure

Mask should be placed with the pointed area over the nasal bridge taking care not to cover the patient's eyes nor extend beyond the chin. Attach tubing to high-flow O_2 at 15 L/min for a FiO_2 of 0.9.

One-Hand Method

- EC clamp method (Figure 6.10A)
  - Thumb and index finger exerts pressure on the proximal and inferior mask, respectively, while the third and fifth fingers grasp mandible body/angle and perform a jaw thrust.
    - Do not clasp the submandibular soft tissue and induce inadvertent tongue occlusion.
  - Though this is touted as the classic method, only use this practice if there are not enough personnel to perform the two-hand method, as one cannot reliably maintain a seal with one hand as this is difficult and fatiguing.

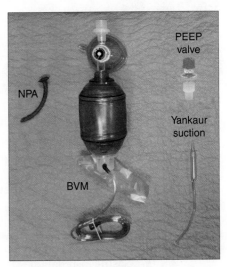

FIGURE 6.9 Bag-valve mask, nasopharyngeal airway, Yankauer, and positive-end-expiratory-pressure valve.

Two-Hand Method

- Thenar eminence method (Figure 6.10B).
  - Place both thenar eminences on each side of the mask parallel to the stretcher and apply downward force while the second to fifth fingers grasp the mandible body/angle and perform a bilateral jaw thrust.
  - Creates a greater seal with considerably less effort.
- This two-handed thenar eminence method is recommended over the two-handed EC clamp method as the thenar muscles are the strongest in the hand.
- With a mask seal assured, squeeze to keep airway pressures < 20 mmHg.
  - Lower esophageal sphincter opens with pressures > 25 mmHg
- Positive end-expiratory-pressure
- TVs of ≤ 6 mL/Kg (500 mL)
  - Even at an FiO_2 of 0.5, only 500 mL/min is needed to maintain O_2 sat.
  - Healthy patients consume 250 mL/min of O_2.
- 8 breaths per minute with each squeeze of 2 seconds duration
  - Rapid inspiratory times increase peak airway pressures and risk gastric distention and aspiration.

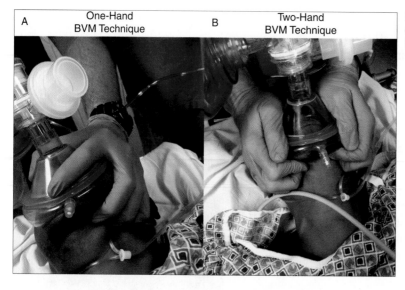

| A | One-Hand BVM Technique | B | Two-Hand BVM Technique |

FIGURE 6.10A and 6.10B One- and two-hand bag-valve mask technique.

Post-Procedure Considerations

- Ensure adequate patient positioning.
- Affirm tubing is attached to a high-flow O_2 source.
- Place an NPA.
- Use the two-person thenar technique when possible.

Complications

- Inability to ventilate (consider LMA)
- Gastric insufflation
  - Maintain airway pressures < 20 mmHg by means of observing the manometer on the device (Figure 6.11).

- Studies have shown that overzealous bagging can impede venous return/cardiac output and induce hypotension by means of increasing mean airway pressure and subsequently induce cerebral anoxia.

LARYNGEAL MASK AIRWAY

This intermediate airway device is increasingly used not only by anesthesiology, but also emergency and prehospital clinicians. The American Heart Association (AHA) states that this is an acceptable devise for use by nonexperts in ETTI when performing advanced airway maneuvers. One can think of this as a small BVM placed over the supraglottic area.

The device is a flexible airway tube 25 cm in length with an inflatable bladder cuff on its distal end. The proximal end has a standard connector that attaches to any ventilating equipment (BVM, ventilator).

Indications include:

- Rescue airway device for failed BVMs
- Rescue airway device for failed ETTIs
  - Should be at an arm's reach when initiating ETTI
- Use by advanced airway providers with inadequate skills in terms of ETTI

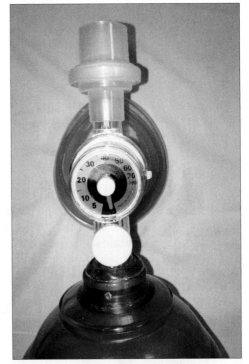

FIGURE 6.11 Bag-valve mask manometer. Keep airway pressure below 20 mmHg during bag ventilations when possible to mitigate risk of opening the lower esophageal sphincter (25 mmHg).

Contraindications and Relative Contraindications

- Because this is a blind insertion device, its use is not recommended in cases with potential upper airway foreign bodies (Figure 6.12).

Special Considerations

- Less gastric distention (aspiration) than BVM as it requires less pressure to achieve effective ventilation.
  - Stone et al. have shown that the incidence of gastric regurgitation was lower when the LMA was used in favor of BVM before ETTI.
- Higher first time success rate than ETTI
- Rapid novice placement
- Allows for minimal/no chest compression interruption

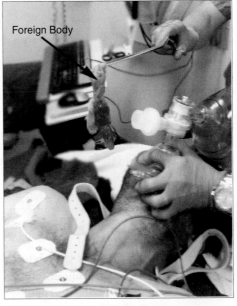

Foreign Body

FIGURE 6.12 Upper-airway foreign-body retrieved after prehospital laryngeal mask airway insertion (blind).

- Easier to ventilate compared with BVM
  - Bypasses tongue and pharyngeal soft tissue and is closer to the glottis
- Placement requires no head movement
- Requires one person as opposed to BVM, which ideally requires two
- Straight and curved devices
- Some provide a separate channel for:
  - Gastric suctioning
  - ETT placement (intubating LMA)
- Five pediatric and three adult sizes
  - #4 sufficient for most adults

Procedure Preparation

- Usually comes in a prepackaged container with all needed equipment (Figure 6.13).
- Remove all air from bladder and check for leaks.
- Lubricate the posterior cuff surface.
  - Opposite surface of where air exchange occurs

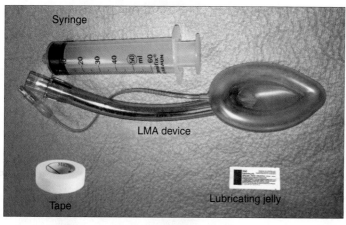

FIGURE 6.13 Laryngeal mask airway set up—syringe, lubricating jelly, tape—usually prepackaged.

Procedure

- Stand at the head of the bed.
- Tilt the head backward (avoid in potential C-spine injuries).
- Hold the LMA with your dominant hand like a pen, with the index finger pointed distally.
- Open the mouth as much as possible and insert against and along the hard and then soft palate and continue this motion until the full cuff is completely beyond the tongue and resistance is felt (Figure 6.14).
  - The final resting position is when the cuff is beyond the inferior/posterior tongue at the laryngeal inlet (hypopharynx) (Figure 6.15).
  - Nondominant hand should grasp and place full downward pressure on the shaft once the dominant distal index finger can go no further.
  - Ensure the leading edge remains firm and flat against the hard palate to prevent it from folding over on itself upon advancing.

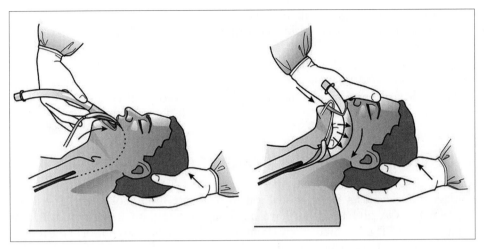

FIGURE 6.14 Laryngeal mask airway placement.

- Inflate cuff with approximately 30 mL of air.
  - During inflation the shaft may move out 1 to 2 cm as the cuff finds its location.
- Connect the device to a positive pressure system.
- Secure with formal strap or tape.

Post-Procedure Considerations
- As in ETTI, capnography is the gold standard for successful placement.
- Unlike ETTI, auscultation over the neck trumps the lateral chest area for assessment of proper placement.
- If an air leak is detected, add 5 to 10 mL of additional air to cuff.
  - If this fails, remove the device and replace it, possibly with a larger device.
- Unlike the ETT, medications should not be delivered via the LMA.
- May be difficult to ventilate:
  - If high-peak airway pressures are encountered
  - Obesity

Complications
- Improper placement can occur and result in a poor seal or obstruction of air flow.
  - In a meta-analysis, Hubble et al. have shown that the common level of obstruction is at the oropharynx.
    - Epiglottis folds down upon itself.
    - Tongue and or pharyngeal soft tissue is pushed into the airway.

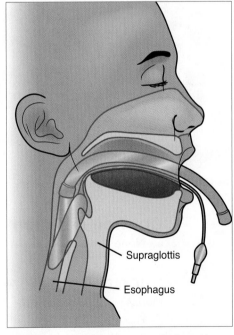

FIGURE 6.15 LMA proper supraglottic position. Note that the distal tip of the cuff sits partially on the esophagus while its anterior surface sits in the supraglottic area. Note the trachea and esophagus are not isolated from each other.

- Gastric distention, regurgitation, and aspiration
  - Only provides partial occlusion of the esophagus and does not isolate the trachea
- In 1% to 5% of the time, the cuff may fold over itself upon insertion
- Upper airway/tooth trauma
- Laryngospasm may occur if the cuff tip comes into contact with the glottis or if aspiration occurs

VIDEO-ASSISTED LARYNGOSCOPY

The typical VAL has a light and an optic magnifier. The GlideScope model has a 60-degree angle on its blade allowing it to negotiate the almost 90-degree angle between the OA and LA (DLs have a 30-degree angle on their curved blades) (Figure 6.16). ETTI is required in any situation in which definitive control of the airway is needed. Indications include, but are not limited to:

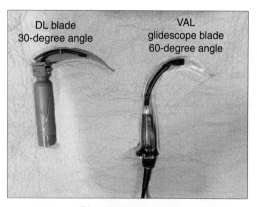

FIGURE 6.16 Direct laryngoscopy versus GlideScope blades.

- Cardiac/respiratory failure
  - 2010 AHA guidelines state that in the cardiac arrest patient, circulation and airway are attended to before breathing.
    - Cardiac airway breathing (CAB) model
- Failure to protect the airway (depressed mentation)
- Inadequate oxygenation and or ventilation
- Impending or existing airway obstruction
- Any critically ill patient with multiple systemic diseases and/or injuries

Contraindication

- None

Special Considerations

Predictors of potential difficult intubations:

- Facial trauma
- Neck tumors
- Burns
- Angioedema
- Infections
  - Pharyngeal
  - Laryngeal
  - Soft tissue
- Mallampati classification
  - A high Mallampati score (Class III or IV) is associated with more difficult intubation as well as a higher incidence of sleep apnea.

- Class I: Soft palate, uvula, fauces, pillars visible
- Class II: Soft palate, uvula, fauces visible
- Class III: Soft palate, base of uvula visible
- Class IV: Only hard palate visible

Procedure Preparation

Ensure the patient is attached to the cardiac monitor, pulse oximeter is on and working, at least one IV is in place and preoxygenation is underway. Patient's positioning should be supine, maximizing the three airway axes described earlier and in 30 degrees reverse Trendelenburg position. Assign any respiratory therapist/assistant to observe the monitor and report any changes immediately. RSI medications should be in syringes with NSS flushes prefilled. The height of the bed should be at the lower sternum of the laryngoscopist.

Back-up airway equipment needs to be available at an arm's reach and one must always assume the procedure may fail. At the least, an LMA should be at the bedside (Figure 6.17).

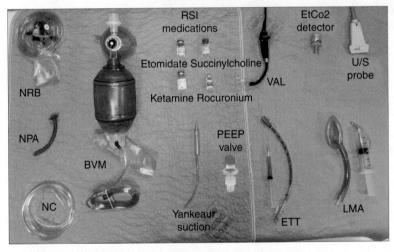

FIGURE 6.17 Backup airway equipment should always be within an arm's reach.

Equipment:

- Gloves
- Eye protection
- Yankauer suction
  - Attach to suction canister, turn on, and secure at rear of stretcher.
  - Copious secretions may interfere with the video camera; therefore, ensure suction is turned to its fullest and have backup clean blades at an arm's reach in such cases.
- VAL (Figure 6.18)
  - Should be on, at the right side of bed with the view screen in line of sight
  - Proper blade size preattached
    - Size 2 in pediatric patients
    - Size 3 in normal size adult
    - Size 4 is recommended in all adults

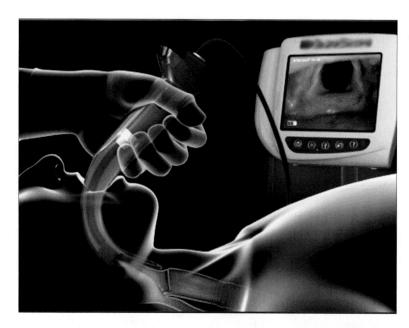

FIGURE 6.18 GlideScope video-assisted laryngoscopy.

- ETT with rigid stylet in place
  - Ensure the tip of the stylet does not propel past the distal tip of the ETT.
  - Requires up to a 60-degree curve at the distal end to negotiate the 60-degree curve of the VAL blade (GlideScope and similar models) and three airway axes.
  - Use the largest ID size possible in order to decrease the airway resistance in intubated patients as it is difficult to "breathe through a straw."
    - Size 8 in most adults
    - Pediatric size
      - Neonate: 3.0 mm
      - 0 to 6 months: 3.5 mm
      - 6 to 12 months: 4.0 mm
      - Older than 12 months: age in years/4) + 4 = ETT size
  - Check the cuff for leak with insufflation of air and then remove all air.
  - Have a smaller size than calculated on table and ready if needed.
- Syringe 10 mL
- BVM attached to high-flow FiO_2 source
- NPA
- Formal oral trachea tube holder/tape/bite block
- ETT confirmation devices
  - Capnography device
  - Bedside ultrasound
  - Stethoscope

PROCEDURE
- Initiate only after proper positioning, preoxygenation, and apneic oxygenation fully utilized as described previously.
- Eyes should be close to the video monitor.
- Hold the VAL in the left hand with the blade facing down.

- Open patient's mouth with your right hand using the scissor technique.
    - Place the thumb and index finger of the right hand into the right side of the patients' mouth. Place the index finger on the patient's upper teeth and the thumb on the lower teeth, using a scissor-like movement, open the mouth *as wide as possible* (Figure 6.19).

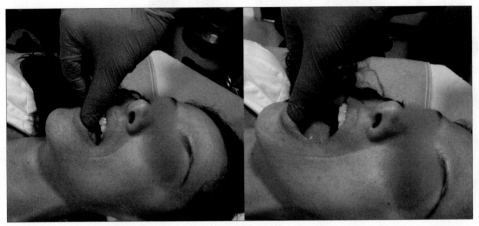

FIGURE 6.19 Scissor technique in opening the mouth.

- Introduce the VAL in the your left hand and introduce the blade into the center of the mouth **(Video 6.1)**.
    - Ensure you are looking at the patient and not the video monitor until the blade is within the mouth over the center of the tongue, not sweeping it to the side as in DL.
- While looking at the video monitor, follow the tongue into the valleculu deep and anterior to the visualized epiglottis (Figure 6.20).
    - In lieu of lifting, use more of a wrist abduction ("cocking of the wrist") movement and the glottis will come into view.
        - Note that in DL one lifts in a 45-degree angle in an attempt to align the three airway axes.

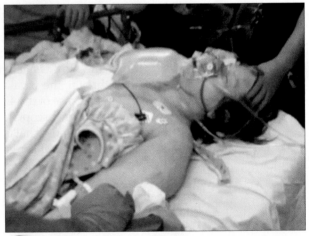

VIDEO 6.1 Video-assisted laryngoscopy. Note that NC/apneic oxygenation is not shown and should be done in all cases of endotracheal tube intubation. Also, for endotracheal tube confirmation, rapid trachea ultrasound exam should be done before ventilations/auscultation.
springerpub.com/campo

- If difficulty seeing the glottis, move blade slightly out of the mouth as sometimes overzealous depth places the blade tip in the esophagus.
    - In this case, one would see the epiglottis "pop" into sight as the blade is withdrawn.

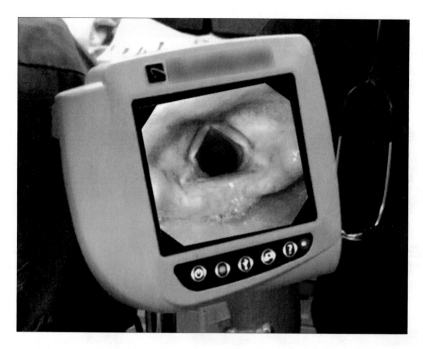

FIGURE 6.20 Video monitor displaying the glottis upon video-assisted laryngoscopy.

- Keep your focus on the video monitor while having an assistant place a finger in patient's mouth pulling the bucca laterally allowing more room for the VAL blade to occupy the mouth to make room for the ETT.
- Grasp and hold the ETT with stylet in place in your right hand and, while looking at mouth, place into the right side of the mouth with the curved side facing up.
  - Upon entry of the ETT into the mouth, focus again on the video monitor.
  - Note that in DL, the most challenging part of ETTI is glottis visualization, as passing the ETT through the vocal cords is relatively easy as it is a more direct straight line; this is because of the 45-degree upward angle that and maintained force applied by the laryngoscopist in decreasing the three airway axes.
  - In contrast, in VAL the most challenging part of ETTI is the actual placement of the ETT through the vocal cords, negotiating the 60-degree angle in which fiberoscopy bypasses in terms of visualization; in other words, glottis visualization is relatively easy while passing the ETT through the glottis may be slightly more challenging.
  - The ETT should be placed 4 to 5 cm past the vocal cords.
    - ETT should be at the lips:
      - 21 cm in adult females
      - 23 cm in adult males
      - Pediatric tube length is age/2 + 12
- Inflate the cuff via the pilot balloon port to the minimum pressure required to prevent an air leak in order to isolate the trachea from the esophagus and prevent aspiration.
  - Keep pilot balloon < 25 mmHg as the tracheal mucosa capillary pressure is 30 mmHg.
  - Usually less than 10 mL of air
- Immediately attach and record capnography.

- Secure the ETT with a bite block and use either:
  - A formal oral trachea tube holder (preferably)
  - Tape
- Restraints
  - Preferably chemical
  - Physical

Post-Procedure Considerations

Though it seems intuitive to know whether the ETT is in the trachea or the esophagus, evidence states the contrary as up to 6% are in erroneous positions in pooled emergent studies. More important, the sequelae of a misplaced ETT can be devastating and significantly increase the morbidity and mortality by means of:

- Hypoxia
- Hypoventilation
- Gastric distension
  - Regurgitation/aspiration
  - Gastric rupture

  There are multiple methods for ensuring proper ETT tracheal placement

- Quantitative capnography
  - 2010 advanced cardiac life support (ACLS) guidelines state this is the most sensitive and the standard of care
    - Only 25% of emergency departments have this.
  - False negatives
    - Requires pulmonary blood flow and so is not sensitive in shock states
  - False positives
    - Supraglottic placement
    - Gastric contents
    - Mucus
    - Drugs (epinephrine)
- Qualitative capnography
  - Inexpensive and widely available
  - Requires up to six ventilations
  - False negatives/positives as described in quantitative capnography
- Direct visualization of the ETT entering the vocal cords.
  - Can dislodge
- Esophageal detector device.
  - Low sensitivity
- CXR (chest x-ray)
  - Depicts height of the ETT through detection of a radiopaque line embedded in the ETT tip above/below the carina (Figure 6.21).
    - Requires time (prolonged ventilations)
    - Transportation of x-ray machine
    - Patient movement
    - Does not decipher if the ETT is in the trachea or the esophagus
  - Displays pulmonary complications.
    - Pneumothorax
    - Aspiration

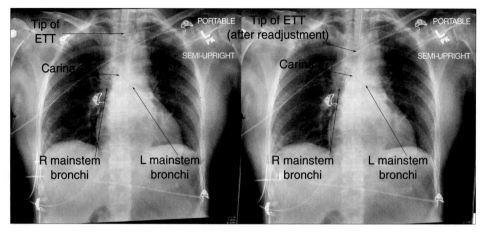

FIGURE 6.21 CXR with endotracheal tube in proper position above the carina. Note that this modality does not rule in/out an esophageal intubation.

■ Auscultation
  ■ Not sensitive
  ■ Depends on ventilations.
    • Gastric distention if an esophageal intubation
  ■ Auscultate over the stomach first and if borborygmi is heard, immediately pull the ETT completely out.
  ■ Auscultate over the midaxillary lines as air sounds from the contralateral lung and the stomach can be transmitted throughout the thoracic cavity.
    • Becuase the right mainstem bronchi is more vertical, wider, and shorter than the left, most endobronchial intubations ("ETT too deep") are placed here so listen on the right lateral chest first (to ensure trachea placement) and then listen to the left side (if no breath sounds, pull back 2 cm and recheck).
  ■ Fogging of the ETT
    • Not sensitive nor specific.
    • Kelly et al. have shown in the canine model that 50% of esophageal intubations may display mist in the ETT.
■ Bedside ultrasound
  ■ As stated previously, ultrasonography is ubiquitous in acute care settings and is immediately available.
  ■ Proper placement can be detected immediately, without administering a single ventilation to the patient, therefore iatrogenic gastric insufflation, is not a concern.
  ■ In the cardiac arrest patient, confirmation can be obtained without interruption of CPR (cardiopulmonary resuscitation).

The following results of using this modality have shown prospectively in the trachea rapid ultrasound exam (TRUE) during emergency intubation (Chou et al.)

Gottlieb et al. (2014) have shown, in a meta-analysis composed of 969 patients, similar results:

■ Sensitivity—98%
■ Specificity—98%

Lema et al. have shown that this technique can be taught to paramedics and new emergency medicine residents with similar results.

The anatomical relationship of the esophagus in relation to the trachea:

- Posterior left—80%
- Directly posterior—16%
- Posterior right—4%

The empty trachea appears sonographically the same as the trachea with the ETT in its lumen because one is essentially placing an air-filled cylindrical tube in another air-filled cylindrical tube and both have the same sonographic appearance.

PERTINENT SONOGRAPHY PRINCIPLES

- Due to the significant difference in acoustic impedance between soft tissue and air, sound waves are strongly reflected, resulting in a hyperechoic (bright) appearance at the A–M interface along the anterior trachea border.
- The air within the tracheal lumen does not permit transmission and return of ultrasound so the lumen and posterior trachea wall are not visualized.
- The A–M interface also induces (through high reactivity between the two densities) characteristic reverberation artifact, which appear as a series of parallel hyperechoic lines that occur at regularly spaced intervals deep to the A–M interface.
- The esophagus is normally collapsed and because of this there is no A–M interface and therefore it is difficult to normally see it as it is homogeneous with the surrounding neck soft tissue (Table 6.5).

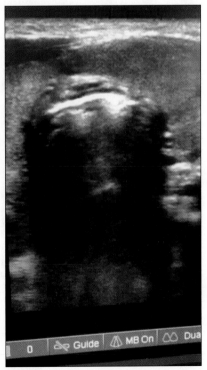

TABLE 6.5 Trachea Rapid Ultrasound Exam (True) During Emergency Intubation

Sensitivity	99%
Specificity	94%
PPV	99%
NPV	94%
Operating time	9 seconds

Adapted from Chou et al. (2011).

Because the esophagus usually lies lateral to the trachea and is not normally visualized, if one sees:

- A single lumen, the ETT is in the trachea
  - A twisting motion of the ETT may add sensitivity **(Video 6.2)**
- A double lumen, the ETT is in the esophagus.
  - Double lumen sign (Figure 6.22)

Detecting sliding of the visceral and parietal pleura/comet tails or diaphragm movement also signifies trachea placement.

- Requires ventilation

VIDEO 6.2 Ultrasound of endotracheal tube in trachea upon twisting the tube.
springerpub.com/campo

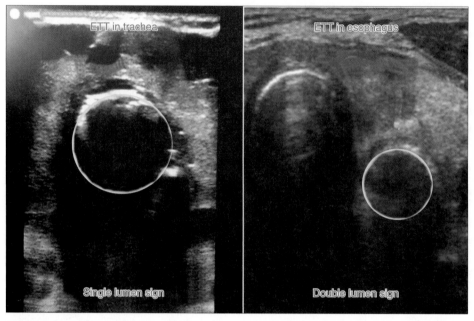

FIGURE 6.22 Ultrasound appearance of anterior neck upon trachea intubation. Note the double lumen sign in the esophageal intubation.

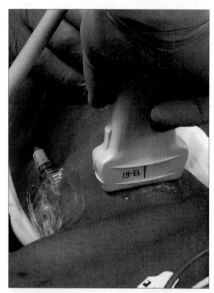

FIGURE 6.23 Trachea rapid ultrasound exam (TRUE).

Place the high-frequency linear probe transversely in the midline, just over the suprasternal notch (Figure 6.23).

- Obese patients may require the lower frequency curvilinear probe.
- In circumstances when the view is equivocal and one is evaluating a possible retro tracheal midline posterior esophagus, a left paramedial approach may be used.

Complications

- Most serious
  - *Unrecognized* esophageal intubation
  - Iatrogenic hypoxia
- Gastric distension
- Trauma
  - Lips
  - Teeth
  - Pharyngeal soft tissue
  - Vocal cords
- Pneumothorax
- Vomiting/aspiration
- Pneumonitis
- Pneumonia
  - 86% of nosocomial pneumonias are associated with mechanical ventilation.
    - Ventilator-associated pneumonia (VAP)

- The ETT itself is a reservoir for potential infection, as one study demonstrated that 84% of endotracheal tubes examined had a biofilm laden with bacteria, usually gram-negative organisms.
- By definition, VAP requires 48 hours of ETTI.
- Aggressive means of treating underlying pulmonary pathology and extubating before this time is critical.
- Exacerbation of cervical spine injuries
- Glottic/subglottic stenosis
  - Incidence ranges from 10% to 22%, but only 1% to 2% of the patients are symptomatic or have severe stenosis.
  - Prolonged intubation, usually longer than 5 days
  - Can occur anywhere from the level of the ETT tip up to the glottis.
  - Most common site is where the ETT cuff has been in contact with the tracheal wall.

Special Considerations
Delayed Sequence Intubation

- Indicated when patients do not cooperate with normal preoxygenation.
- If one cannot preoxygenate for 3 minutes to the point of full denitrogenation, then there will be minimal, if any, safe apnea time.
- Think of this technique as a conscious sedation procedure in which the procedure to be performed is that of proper preoxygenation.
- Accomplished by the clinician delivering the sedative *without* simultaneous administration of the paralytic agent.
  - Ketamine is the ideal agent at 1.5 mg/kg IV
  - Dissociative anesthetic maintains protective airway reflexes
  - Preoxygenation can now occur for 3 minutes
- Paralytic agent can now be administered and RSI/VAL can be carried out as previously outlined.

VAL can also be used to retrieve upper airway foreign bodies (see Chapter 5, Figure 5.13).

EDUCATIONAL POINTS

- A failed airway is not defined by the inability to place an ETT but rather by not alleviating or inducing hypoxia via improper BVM ventilation.
- Use of the Sellick maneuver in preventing aspiration has never been proven but it has been confirmed in increasing airway resistance and decreasing TVs.
- The head should not be posterior to the sternum upon airway positioning.
- There are currently no prospective studies on which particular airway device is best used for the cardiac arrest patient; however, the literature is clear on the significant decrease in morbidity and mortality when CPR is interrupted for any reason.
- O_2 consumption is two times higher in the pediatric patient and because of such, the O_2 sat can drop precipitously with little warning, resulting in a shorter safe apnea time.
- Capnography is the gold standard for confirmation of proper ETT placement though bedside transverse ultrasound of the neck should be the true secondary confirmation modality, especially in cases of low/no pulmonary blood flow.
- Patients in shock state have lower VO_2 sat and therefore typically require volume resuscitation to improve their cardiac output which in turn increases their VO_2 sat resulting in a higher AO_2 sat.
- If after 3 minutes of preoxygenation the O_2 sat is less than 95%, the patient is displaying physiologic shunting and needs PPV with PEEP for 3 minutes.

- Patients with physiologic shunts require PEEP in order to oxygenate as close to 100% as possible.
- Ventilating a patient faster will not raise the O_2 sat any higher than a controlled slower rate; using a faster rate has detrimental effects on cardiac physiology and cerebral blood flow.
- A PEEP valve can be added to the exhalation port of standard BVM devices but only works if a continuous mask seal is maintained.
- BIPAP may be used as a bridge to extubation in potentially COPD ventilator-dependent patients in an effort to decrease ventilatory dependency.
- Any airway device that is not secured (those that are not an ETT) may lead to inadvertent gastric distention.
- PEEP valves can decrease the incidence of gastric distention by means of a visual manometer and, hence, keep insufflation pressures below that of the opening pressure of the lower esophageal sphincter (LES).

PEARLS

- All unconscious patients are assumed to have a partial airway obstruction and chin lift/jaw thrust maneuvers are in order, along with an NPA.
- All unconscious patients are assumed to be hypoglycemic, opioid toxic, hypoxic, or hypercapnic until proven otherwise.
- Think of the sniffing position as the neck/head position that occurs when crossing a finish line in a close race; win with your chin.
- Impending respiratory failure is a clinical diagnosis, not based upon imaging or blood testing.
- At a minimum, always have an NPA and Yankauer suction ready.
- Think about extubation the moment the ETT is secure in order to mitigate prolonged ventilator time and its daily additive and inherent complication rate.
- Preparation is everything; check all equipment before its use and have backup airway devices within arm's reach.
- Never intubate without preoxygenation (unless a crash airway).
- NRB do not have one-way valves on their exhalation ports and therefore cannot get to an FiO_2 of 1.0.
- BVM ventilation is a two-person procedure.
- Only after correct airway positioning and use of an NPA, can one proficiently apply proper BVM technique.
- It is easier to make a seal with a larger mask than a smaller mask.
- If the mask seal leaks in BVM, ambient air entrains the face and, in essence, the patient is receiving room air O_2.
- The most common leak site in BVM ventilation is over the nasal bone.
- Hovering a BVM over a patient's mouth and/or nose essentially provides only ambient air flow.
- Keep dentures in place during BVM ventilation and only remove upon laryngoscopy as they help maintain the mandible in an anterior position and, in doing so, displace the tongue away from the pharyngeal wall.
- Partial inflation of the LMA cuff before insertion may prevent it from folding upon itself upon insertion.
- After insertion of the LMA if the cuff is visible it is not in the proper position.

- Usage of a tongue depressor before insertion of the LMA helps prevent the tongue from being pushed into the posterior pharynx by the LMA upon insertion.
- All patients undergoing RSI should have O_2 administered simultaneously via an NC and NRB/BVM with both sources of O_2 emanating from two different tanks.
- Use of sedative/paralytic agents greatly enhances the success rate of ETTI.
- Twenty degrees of head/torso elevation or 30 degrees of reverse Trendelenburg prevent posterior lung alveoli atelectasis and increases FRC by 20%, thereby improving and maintaining oxygenation.
- Bedside ultrasound should be in one's armamentarium in cases of ETTI and should be performed periodically after patient movement/transfer.
- VAL improves success rate and glottic visualization compared with DL.
- Practice makes perfect, though VAL requires much less practice than DL in acquiring and maintaining this critical airway skill **(Video 6.3)**.

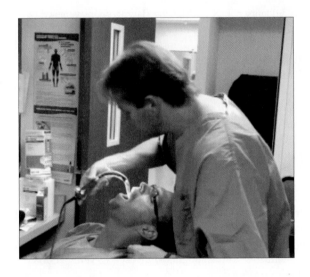

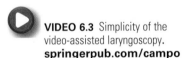

VIDEO 6.3 Simplicity of the video-assisted laryngoscopy.
springerpub.com/campo

RESOURCES

Adhikari, S., Farrell, I., & Stolz, U. (2012). How accurate is ultrasonography in confirming endotracheal tube placement? A meta-analysis. *Annals of Emergency Medicine, 60*(45), S18.

Adnet, F., Baillard, C., Borron, S. W., Denantes, C., Lefebvre, L., Galinski, M., . . . Lapostolle, F. (2001). Randomized study comparing the "sniffing position" with simple head extension for laryngoscopic view in elective surgery patients. *Anesthesiology, 95*(4), 836–841.

Akihisha, Y., Hoshijma, H., Maruyama, K., Koyama, Y., & Andoh, T. (in press). Effects of sniffing position for tracheal intubation" a meta-analysis of randomized controlled trials. *American Journal of Emergency Medicine*.

Ambrosio, A., Pfannenstiel, T., Bach, K., Cornelissen, C., Gaconnet, C., & Brigger, M. T. (2014). Difficult airway management for novice physicians: A randomized trial comparing direct and video assisted laryngoscopy. *Otolaryngology Head & Neck Surgery, 150*(5), 775–778.

Baillard, C., Fosse, J. P., Sebbane, M., Chanques, G., Vincent, F., Courouble, P., . . . Jaber, S. (2006). Noninvasive ventilation improves preoxygenation before intubation of hypoxic patients. *American Journal of Respiratory Critical Care Medicine, 174*, 171–177.

Baraka, A. S., Taha, S. K., Siddik-Sayyid, S. M., Kanazi, G. E., El-Khatib, M. F., Dagher, C. M., . . . Hajj, R. E. (2007). Supplementation of preoxygenation in morbidly obese patients using nasopharyngeal oxygen insufflation. *Anesthesia, 62*, 769.

Brindley, P. G. (2008). "Win with your chin": An alternative to the "sniffing position" analogy for teaching optimal head-positioning with intubation. *Resuscitation, 78*(2), 242.

Burlke, C. M., Zepeda, F. A., Bacon, D. R., & Rose, S. H. (2004). A historical perspective on use of the laryngoscope as a tool in anesthesiology. *Anesthesiology, 100*(4), 1003–1007.

Byars, D., Lo, B., Evans, D., Schott, C., Deljoui, K., & Haroutunian, M. (2011). Video-assisted laryngoscopy as the "great equalizer" in the management of the simulated difficult adult airway. *Annals of Emergency Medicine, 58*(45). doi:10.1016/j.annemergmed.2011.06.227

Chou, H. C., Tseng, W. P., Wang, C. H., Ma, M. H., Wang, H. P., Huang, P. C., . . . Chen, S. C. (2011). Tracheal rapid ultrasound (T.R.U.E.) for confirming endotracheal tube placement during emergency intubation. *Resuscitation, 82*(10), 1279–1284.

Cooney, D. R., Cooney, N. L., Wojok, S., & Wallus, H. (2011). Success and satisfaction of emergency physicians using a video-assisted semi rigid fiber optic stylet for intubation of a difficult airway model. *Annals of Emergency Medicine, 58*(Suppl. 4), S307.

Dibble, C., & Maloba, M. (2006). Best evidence topic report. Rapid sequence induction in the emergency department by emergency medicine personnel. *Emergency Medicine Journal, 23*(1), 62–64.

Donoghue, A. J., Ades, A. M., Nishiske, A., & Deutsch, E. S. (2013). Video laryngoscopy versus direct laryngoscopy in simulated pediatric intubation. *Annals of Emergency Medicine, 61*(3), 271–277.

Drenguis, A. S., & Carlson, J. N. (2015). GlideScope vs. C-MAC for awake upright laryngoscopy. *Journal of Emergency Medicine, 49*(9), 361–368.

Engstrom, J., Hedenstierna, G., & Larsson, A. (2010). Pharyngeal oxygen administration increases the time to serious desaturation at intubation in acute lung injury: An experimental study. *Critical Care, 14*, R93.

Farmery, A. D., & Roe, P. G. (1996). A model to describe the rate of oxyhaemoglobin desaturation during apnoea. *British Journal of Anaesthesia, 76*(2), 284–291.

Girou, E., Brun-Buisson, C., Taille, S., Lemaire, F., & Brochard, L. (2003). Secular trends in nosocomial infections and mortality associated with noninvasive ventilation patients with exacerbation of COPD and pulmonary edema. *Journal of the American Medical Association, 290*(22), 2985–2991.

Girou, E., Schortgen, F., Delclaux, C., Brun-Buisson, C., Blot, F., Lefort, Y., . . . Brochard, L. (2000). Association of noninvasive ventilation with nosocomial infections and survival in critically ill patients. *Journal of the American Medical Association, 284*(18), 2361–2367.

Gottlieb, M., & Bailitz, J. (2015). Can transtracheal ultrasonography be used to verify endotracheal tube placement? *Annals of Emergency Medicine, 66*(1), 67–68.

Gottlieb, M., Balilitz, J. M., Christian, E., Russell, F. M., Ehrman, R. R., Khishfe, B., . . . Ross, C. (2014). Accuracy of a novel ultrasound technique for confirmation of endotracheal intubation by expert and novice emergency physicians. *Western Journal of Emergency Medicine, XV*(7), 834–839.

Griesdale, D. E., Liu, D., McKinney, J., & Choi P. T. (2012). GlideScope video-laryngoscopy versus direct laryngoscopy for endotracheal intubation: A systematic review and meta-analysis. *Canandian Journal of Anaesthesia, 59*(1), 41–52.

Hawkins, E., Philip, M., & Brice, J. (2013). Critical airway skills and procedures. *Emergency Medical Clinics of North America, 31*, 1–28.

Howard-Quijano, K. J., Huang, Y. M., Matevosian, R., Kaplan, M. B., & Steadman, R. H. (2008). Video-assisted instruction improves the success rate for tracheal intubation by novices. *British Journal of Anesthesia, 101*(4), 568–572.

Hubble, M. W., Brown, L., Wilfong, D. A., Hertelendy, A., Benner, R. W., & Richards, M. E. (2010). A meta-analysis of prehospital airway control techniques part I: Orotracheal and nasotracheal intubation success rates. *Prehospital Emergency Care, 14*(3), 377–401. doi: 10.3109/10903121003790173

Javre, P., Combes, X., Lapostolle, F., Dhaouadi, M., Ricard-Hibon, A., Vivien, B., . . . KETASED Collaborative Study Group. (2009). Etomidate versus ketamine for rapid sequence intubation in acutely ill patients: A multicenter randomized controlled trial. *Lancet, 374*(9686), 293–300.

Je, S. M., Kim, M. J., Chung, S. P., & Chung, J. S. (2012). Comparison of GlideScope versus Macintosh laryngoscope for the removal of a hypopharyngeal foreign body: A randomized cross-over cadaver study. *Resuscitation, 83,* 1277–1280.

Keenan, S. P., Sinuff, T., Cook, D. J., & Hill, N. S. (2003). Which patients with acute exacerbation of chronic obstructive pulmonary disease benefit from noninvasive positive-pressure ventilation? A systematic review of the literature. *Annals of Internal Medicine, 138*(11), 861–870.

Kelly, J. J., Eynon, C. A., Kaplan, J. L., de Garavilla, L., & Dalsey, W. C. (1998). Use of tube condensation as an indicator of endotracheal tube placement. *Annals of Emergency Medicine, 31*(5), 575–578.

Kilic, T., Goksu, E., Durmaz, D., & Yildiz, G. (2013). Upper cervical spine movement during intubation with different airway devices. *American Journal of Emergency Medicine, 31,* 1034–1036.

King. B. R., & Hagberg, C. (2007). Management of the difficult airway. In C. King & F. M. Henretig (Eds.), *Textbook of pediatric emergency procedures* (2nd ed., pp. 191–246). Philadelphia, PA: Wolters Kluwer/Lippincott Williams & Williams.

King, C., & Rappaport, L. D. (2007). Emergent endotracheal intubation. In C. King & F. M. Henretig (Eds.), *Textbook of pediatric emergency procedures* (2nd ed., pp. 146–189). Philadelphia, PA: Wolters Kluwer/Lippincott Williams & Williams.

King, C., & Reynolds, S. L. (2007). Bag-valve-mask ventilation. In C. King & F. M. Henretig (Eds.), *Textbook of pediatric emergency procedures* (2nd ed., pp. 109–126). Philadelphia, PA: Wolters Kluwer/Lippincott Williams & Williams.

Konrad, C., Schüpfer, G., Wietlisbach, M., & Gerber, H. (1998). Learning manual skills in anesthesiology: Is there a recommended number of cases for anesthetic procedures? *Anesthesiology Analgesia, 86,* 635–639.

Lafferty, K. (2014). *Medications for rapid sequence endotracheal intubation.* Retrieved from http://emedicine.medscape.com/article/109739-overview

Lane, S., Saunders, D., Schofield, A., Padmanabhan, R., Hildreth, A., & Laws, D. (2005). A prospective, randomized controlled trial comparing the efficacy of preoxygenation in the 20 degrees head up vs supine position. *Anesthesiology, 60,* 1064–1067.

Lawes, E. G., Campbell, I., & Mercer, D. (1987). Inflation pressure, gastric insufflation and rapid sequence induction. *British Journal of Anaesthesia, 59,* 315–318.

Lema, P. C., Wilson, J., O'Brien, M., Lindstrom, H., Tanski, C., Consiglio, J., Clemency, B. (2014). Ultrasound identification of successful endotracheal tube placement by paramedics and residents. *Annals of Emergency Medicine, 64*(4S), S8.

Levitan, R. M. (2013). Video laryngoscopy, regardless of blade shape, still requires a backup plan. *Annals of Emergency Medicine, 61,* 421–422.

Levitan, R. M., Everett, W. W., & Ochroch, E. A. (2004). Limitations of difficult airway prediction in patients intubated in the emergency department. *Annals of Emergency Medicine, 44,* 307.

Levitan, R. M., Jeitz, J. W., Sweeney, M., & Cooper, R. M. (2011). The complexities of tracheal intubation with direct laryngoscopy and alternative intubation devices. *Annals of Emergency Medicine, 57*(3), 240–247.

Li, H., Hu, C., Xia, J., Li, X., Wei, H., Zeng, X., & Jing, X. (2013). A comparison of bilevel and continuous positive airway pressure noninvasive ventilation in acute cardiogenic pulmonary edema. *American Journal of Emergency Medicine, 31,* 1322–1327.

Liesching, T., Nelson, D., Cormier, K. L., Sucov, A., Short, K., Warburton, R., & Hill, N. S. (2014). Randomized trial of bilevel verses continuous positive airway pressure for acute pulmonary edema. *Journal of Emergency Medicine, 46*(1), 130–140.

Lisa, M. M., Makr, K. W., & Stephen, M. W. (2009). Removal of hypopharyngeal foreign body with the GlideScope video laryngoscope. *Otolaryngology Head & Neck Surgery, 141,* 416–417.

Maassen, R., Lee, R., Hermans, B., Marcus, M., & van Zundert, A. (2009). A comparison of three ideolaryngoscopes: The Macintosh laryngoscope blade reduces, but does not replace, routine stylet use for intubation in morbidly obese patients. *Anesthesiology Analgesia, 109*, 1560–1565.

Mace, S. E. (2006). Challenges and advances in intubation: Airway evaluation and controversies with intubation. *Emergency Medicine Clinics of North America, 26*, 977–1000.

Malki, M. A., Hassett, P. C., Jiggins, B. D., Harte, B. H., & Laffey, J. G. (2009). A comparison of the GlideScope, Pentaz AWS, and Macintosh laryngoscopes when used by novice personnel: A manikin study. *Anaesthesioloy, 65*(11), 802–811.

Milling, T. J., Jones, M., Khan, T., Tad-y, D., Melniker, L. A., Bove, J., . . . SchianodiCola, J. (2007). Transtracheal ultrasound for identification of esophageal intubation. *Journal of Emergency Medicine, 32*(4), 409–414.

Mills, P. J., Baptiset, J., Preston, J., & Barnas, G. M. (1991). Manual resuscitators and spontaneous ventilation-an evaluation. *Critical Care Medicine, 19*, 1425–1431.

Mort, T. C. (2005). Preoxygenation in critically ill patients requiring emergency tracheal intubation. *Critical Care Medicine, 33*, 2672–2675.

Mosier, J., Chiu, S., Patanwala, A. E., & Sakles, J. C. (2013). A comparison of the GlideScope video laryngoscope to the C-MAC video laryngoscope for intubation in the emergency department. *Annals of Emergency Medicine, 61*(4), 414–420.

Mulcaster, J. T., Mills, J., Hung, O. R., MacQuarrie, K., Law, J. A., Pytka, S., . . . Field, C. (2003). Laryngoscopic intubation: Learning and performance. *Anesthesiology, 98*, 23–27.

Murphy, L. D., Kovacs, G. J., Reardon, P. M., & Law, J. A. (2014). Comparison of the king vision video laryngoscope with the Macintosh laryngoscope. *Journal of Emergency Medicine. 47*(2), 239–246.

Nagler, J., & Krauss, B. Devices for assessing oxygenation and ventilation. In J. R. Roberts & J. R. Hedges (Eds.), *Clinical procedures in emergency medicine* (6th ed). Philadelphia, PA: Saunders Elsevier.

Nimmagadda, U., Salem, M. R., Joseph, N. J., Lopez, G., Megally, M., Lang, D. J., & Wafai, Y. (2000). Efficacy of preoxygenation with tidal volume breathing. Comparison of breathing systems. *Anesthesiology, 93*, 693–698.

Nouruzi-Sedeh, P., Schumann, M., & Growben, H. (2009). Laryngoscopy via Macintosh blade versus GlideScope: Success rate and time for endotracheal intubation in untrained medical personnel. *Anesthesiology, 110*, 32–37.

Nur Hafiizhoh, A. H., & Choy, C. Y. (2014). Comparison of the "sniffing the morning air" position and simple head extension for glottic visualization during direct laryngoscopy. *Middle East Journal of Anaesthesiology, 22*(4), 399–405.

Oto, B. (2012). Mastering BLS ventilation: Core techniques. *Medscape Reference. Drugs, Diseases & Procedures*. EMS basics: fundamentals of care for the working EMT. Retrieved from emsbasics.com/tag/respiration

Peipho, T., Fortmueller, K., Heid, F. M., Schmidtmann, I., Werner, C., & Noppens, R. R. (2011). Performance of the C-MAC video laryngoscope in patients after a limited glottis view using Macintosh laryngoscopy. *Anaesthesiology, 66*(12), 1101–1105.

Ramkumar, V., Umesh, G., & Phillip, F. A. (2011). Preoxygenation with 20 degree head up tilt provides longer duration of non-hypoxic apnea than conventional preoxygenation in non-obese health adults. *Journal of Anesthesia, 25*, 189–194. Retrieved from http://criticalcare-medicine.pbworks.com/f/Ram+Cochrane+Database+Syst+Rev+2004.pdf

Reardon R. F., Mason, P. E., & Clinton, J. E. (2014). Basic airway management and decision making. In J. R. Roberts & J. R. Hedges (Eds.), *Clinical procedures in emergency medicine* (6th ed., pp. 39–61). Philadelphia, PA: Saunders Elsevier.

Reardon, R. F., McGill. J. W., & Clinton. J. E. (2014). Tracheal Intubation. In J. R. Roberts & J. R. Hedges (Eds.), *Clinical procedures in emergency medicine* (6th ed.). Philadelphia, PA: Saunders Elsevier.

Ruben, H., Knudsen, E. J., & Carugati, G. (1961). Gastric inflation in relation to airway pressure. *Acta Anaesthesiologica Scandinavica, 5*, 107–114.

Sakles, J. C., Mosier, J., Chiu, S., Cosentino, M., & Kalin, L. (2012). A comparison of the C-MAC video laryngoscope to the Macintosh direct laryngoscope for Intubation in the emergency department. *Annals of Emergency Medicine, 60*(6), 739–748.

Serocki, G., Bein, B., Scholz, J., & Dorges, V. (2010). Management of the predicted difficult airway: A comparison of conventional blade laryngoscopy with video assisted blade laryngoscopy and the GlideScope. *European Journal of Anaesthesiology, 27*(1), 24–30.

Silverton, N. A., Youngquist, S. T., Mallin, M. P., Bledsoe, J. R., Barton, E. D., Schroeder, E. D., . . . Axelrod, D. A. (2012). GlideScope versus flexible fiber optic for awake upright laryngoscopy. *Annals of Emergency Medicine, 43*, 1188–1195.

Stone, B. J., Chantler, P. J., Baskett, P. J., & Department of Resuscitation, Conquest Hospital, Hastings, E. Sussex, UK. (1998). The incidence of regurgitation during cardiopulmonary resuscitation: A comparison between the bag valve mask and laryngeal mask airway. *Resuscitation, 38*(1), 3–6.

Swaminathan, A. K., Berkowitz, R., Baker, A., & Spyres, M. (2015). Do emergency medicine residents receive appropriate video laryngoscopy training? A survey to compare the utilization of video laryngoscopy devices in emergency medicine residency programs and community emergency departments. *Journal of Emergency Medicine, 48*(5), 613–619.

Taha, S. K., Siddik-Sayyid, S. M., El-Khatib, M. F., Dagher, C. M., Hakki, M. A., & Baraka, A. S. (2006). Nasopharyngeal oxygen insufflation following pre-oxygenation using the four deep breath technique. *Anesthesia, 61*, 427.

Vender, J. S., & Szokol, J. W. (2007). Oxygen delivery systems, inhalation therapy, and respiratory therapy. In C. A. Hagberg (Ed.), *Benumof's airway management: Principles and practice* (2nd ed., pp. 321–345). Philadelphia, PA: Mosby.

Vissers, R. J., & Gibbs, M. A. (2010). The high-risk airway. *Emergency Medical Clinics of North American, 28*, 201–217.

Vyas, J., Milner, A. D., & Hopkin, I. E. (1993). Face mask resuscitation: Does it lead to gastric distension? *Archives of Disease in Children, 58*, 373–375.

Weingart, S. D. (2010). Preoxygenation, reoxygenation and delayed sequence intubation in the emergency department. *Journal of Emergency Medicine, 40*(6), 661–667.

Weiss, A. M., & Lutes, M. (2008, September). Focus on-bag-valve mask ventilation. *ACEP News*.

Xanthos, T., Stroumpoulis, K., Bassiakou, E., Koudouna, E., Pantazopoulos, I., Mazarakis, A., . . . Iacovidou, N. (2011). GlideScope videolaryngoscope improves intubation success rate in cardiac arrest scenarios without chest compressions interruption: A randomized crossover manikin study. *Resuscitation, 82*, 464–467.

Zuckerbraun, N., & Pitetti, R. D. (2007). Rapid sequence induction. In C. King & F. M. Henretig (Eds.), *Textbook of pediatric emergency procedures* (2nd ed., pp. 127–144). Philadelphia, PA: Wolters Kluwer/Lippincott Williams & Williams.

UNIT **IV**

Intravenous Access

CHAPTER **7**

Ultrasound-Guided Peripheral Intravenous Access

Theresa M. Campo

VASCULAR ANATOMY

Antecubital Fossa (Figure 7.1)

- Median cubital—first choice because of its large diameter, inherent anchoring to surrounding tissue, its relatively easy access, and it is interpreted as the least painful.
- Cephalic—second choice as it may be difficult to palpate, but is well anchored to surrounding tissue.
- Basilic—third choice because of the proximity to the brachial artery and two nerve branches. This vessel is easy to palpate but not well anchored to surrounding tissue and can be more painful then other vessel locations.

> **NOTE** *The cephalic and basilic veins are also located in the upper arm and forearm but are more difficult to palpate because of their location deep within the muscle and proximity to bone structures.*

BACKGROUND

Ultrasound-guided peripheral vascular access (PVA) is an easy and readily available method that can be used in various settings. Ultrasound-guided PVA has numerous advantages, including cannulation of veins that are nonvisible or palpable, decreasing the need for central line placement, prevention of complications from multiple attempts, and increased patient satisfaction. PVA is indicated for infusion of fluids, medications, blood, and contrast material. Traditionally, PVA is performed using knowledge of vascular anatomy, visualization, and/or palpation of a vessel for cannulation. However, problems arise when veins are distorted, rolling, sclerosed, and/or scarred; also abnormal anatomy makes cannulation very difficult. The inability to properly cannulate can lead to central line placement or multiple attempts, including "blind" attempts that are painful and upsetting to both the patient and health care professional.

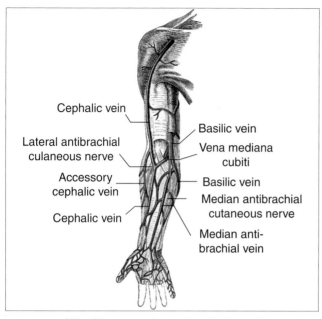

Cephalic vein

Lateral antibrachial culaneous nerve

Accessory cephalic vein

Cephalic vein

Basilic vein

Vena mediana cubiti

Basilic vein

Median antibrachial cutaneous nerve

Median anti-brachial vein

FIGURE 7.1 Vascular anatomy of upper extremity.

Ultrasound has helped to minimize complications and increase patient satisfaction among adult and pediatric patients. Studies have shown positive results regarding higher first-pass success rates, decreased complications, and rapid and safe success overall. Ultrasound has been shown to facilitate decreased length of stay in the emergency and urgent care settings with rapid and uncomplicated PVA. Delay in PVA can lead to delay in medical diagnosis and delay in the administration of necessary fluids, medications, and blood transfusions. In a multicenter prospective study, Au et al. have shown that the use of ultrasound-guided peripheral IV placement in those persons who have difficultly with IV access prevented the need for central venous cannula (CVC) placement in 85% of these patients. There is also a statistically significant decrease in length of stay.

Indications

- Blood sampling
- Blood transfusion
- Burns
- Chronic conditions requiring multiple PVA
- Dehydration
- Failure to cannulate with traditional techniques
- Infusion of fluid, medication, and/or contrast material
- Intravenous drug users
- Obesity
- Peripheral edema
- Sclerosis
- Steroid use
- Trauma

Contraindications/Relative Contraindications

- Cellulitis
- Ipsilateral radical mastectomy
- Phlebitis
- Sclerosis
- Severe burns
- Significant peripheral edema
- Thrombosis

Procedure Preparation

- Intravenous initiation kit:
  - Tourniquet
  - Skin prep
  - Gauze
  - OpSite/clear adhesive cover
  - Extension tubing

- Angiocatheter (16 gauge, 18 gauge, 20 gauge):
  - Standard length of 1.18 in.
  - Long would be 1.25 to 2.0 in.
    - Longer catheters are needed for deeper veins in the antecubital fossa.

- Sterile gel—prepackaged water-based lubricant is preferred (ultrasound gel is not sterile, especially multiple-use bottles):
  - Saline syringe flush
  - Blood sampling vials as needed
  - Transducer cover
  - Ultrasound machine

- Linear, curvilinear, or intracavity probe attachment:
  - Linear probe—most preferred for high resolution of superficial structures. High frequency, 7.5 to 10 MHz.
  - Curvilinear probe—preferred for deeper structures. The probe is low frequency, 2 to 5 MHz. Use the highest frequency of 5 MHz for greater resolution.
  - Intracavity probe—can be used if linear probe is not available. Can view up to 180 degrees. High frequency, 8 to 13 MHz; provides improved resolution but at the expense of depth penetration.

- Anesthesia:
  - Topical can be used but consideration for time to initiation of action must be taken into account, especially if the patient is not stable.
  - Local infiltration can also be utilized. Swelling from infiltration can make traditional cannulation difficult but not with ultrasound-guided PVA.

Procedure

As with any procedure it is important that both the patient and provider are comfortable. The patient can be either supine or sitting, and the provider should sit at the bedside of the upper extremity intended for PVA. The ultrasound machine should be either directly in front of the provider for easy viewing or on the other side of the stretcher/bed/table with the screen facing the provider.

- The patient's arm should be abducted and externally rotated (Figure 7.2).

Survey the venous anatomy:

- Starting at the antecubital fossa, slide the transducer up and down the humerus, identifying the target veins (basilica, brachial, cephalic).
- Position the transducer in the transverse position with the probe indicator pointing to the patient's right side; this will allow for the provider's left side to correspond to the left side of the screen for best orientation and imaging (Figure 7.3).

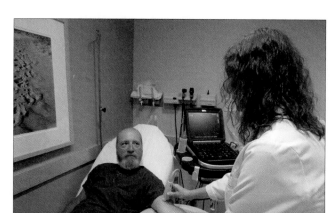

FIGURE 7.2 Position of patient and provider for conducting an ultrasound.

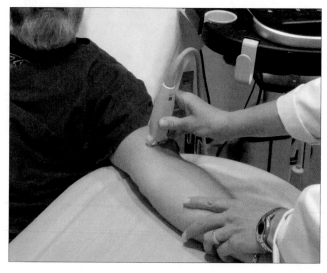

FIGURE 7.3 Position of the transducer.

- Compress the vessels to easily and completely collapse, identifying the vessel as a vein (arteries do not completely collapse). Color Doppler flow can be utilized to aid in the identification of the vessel as vein or artery.
- Slide the transducer up and down the target vein to determine the direction and depth of the vessel (**Video 7.1**).
- Choosing a target vessel is dependent on the following:
  - Diameter (0.4–1.5 cm)
  - Depth (distance from the skin surface to the vessel)
  - Path (straight or tortuous)

DYNAMIC METHOD
- Place the transducer cover over the transducer.
- Apply the tourniquet proximal to the access site.
- Prepare the site with skin prep.

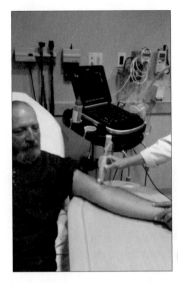

 VIDEO 7.1 Locating a vessel.
springerpub.com/campo

- Apply gel to the transducer and arm.
- Hold the transducer probe with your nondominant hand over the target vessel.
- Hold the angiocatheter with your dominant hand.
- Center the probe over the vessel so it is also centered on the screen.
- Notice the depth of the target vessel by using the marking on the side of the screen.
- Prior to insertion of the needle for cannulation, slide the catheter between the transducer and skin and look for shadow artifact.
- Insert the needle at a 45-degree angle the same distance in front of the transducer as the depth of the vessel.
- After puncturing the skin, identify the tip of the needle by scanning back and forth in a fanning pattern. Follow the tip of the needle into the vessel on the screen, similar to Figure 8.8.
- Look for a "flash" of blood to confirm placement in the vessel.
- For added ability to follow the needle tip directly into the veins outer wall, and continue cannulation into the lumen, turn the linear probe 90 degrees clockwise for a longitudinal view.
- Cannulate the vessel.
- Place the transducer probe aside.
- Follow the traditional technique for blood draw and intravenous line connection based on your institution's protocol.

STATIC METHOD

- You can use ultrasound to identify the vascular structures and relation to the external landmarks and then cannulate the vessel using the traditional method. The authors recommend the dynamic method.

TWO-PERSON METHOD

- You can have an assistant manage the transducer probe while you cannulate the vessel.

Complications

- Air embolism
- Arterial puncture
- Bruising
- infection
- Infiltration
- Nerve damage
- Phlebitis
- Thrombosis

PEARLS

- Look for larger, straighter veins for cannulation.
- When viewing vessels in the transverse view it may be difficult to visualize the needle tip directly entering the lumen. Often one will see an indentation, which represents the needle tip out of the visual plane depressing the outer vessel wall.
- For improved visualization after the vein is seen in the transverse plane, rotate the probe 90 degrees clockwise in order to directly envision the needle entering the vessel lumen.
- Shokoohi et al. have recently shown that, after a minimal training session, the use of ultrasound-guided peripheral IV access in the "difficult stick" patient reduces the use of central venous catheterization 85% of the time.

RESOURCES

Au, A. K., Rotte, M. J., Grzybowski, R. J., Ku, B. S., & Fields, J. M. (2012). Decrease in central venous placement due to use of ultrasound guidance for peripheral intravenous catheters. *American Journal of Emergency Medicine, 30*(9), 1950–1954.

Arbique, D., Bordelon, M., Dragoo, R., & Huckaby. (2014). Ultrasound-guided access forperipheral intravenous therapy. *Academy of Medical–Surgical Nurses, 23*(3), 1, 10–15.

Bartlby.com. *Superficial veins of the upper extremity plate #574.* Retrieved from https://commons .wikimedia.org/wiki/File%3AGray574.png

Benkhadra, M., Collignon, M., Fournel, I., Oeuvrard, C., Rollin, P., Perrin, M., ... Girard, C. (2012). Ultrasound guidance allows faster peripheral IV cannulation in children under 3 years of age with difficult venous access: A prospective randomized study. *Pediatric Anesthesia, 22,* 449–454.

Liu, S. W., & Zane, R. D. (2014). Peripheral intravenous access. In J. R. Roberts & J. R. Hedges (Eds.), *Clinical procedures in emergency medicine* (6th ed). Philadelphia, PA: Saunders Elsevier. Retrieved from https://www.clinicalkey.com/#!/content/book/3-s2.0-B9781455706068000215

Oakley, E., & Wong, A. (2010). Ultrasound-assisted peripheral vascular access in a paediatric ED. *Paediatric Emergency Medicine, 22,* 166–170.

Schoenfeld, E., Shokoohi, H., & Boniface, K. (2011). Ultrasound-guided peripheral intravenous access in the emergency department: Patient-centered survey. *Western Journal of Emergency Medicine, 12*(4), 475–477.

Shannon, A. W., Butts, C., & Cook, J. (2013). Ultrasound-guided vascular access. In *Emergency Medicine* (2nd ed.). Philadelphia, PA: Saunders Elsevier. Retrieved from https://www .clinicalkey.com/#!/content/book/3-s2.0-B9781437735482000069

Shokoohi, H., Boniface, K., & McCarthy, M. (2013). Ultrasound-guided peripheral intravenous access program is associated with a marked reduction in central venous catheter use in non-critically ill emergency department patients. *Annals of Emergency Medicine, 61*(2), 198–203.

CHAPTER 8

Ultrasound-Guided Central Venous Access

Keith A. Lafferty

BACKGROUND

Intravenous (IV) access is paramount to patient care and central venous access. Along with airway management, venous access is an important procedural skill needed in managing critical emergency patients. There are over 5,000,000 central lines placed annually in the United States. Mastery of this critical skill demands not only an appreciation of regional anatomy but also dexterity and competence in performing the Seldinger technique (this technique is described here). The use of ultrasound (US)-guided central venous access is currently the standard of care for performing this invasive procedure. Its use has greatly reduced inherent complication rates.

Central venous catheterization (CVC) access can be accomplished via the internal jugular vein (IJV), the subclavian vein (SCV), or femoral vein (FV). Recent evidence demonstrates no statistical difference in the infection rates in access through the FV versus other supradiaphragmatic sites. A Cochrane review found increased rates of CVC colonization with femoral versus supradiaphragmatic CVCs, but, more importantly, there was no statistically significant difference among catheter-related bloodstream infection (CRBI) rates when strict protocols were followed.

Regional anatomy impacts the use of US-assisted CVC access. For example, because the IJV has no bony structure overlay, is proximally located, and is relatively superficial, it is easily accessed using US guidance. In contrast, the SCV is not favorable for US guidance because of its deep placement within the upper chest and bony surroundings (lies between the clavicle and the first rib). Furthermore, the CVC technique described can be performed in other anatomical locations and may require modifications in insertion site according to regional anatomy and body habitus characteristics.

No discussion of CVC would be complete without briefly describing the work of Sven Seldinger. In 1953, Sven Seldinger, a Swedish radiologist, developed and pioneered a way of assessing and cannulating large vessels deep within the body that is still used today. Using a finder needle to identify the vessel, he inserted a guide

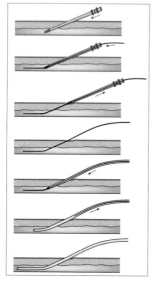

FIGURE 8.1 Seldinger technique.

wire into the vessel through the finder needle, then, by placing a catheter over the proximal end of the guide wire, he was able to insert the catheter distally into the vessel in a progressive manner, finally removing the guide wire after the catheter was advanced deep into the vessel. This landmark-guided technique eliminated the surgical cut-down approaches previously required for CVC placement (Figure 8.1).

> **NOTE** *Just as the Seldinger technique eliminates the time and inherent complications of deep surgical vessel exploration, US-guided CVC placement now eliminates much of the inherent anatomical aberrancy and complications of the landmark technique.*

ANATOMY

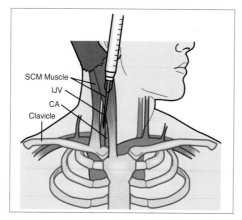

FIGURE 8.2 Needle placement in the internal jugular vein and surrounding anatomy.

The IJV lies in the carotid sheath adjacent to the carotid artery (CA) and vagus nerve, located in a triangle formed by the sternal and clavicular heads of the sternocleidomastoid muscle (SCM) at its superior apex and the clavicle bone inferiorly. It runs vertically down the neck and empties into the supraclavicular vein (SCV). The right IJV is easier to cannulate compared to the left IJV because of its inherent straight trajectory to the SCV, whereas the left IJV joins at a more acute angle. Additionally, the right pleural dome is smaller in diameter and lies more inferiorly compared to the left, reducing the risk of procedure-associated pneumo-hemothorax. In general, the IJV is superficial and lateral to the CA but aberrancy is the rule (Figure 8.2).

Studies have shown that 11% of right IJVs and 24% of left IJVs are actually medial to the CA. Troianos et al. found the right IJV to overlie most (75%) of the CA in 54% of patients, and is anterior to the CA in a majority of cases. Because of these anatomical aberrancies there is a 9% to 11% greater risk of CA puncture when inadvertently traversing the posterior IJV wall when using the CVC landmark technique without the use of US guidance to confirm the vascular anatomy (Figure 8.3).

Balls, LoVecchio, Kroeger, and Stapczynski (2010) found that US guidance also reduces the number of total punctures per attempt, therefore decreasing complication risks including CVC associated blood stream infection which is known to be correlated with the number of skin puncture attempts.

Karakitsos, Labropoulos, and De Groot (2006) compared CVC insertion via the landmark and US methods. Outcomes associated with using the landmark- versus US-guided CVC approach are found in Table 8.1.

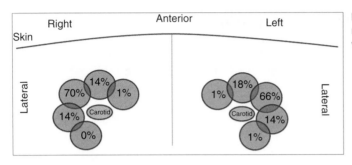

FIGURE 8.3 Aberrant relationships of the internal jugular vein and the carotid artery.

NOTE *Many advisory groups, including the National Institute for Clinical Excellence (NICE), have recommended the use of US guidance as the preferred method for elective CVC insertion for children and adults.*

TABLE 8.1 Ultrasound- Versus Landmark-Guided Central Vein Catheter Technique Outcomes

Study Results	Ultrasound	Landmark
Arterial Sticks	0%	54%
Needle Attempts	1.5	10.4
Needle to Vein Time	58 sec	338 sec
Success Rate	100%	42.8%

PATIENT PRESENTATION

Procedure Indications

In general, placement of a CVC is indicated in the following:

- Delivery of critical and or caustic medications
- Emergency resuscitation
- Monitoring of CVP
- Emergency venous access after inability to achieve a peripheral intravenous (IV) line
- Insertion of a transvenous pacemaker/pulmonary artery catheter
- Hemodialysis

CONTRAINDICATIONS AND RELATIVE CONTRAINDICATIONS

- Infection of the area overlying the deep vein
- Thrombosis of the deep vein
- Coagulopathy (relative)

PROCEDURE PREPARATION

Most supplies listed are available in commercially packaged kits (Figure 8.4).

- Full sterile barrier (sterile gloves, gown, cap, mask, and face shield)
- Chlorhexidine
- Sterile drapes to cover top half of body
- Topical anesthetic
- Syringes
- #11 blade scalpel
- Sterile gauze
- Catheter dilator (1 Fr. larger than the CVC)
- Needle and wire
- CVC (single or multiple lumen)
- Silk suture
- Sterile saline flushes
- Antibiotic dressing (preferably impregnated antibiotic sponge)
- Ensure proper CVC size based on clinical scenario. In general, for resuscitation or dialysis purposes, an 8.5 to 11.5 Fr. is preferable. Otherwise, the standard triple-lumen 7 Fr. can be used for multiple port access. Poiseuille's law dictates that the flow rate of a liquid is directly proportional to the fourth power of the conduit's radius and is inversely proportional to the conduit's length by a factor of 8 (*flow rate = radius⁴/length[8]*). In other words, use shorter, larger diameter catheters for fluid resuscitation (Figure 8.5).

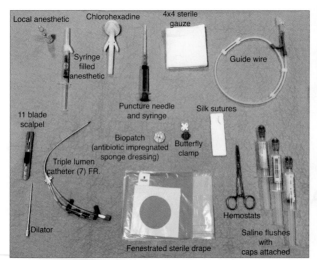

FIGURE 8.4 Open CVC kit.

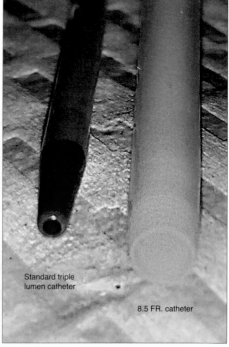

FIGURE 8.5 Comparison of standard 7.0 triple lumen and an 8.5 Fr. catheter.

PROCEDURE

- Place patient in at least a 20-degree Trendelenburg position to engorge the IJV and to decrease the risk of an air embolism.
- Turn chin away from vein to be accessed.
- Use the right IJV to obtain a more direct approach to the SVC.
- Identify the apex of the triangle formed by the sterno and clavicular heads of the SCM and aim the needle toward the ipsilateral nipple.

Anatomical landmarks are used for initial probe placement, not for needle insertion and trajectory.

- Put on full sterile barrier (Figure 8.6).
- Cleanse the skin with a skin cleanser, such as chlorhexidine.
- Drape the skin.
- Using an assistant, place sterile, long US sleeve with gel over probe.
- Using your nondominant hand, place US probe directly over landmark needle insertion site using the transverse plane **(Video 8.1)**.

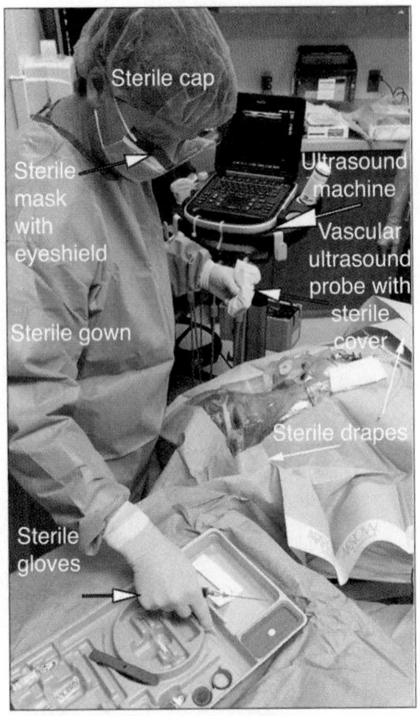

FIGURE 8.6 Clinician and patient barriers.

Using the ultrasound probe, first identify two circular hypoechoic areas that represent the IJV and the CA. The IJV is more oval in shape and thinly walled, making it compressible. It is also usually superior and lateral to the CA (remember aberrancy is the rule). The CA is always circular, consists of a thicker muscular wall, and is not compressible (Figure 8.7).

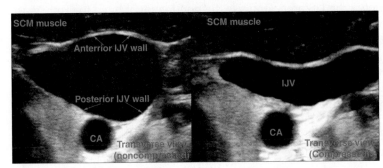

FIGURE 8.7
Ultrasound appearance of the internal jugular vein and carotid artery. Notice the carotid artery is noncompressible and maintains its circular form.

- Apply topical anesthetic.
- Remove the cap from the port in which the guide wire will be threaded (the longest lumen).
- Using your dominant hand, enter the insertion site at a 45-degree angle from the coronal plane with the long access of the needle pointing toward the ipsilateral nipple (after penetrating skin, apply gentle suction).
- Ensure needle entry site is just proximal and in the exact middle portion of the US probe.
  - Avoid penetration into the deep tissues of the neck.
  - Realize that the IJV technically is a deep vein but, in reality, it lies relatively superficially in the neck; because of this the puncture depth is rarely greater than 1.5 cm.
- Observe the needle shadow as it appears in the image (Figure 8.8), puncturing the vessel wall by first depressing the needle and then noticing a "bounce back return"

of the vessel's original shape, followed by flash of venous blood (darker and non-pulsatile as opposed to the CA).

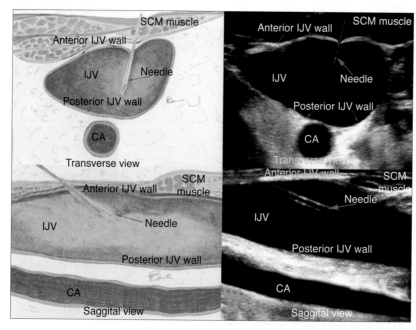

FIGURE 8.8 Ultrasound appearance of needle-vein cannulation.

- Once the IJV is cannulated by the needle and return of blood via the syringe is constant, put down the US probe and use the nondominant hand to firmly grasp the hub of the needle with the thumb and index finger while the rest of the hand lies firmly on the patients neck (diminishes distal needle migration).
- Remove the syringe; you should notice a slow drip of venous blood.
- Place the distal/curved end of the guide wire into and through the hub and needle and advance the guide wire to proper length (usually the proximal/straight end of the guide wire will not surpass the patient's head).
  - If a dysrhythmia occurs during the procedure, the guide wire may be irritating the myocardium and should be withdrawn slowly until the dysrhythmia reverses.
  - If unable to pass the guide wire through the needle, the needle may have inadvertently pierced the posterior IJV wall. In this case, the wire should be removed, placing a syringe on the needle hub and withdrawing the needle with slight suction until blood returns again.
- **Never let go of the guide wire.**
- Withdraw the needle leaving the guide wire in place by retracting the needle out of the skin with the nondominant hand, using the dominant hand to hold the proximal end of the guide wire.
  - If resistance is encountered when removing the guide wire through the needle, remove both as one unit to reduce the risk of shearing and creating a guide wire embolism.
- Once the needle is completely out of the skin, use the nondominant hand to grasp the distal end of the guide wire while the dominant hand retracts the needle fully off the guide wire.

- Using the scalpel with the sharp end caudal, make a small catheter-sized incision at the point of the guide wire–skin interface in a vertical plane through the dermal tissue but not into the carotid sheath.
- Place the dilator over the guide wire and via a twisting motion pass it through the skin to an approximate depth of 2 cm.
  - Use the nondominant hand now to hold the proximal end of the guide wire as the dilator penetrates the skin.
- Remove the dilator while always having a hand on the guide wire.
- Apply gauze to minimize bleeding after dilator removal.
- Place the CVC over the guide wire just until it is proximal to the skin. (If the guide wire was initially advanced too far, use the nondominant hand and retract the guide wire until it appears in the open proximal port of the CVC.)
- Using the dominant hand, grasp proximal end of the guide wire and insert the CVC to the appropriate depth in as twisting fashion through the skin.
  - Ideal catheter tip position is in the SVC proximal to the right atrium.
- Check for blood return and flush all ports with normal saline syringes and ensure caps are secure on all hubs.
- Apply impregnated antibiotic sponge and secure CVC using silk sutures.
- Apply sterile dressing (Figure 8.9).
- Order a chest x-ray to ensure proper tip depth and to ensure there is no iatrogenic pneumo/hemothorax.

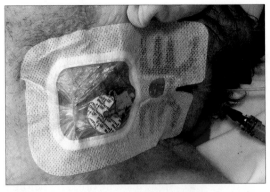

FIGURE 8.9 Impregnated antibiotic sponge under sterile dressing.

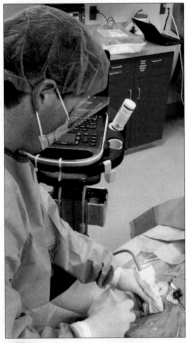

VIDEO 8.1 Central venous catheter insertion.
springerpub.com/campo

POST-PROCEDURE CONSIDERATIONS

Educational Points

- Using the US, try to visualize the tip of the needle at all times; the transverse view, while excellent for lateral/medial orientation, is not as good as the sagittal/longitudinal view in assessing for needle depth to avoid penetration through the IJV posterior wall and inadvertent CA puncture.
- If arterial puncture occurs, remove the needle and place firm pressure for 10 minutes or until there is no bleeding.
- Curved or "J" guide wires are used to negotiate the tortuous turns of vessels.

- Miles et al. has prospectively shown that regardless of past experience, with proper guidance a 2-hour training session on the use of US-guided CVC placement promotes clinical proficiency in this skill.
- A 13-year observational study has shown that nurse practitioners and physician assistants can perform CVC placement with success; their complication rates are similar to those of physicians.
- Since 1996, US-guided CVC placement has been shown consistently to be superior to the landmark technique in decreasing complications and procedure duration.
- IJV clots have been incidentally identified in 2% to 4% of patients undergoing US-guided CVC upon initiation of the procedure.
- Apply a sterile dressing before removing the sterile field.
- With the application of strict protocols, ICU CRBIs have decreased from 2001 to the time of this printing from 49,000 to 16,000 cases annually.
  - Each CRBI is associated with increased hospital length of stay (22 days) and increased mortality rates of 12% to 25% (4,000 patients die annually).
- LeMaster et al. found that emergency department–placed CVCs have similar infection rates (< 2 per 1,000 catheter days) when compared to those placed in ICUs. Therefore, when proper aseptic insertion techniques are followed within the emergency department it is not recommended that emergency department–placed CVCs be removed upon transfer to the ICU.
- Antiseptic-impregnated CVCs have been shown to induce a fivefold decrease in CRBI as compared to normal CVCs and are recommended when the CVC is to remain in place for longer than 5 days.

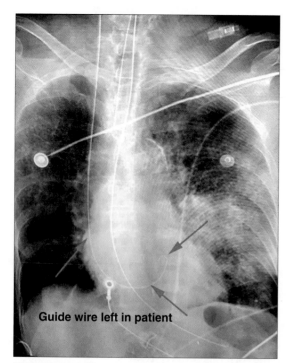

FIGURE 8.10 Chest x-ray of guide wire embolism.

COMPLICATIONS

Leung et al. (2006) found that ultrasound not only increased the success rate of IJV placement by 15.4% but also decreased the overall complication rate by 12.3% as compared to the landmark technique (15%–2.7%). Complications are classified as immediate or delayed.

Immediate

- Arterial puncture (4.2%)
- Hematoma (0.72%)
- Pneumothorax (0.67%)
- Hemothorax (0.05%)
- Air embolism (0.1%)
- Guide wire embolism (Figure 8.10)
- Dysrhythmia (0.3%)

Delayed

- Infection
  - CRBI
  - Local cellulitis

- Deep vein thrombosis (0.2%)
- In a landmark perspective study, Pronovost et al. (2006) evaluated 103 ICUs, including 1,981 months of data, and concluded that the following practices decrease rates of CRBIs:
  - Handwashing
  - Full-body precautions during insertion (repetitive studies have shown that this is one of the most effective practices in preventing CRBI)
  - Chlorhexidine skin cleansing (numerous studies have shown its effectiveness in preventing CRBI)
  - Removal of unnecessary catheters (decreases bacteremia rate and possible seeding of other catheters)
  - Utilizing a daily checklist
  - Avoidance of the femoral site when possible (other studies, such as the Cochrane Review, have shown that this insertion site is not independently associated with development of CRBI when a strict protocol is followed)
- Other practices associated with decreasing CRBI rates to less than 1 per 1,000 catheter days include:
  - Use of a checklist
  - Daily assessment of the continued need of the CVC
  - Daily assessment of the insertion site
  - Handwashing and cleansing hub with alcohol before use

PEARLS

- Never let go of the wire during the procedure.
- If one should encounter resistance, never force the guide wire through the needle.
- Have an assistant prearrange sterile flushes with caps already placed on tray at start of procedure.
- The straight end of the guide wire often has a soft tip (avoids vessel wall injury) and may be used if one encounters difficulty passing the curved end.
- If there is continued difficulty obtaining blood return through the needle in the initial puncture, flush the needle with sterile saline as a blood clot may have formed in the needle itself.
- Studies have shown that the use of US for peripheral IV placement in "difficult stick" patients can decrease the need for CVC placement in up to 80% of the time.
- Turning the patient's head 45 degrees or greater increases the overlap of the IJV in relation to the underlying CA.
- US has been shown to decrease the risk of pneumothorax to almost 0%.
- The more obese the patient the more likely the landmark technique will result in inaccurate placement.
- Having the patient in the Trendelenburg position and/or performing a Valsalva maneuver increases the IJV size.
- In hypotensive or hypoxic patients, pulsatile or red blood flow return may not be apparent following arterial puncture.

(continued)

- The post-procedure chest x-ray is not used in determinating CVC use, but rather for its tip anatomical position and to assess immediate complications.
- IJV depth is rarely greater than 1.5 cm below the surface of the neck.
- One should consider removal of the CVC after confirmation of successful placement in order to decrease ongoing risk of CRBI.
- Generally, one does not need to pass the guide wire further than the patient's head during the entire procedure, as it needs to be advanced only far enough to maintain reliable control of the tract from the skin surface to the intravascular space (if the guide wire requires withdrawal through the catheter for control of the proximal/rigid end, the guide wire was inserted too far).
- After the syringe is removed and before the wire is inserted (and the same goes for when the CVC is placed and the guide wire is removed), one should occlude the catheter by placing the thumb over the needle hub in order to prevent an air embolism.
- Teismann, Knight, and Rehrer (2013) found that when using an 18-gauge, 21/2 peripheral intravenous catheter (IVC), one can cannulate the IJV using US guidance and in essence have a "peripheral IJ" with no reports of spontaneous IVC migration out of the vein lumen (Figure 8.11 and **Video 8.2**).

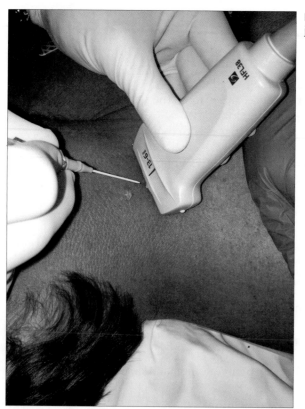

FIGURE 8.11 Peripheral internal jugular insertion.

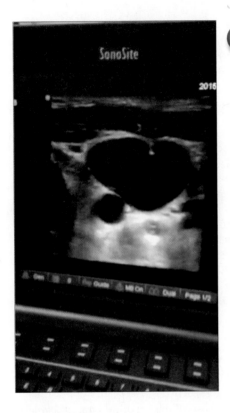

 VIDEO 8.2 Peripheral internal jugular insertion.
springerpub.com/campo

RESOURCES

Akhter, M., Runde, D., & Lee, J. (2013). Which central line insertion site is the least prone to infection? *Annals of Emergency Medicine, 61*(3), 362–363.

Alexandrou, E., Spencer, T. R., Frost, S. A., Mifflin, N., Davidson, P. M., & Hillman, K. M. (2014). Central venous catheter placement by advanced practice nurses demonstrates low procedural complication and infection rates—A report from 13 years of service. *Critical Care Medicine, 42*(3), 536–543.

Arai, T., &Yamashita, M. (2005). Central venous catheterization in infants and children-small caliber audio-Doppler probe versus ultrasound scanner. *Pediatric Anesthesia, 15*(10), 858–861.

Au, A. K., Rotte, M. J., & Grzybowski, R. J. (2012). Decrease in central venous catheter placement due to use of ultrasound guidance for peripheral intravenous catheters. *American Journal of Emergency Medicine, 30,* 1950–1954.

Bailey, P. L., Whitaker, E. E., Palmer, L. S., & Glance, L. G. (2006). The accuracy of the central landmark used for central venous catheterization of the internal jugular vein. *Anesthesia Analgesia, 102*(5), 1327–1332.

Balls, A., LoVecchio, F., Kroeger, A., & Stapczynski, J. S. (2010). Ultrasound guidance for central venous catheter placement: Results from the central line emergency access registry database. *American Journal of Emergency Medicine, 28*(5), 561–567.

Bauman, M., Braude, D., & Crandall, C. (2009). Ultrasound-guidance vs. standard technique in difficult vascular access patients by ED technicians. *American Journal of Emergency Medicine, 27*(2), 135–140.

Brannam, L., Blavias, M., Lyon, M., & Flake, M. (2004). Emergency nurses' utilization of ultrasound guidance for placement of peripheral intravenous lines in difficult-access patients. *Academy of Emergency Medicine, 11*(12), 1361–1363.

Deshpande, K. S., Hatem, C., Ulrich, H. L. Currie, B. P., Aldrich, T. K., Bryan-Brown, C. W., & Kvetan, V. (2005). The incidence of infectious complications of central venous catheters at the subclavian, internal jugular and femoral sites in an intensive care unit population. *Critical Care Medicine, 33*, 13–20.

Domino, K. B., Bowdle, T. A., Posner, K. L., Spitellie, P. H., Lee, L. A., & Cheney, F. W. (2004). Injuries and liability related to central vascular catheters. *Anesthesiology, 100*, 1411–1418.

Gekle, R., Dubensky, L., Haddad, S., Bramante, R., Cirilli, A., Catlin, T., … Nelson, M. (2013). Can bedside sonography replace conventional radiography for confirmation of above-the-diaphram central venous catheter placement? *Annals of Emergency Medicine, 62*(45), S34.

Gillman, L. M., Blaivas, M., Lord, J., & Al-Kadi, A. (2010). Ultrasound confirmation of guidewire position may eliminate accidental arterial dilatation during central venous cannulation. *Scandinavian Journal of Trauma Resuscitation Emergency Medicine, 18*, 39.

Griswold-Theodorson, S., Hannan, J., & Handly, N. (2008). *419: Improving patient safety using ultrasound guidance during internal jugular central venous catheter placement by novice practitioners.* Retrieved from https://www.clinicalkey.com/-!/search/Griswold-Theodorson%20S./%7B%22type%22:%22author%22%7D

Harnage, S. (2012). Seven years of zero central-line-associated bloodstream infections. *British Journal of Nursing, 21*(21), S6, S8, S10–S12.

Karakitsos, D., Labropoulos, N., & De Groot, E. (2006). Real-time ultrasound-guided catheterization of the internal jugular vein: A prospective comparison with the landmark technique in critical care patients. *Critical Care, 10*(6), R162.

Kucher, N. (2011). Clinical practice. Deep-vein thrombosis of the upper extremities. *Journal of Medicine, 364*, 861–869.

LeMaster, C. H., Schuur, J. D., Pandya, D., Pallin, D. J., Silvia, J., Yokoe, D., … Hou, P. C. (2010). Infection and natural history of emergency department-placed central venous catheters. *Annals of Emergency Medicine, 56*, 492–497.

Leung, J., Duffy, M., & Finckh, A. (2006). Real-time ultrasonographically-guided internal jugular vein catheterization in the emergency department increases success rates and reduces complications: A randomized, prospective study. *Annals of Emergency Medicine, 48*(5), 540–547.

Lewis, G., Crapo, S. A., & Williams, J. G. (2013). Critical skills and procedures in emergency medicine vascular access skills and procedures. *Emergency Medicine Clinics of North America, 31*(1), 59–86.

Maki, D. G., Stolz, S. M., Wheeler, S., & Mermel, L. A. (1997). Prevention of central venous catheter-related bloodstream infection by use of an antiseptic-impregnated catheter. A randomized, controlled trial. *Annals Internal Medicine, 127*(4), 257–266.

McNeil, C. R., & Adams, B. D. Central venous catheterization and central venous pressure monitoring. In J. Roberts & J. Hedges (Eds.), *Clinical procedures in emergency medicine* (pp. 397–431). Philadelphia, PA: Saunders.

Miles, G., Salcedo, A., & Spear, D. (2012). Implementation of a successful registered nurse peripheral ultrasound-guided intravenous catheter program in an emergency department. *Journal of Emergency Nursing, 38*(4), 353–356.

Montecalvo, M. A., McKenna, D., & Yarrish, R. (2012). Chlorhexidine bathing to reduce central venous catheter-associated bloodstream infection: Impact and sustainability. *American Journal of Medicine, 125*(5), 505–511.

Mukherji, J., Ural, N., & Sheikh, T. (2013). Teaching ultrasound imaging for central line placement—A resident's perspective. *Open Journal of Anesthesiology, 3*, 263–227.

Nadel, F. M. (2008). Vascular access. In J. M. Baren, S. G. Rothrock, J. A. Brennan, & L. Brown (Eds.), *Pediatric emergency medicine* (pp. 1147–1156). Philadelphia, PA: Saunders Elsevier.

Pronovost, P., Needham, D., Berenholtz, S., Sinopoli, D., Chu, H., Cosgrove, S., … Goeschel, C. (2006). An intervention to decrease catheter-related bloodstream infections in the ICU. *New England Journal of Medicine, 26,* 2723–2732.

Schoenfeld, E., Boniface, K., & Shokoohi, H. (2011). ED technicians can successfully place ultrasound-guided intravenous catheters in patients with poor vascular access. *American Journal of Emergency Medicine, 29*(5), 496–501.

Shannon, A. W., Butts, C., & Cook, J. (2008) Ultrasound-guided vascular access. *Emergency Medicine, 6,* 50–54.

Shokoohi, H., Boniface, K., & McCarthy, M. (2013). Ultrasound-guided peripheral intravenous access program is associated with a marked reduction in central venous catheter use in noncritically ill emergency department patients. *Annals of Emergency Medicine, 61*(2), 198–203.

Stone, M. B., Nagdev, A., Murphy, M. C., & Sisson, C. A. (2010). Ultrasound detection of guidewire position during central venous catheterization. *American Journal of Emergency Medicine, 28,* 82–84.

Tang, H. J., Lin, H. L., Lin, Y. H., Leung, P. O., Chuang, Y. C., & Lai, C. C. (2014). The impact of central line insertion bundle on central line-associated bloodstream infection. *Bio-Med Central Infectious Disease, 14,* 356.

Teismann, N. A., Knight, R. S., & Rehrer, M. (2013). The ultrasound-guided "peripheral IJ": Internal jugular vein catheterization using a standard intravenous catheter. *Journal of Emergency Medicine, 44*(1), 150–154.

Troianos, C. A., Kuwik, R. J., Pasqual, J. R., Lim, A. J., & Odasso, D. P. (1996). Internal jugular vein and carotid artery anatomic relation as determined by ultrasonography. *Anesthesiology, 85*(1), 43–48. http://anesthesiology.pubs.asahq.org/article.aspx?articleid=2028955

Udy, A., Senthuran, S., & Lipman, J. (2009). Airway obstruction due to a pre-vertebral haematoma following difficult central line insertion—Implications for ultrasound guidance and review of the literature. *Anaesthesia Intensive Care, 37*(2), 309–313.

Wright, S. W., Conine, B., Lindsell, C. J., Yamin, C., Smith, C., Hart, K., & Trott, A. (2013). Mechanical and thrombotic complication rates for central line insertion in emergency medicine: A multi-center cohort study. *Annals of Emergency Medicine, 62*(45), S83.

UNIT V

Managing Pain Using Injectable Anesthetics

CHAPTER 9

Anesthetic Agents and Procedures for Local and Field Infiltration

Keith A. Lafferty

BACKGROUND

The success rate of any procedure depends largely on the modulation of pain. Ever since the first anesthetic agent was introduced in the late 1800s (cocaine), emergent procedures have progressed exponentially.

Pain fibers are peripheral nerves that begin at a receptor in the dermis and travel the length of the neuron ending at the spinal cord. Unlike thick, type A motor/pressure/proprioception nerve fibers, these thin type C pain fibers have no myelin sheath coverage and therefore are more susceptible to blockade by local anesthetics (LAs).

Although not fully understood, the mechanism of action of LAs has to do with the blockade of axonal nerve conduction. Normal neurons conduct an impulse by sodium influx via a specific sodium gate causing depolarization of the neuronal cell membrane, in a distal to proximal direction, to its articulation in the spinal cord. LAs, by either directly blocking sodium entry into the gate or by inducing swelling of the gate itself, do not allow depolarization and, therefore, no signal gets to the spinal cord and hence the brain (Figure 9.1).

Anesthetics are classified into two groups based on an intermediate chain that is either an esther or an amide. This intermediate chain is linked to an aromatic and a hydrophilic segment. The efficacy of each compound is directly related to the slight biochemical changes of these segments and dictates the time of onset, potency, and duration of actions of all the different agents. Metabolism occurs in esters via hydrolysis by plasma cholinesterases, whereas amides are degraded in the liver by microsomal enzymes.

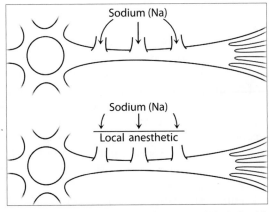

FIGURE 9.1 Neuron action potential; normal blockade with local anesthetic.

Potency is directly proportional to liposolubility as the cell membranes that must penetrate and interact with the sodium channels are mostly composed of phospholipids. Time of onset has to do with how long it takes for an agent to reach the sodium channel. This is a property of its pK_a, which is defined as the pH at which 50% of a structure is in both an ionized and a unionized form. So, the lower the pK_a for a given LA, and the higher the pH of the tissue it enters, the more availability of unionized molecules for cell membrane penetration. Finally, the duration of action relates to the level of protein binding that occurs at the receptor (see Table 9.1).

TABLE 9.1 Anesthetic Agents—Onset, Duration, and Maximum Dose

Drug	Onset (minutes)	Duration (minutes)	Maximum Dose (mg/kg)
Procaine	5–10	30–60	7
Lidocaine	2–5	30–120	4
Without epinephrine With epinephrine	2–5	60–180	7
Bupivicaine	5–10	180–360	2
Without epinephrine With epinephrine	5–10	240–600	3
Mepivacaine	2–5	90–180	6
Diphenhydramine	2–5	20–30	1.5

Certain characteristics have been shown to decrease injection pain:

- Slow injection (causes less distention of tissue)
- Keeping the solution warm (40°C)
- Adding a bicarbonate buffer in a 1:10 ratio with the amides (the esters will precipitate)

Adding epinephrine to the LA allows a larger dose to be used, as epinephrine induces local vasoconstriction and decreases systemic absorption. Note that there is no evidence that this has any negative effect on end arterial areas.

LAs interact with sodium gates of neuronal tissue and all excitable tissues (any cell membrane possessing the ability to depolarize). The central nervous system (CNS), cardiovascular (CV) system, and neuromuscular junction (NMJ) are susceptible to LAs' action and toxicity, especially when high plasma levels are reached. Adding to the CNS susceptibility is the fact that these agents are so lipophilic and cross the blood–brain barrier easily. Another contributor to CV toxicity is the fact that LAs are negative inotropes and they decrease the peripheral vascular resistance. Note that many antidysrhythmics interacting with sodium gates should not be used in cases of CV toxicity. Amiodarone is the antidysrhythmic drug of choice. If seizures develop, lesion-specific anticonvultants like phenytoin are ineffective, as benzodiazipines should be used secondary to their sympatholytic effects. Though convincing evidence is lacking, case reports and in vitro studies indicate that intravenous lipid emulsion therapy may have a role in creating a "lipid sink" and, hence, decrease the amount of free drug available at the cardiac receptor. Signs and symptoms of toxicity do occur in a stepwise manner for the given organ system involved (see Table 9.2).

TABLE 9.2 Signs and Symptoms of Toxicity

Central Nervous System	Cardiovascular System	Neuromuscular Junction
Slurring	Premature ventricular contractions	Paresthesias
Tinnitus	Bradydysarhythmias	Tremor
Confusion	Heart blocks	Twitching
Seizures	Hypotension	Myoclonic jerks

Although much talked about, true allergic reactions are extremely rare. If they do occur, they usually result from an ester compound. A degradation product of the esters is para-amino benzoic acid (PABA), which is responsible for the majority of allergic reactions. Amides are stored in a solution containing methylparaben, which is similar in composition and antigenicity to PABA. If one truly has an ester allergy, use of the code-cart lidocaine, which is devoid of methylparaben, can be an option. Also, if unsure of the class to which a patient is allergic, diphenhydramine can be used for injection after diluting to a 1% solution (10 mg/mL).

TREATMENT

Local anesthesia for wound management is delivered via three different techniques:

- Topical anesthesia (TA)
- Infiltrative anesthesia
- Field-block anesthesia

Topical Anesthesia

This can be applied on arrival while the patient is awaiting evaluation and treatment by the provider. TA has been shown to decrease the need for infiltrative anesthesia. Smaller lacerations or multiple localized abrasions (road rash) may be amenable to this therapy. Although this displays a low potency and a delayed onset, its attributes include easy application, potential decrease in need for child restraints, and no distortion of wound edges.

- TAC (tetracaine, adrenaline, cocaine)—replaced by less toxic preparations
- LET (lidocaine, epinephrine, tetracaine)—as effective as TAC

- Ethyl chloride and fluori-methane sprays—vapor coolants; on topical application, the skin is cooled to −20°C, temporarily freezing the skin (less than 1 minute)
- Benzocaine—highly insoluble in water; used on the mucous membranes

Infiltrative Anesthesia

This is the mainstay of wound anesthesia. It has rapid onset with low systemic toxicity. Injection at the wound margin induces less pain than through the epidermis without an increase in the infection rate. Pinching of the skin at the time of injection has been shown to decrease the pain. A 25- or 27-gauge needle should be used as smaller lumens induce too much injection resistance. Placement of the needle just below the dermis at the level of the superficial fascia is less painful than placement in the dermis, and offers less tissue resistance as the fascia is composed of loose connective and adipose tissue.

Field-Block Anesthesia

A subcutaneous layer of LA is placed at an area away from the wound, surrounding the wound with a linear parallel wall of the agent. This can be used in areas such as the ear, where infiltrative anesthesia would be an anatomical challenge. This may also be used in largely contaminated wounds. Although multiple needle sticks through the epidermis are required, pain can be decreased by administration of subsequent LA through previously anesthetized skin.

The maximal dose of the LA can be calculated as follows: For a 70-kg patient being given lidocaine with epinephrine (max. dose is 7 mg/kg):

- A 100% solution is 1 g/mL or 1,000 mg/mL so a 1% solution is 10 mg/mL.
- Maximal dose is 490 mg or 49 mL.

CONTRAINDICATIONS
- Allergy

PROCEDURE PREPARATION
- Supine or comfortable position of the patient.
- LA should be administered before formal wound irrigation/cleansing.

Topical Anesthesia
- Gloves
- Sterile cotton ball or gauze
- LET (lidocaine 4%, epinephrine 0.1%, tetracaine 0.5%)

Infiltrative Anesthesia and Field-Block Anesthesia
- Gloves
- Skin cleanser
- LA
- Syringe
- 25- or 27-gauge needle

PROCEDURE

Topical Anesthesia

- Remove gross decontaminants.
- Soak cotton ball or gauze and sprinkle drops over the wound.
- Apply anesthetic with an occlusive dressing.
- Allow at least 30 minutes for effect.

Infiltrative Anesthesia

- Direct the needle into the wound margin just below the dermis at the level of the superficial fascia (Figure 9.2).
- Insert the needle two thirds of its length and advance in a direction that is parallel to the wound edge.
- Inject the LA upon slow withdrawal of the needle.
- Repeat this step in an area where the LA was previously deposited.

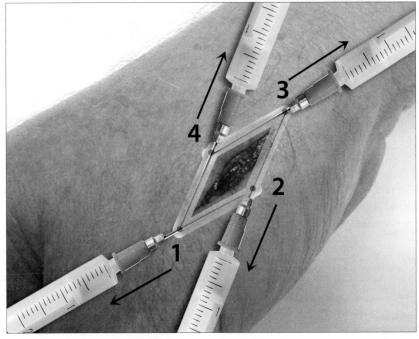

FIGURE 9.2 Infiltrative anesthesia technique.

Field-Block Anesthesia

- Insert the needle 1 cm away from the wound or structure through the epidermis to the level of the subcutaneous tissue (superficial fascia).
- Insert the needle two thirds of its length and advance in a direction that is parallel to the wound edge.
- Inject the LA upon slow withdrawal of the needle.
- Continue repetition of the previous step until a wall of LA is deposited around the wound or a diamond shape surrounds the structure (e.g., when applying to the ear).
- Repeated injections should be placed in an area where the LA was previously deposited (Figure 9.3).

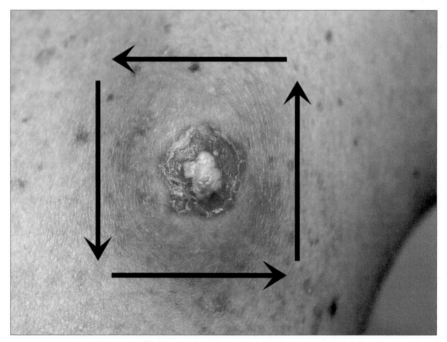

FIGURE 9.3 Field-block anesthesia technique.

COMPLICATIONS

- Infection
- Bleeding
- CV toxicity
- CNS toxicity
- Vasovagal syncope

PEARLS

- Bupivicaine lasts longer than lidocaine.
- True allergic reaction consists of urticaria, pruritis, wheezing, and so on, and not vasovagal symptoms.
- Use LA liberally, even in wounds without a closure, as there is no reason to inflict unnecessary pain on patients.
- Injection through the wound edges is less painful than through the epidermis.
- Topical agents are well tolerated and effective in children.
- Though most cases of systemic toxicity are caused by inadvertent intravenous injection, calculate the maximal dose for large wounds.
- A quick method for converting any LA concentration is to add a zero after the numerical percentage—a 1% solution is 10 mg/mL.

RESOURCES

Cave, G., & Harvey, M. (2009). Intravenous lipid emulsion as antidote beyond local anesthetic toxicity: A systematic review. *Academy of Emergency Medicine, 16*(9), 815–24. doi: 10.1111/j.1553-2712.2009.00499.x

Crystal, C. S. (2007). Anesthetic and procedural sedation techniques for wound management. *Emergency Medical Clinics of North America, 25*(1), 41–71.

Harmatz, A. (2009). Local anesthetics: Uses and toxicities. *Surgery Clinics of North America, 89*(3), 587–598.

Higginbothan, E., & Vissers, R. J. (2004). Local and regional anesthesia. In J. Tintinalli & G. Kelen (Eds.), *Emergency medicine: A comprehensive study guide* (pp. 264–274). New York, NY: McGraw-Hill.

Jackson, T. (2006). Pharmacology of local anesthetics. *Ophthalmologic Clinics of North America, 19*(2), 155–161.

Kapitanyan, R., & Su, M. (2009). *Toxicity, local anesthetics.* Retrieved from http://emedicine.medscape.com/article/819628-overview

McCreight, A., & Stephan, M. (2008). Local and regional anesthesia. In C. King & F. Henretig (Eds.), *Textbook of pediatric emergency procedures* (pp. 439–469). Philadelphia, PA: Lippincott Williams & Wilkins.

Paris, P. M., & Yealy, D. M. (2006). Pain management. In J. Marx, R. Hockberger, & R. Walls (Eds.), *Rosen's emergency medicine concepts and clinical practice* (pp. 2913–2937). Philadelphia, PA: Mosby, Elsevier.

CHAPTER 10

Procedures for Performing Regional Anesthesia

Keith A. Lafferty

BACKGROUND

Blocking a peripheral nerve is intuitively more advantageous because the nerve is inhibited before its distal tributaries. A digital nerve block is the most common use of this technique and is discussed in Chapter 11.

Advantages of regional anesthesia over infiltrative anesthesia include the following:

- Broad area covered
- Less local anesthetic (LA) administered

Also, some areas of the body, such as the ear, palm, sole, and so on, are not amenable to infiltrative anesthesia. In the case of the plantar foot, the large amount of sensory fibers combined with the difficulty of injecting through the dense, septated connective tissue makes regional anesthesia a prudent choice.

These nerve blocks are not as easily mastered as the infiltrative anesthesia technique. However, with repetition, a continued review of the peripheral neuroanatomy, and proper training and supervision, one can gain comfort and success with such procedures. The reader should note the use of ultrasound-guided regional nerve anesthesia has greatly enhanced the accuracy of various peripheral nerve blocks, including those listed in this chapter. Though the use of ultrasound is described in various procedures throughout this book, it has been purposely omitted in this chapter in order to emphasize its use in more commonly performed sonographically guided procedures.

Nerve blocks more proximal to the wrist and ankle, with the exception of an intercostal and penile block, will not be discussed as they are more often used in the operating room and may require a nerve stimulator or an ultrasound machine to precisely localize them. Also, bupivicaine is recommended over lidocaine because of its longer duration of action in general.

PATIENT PRESENTATION

Use with any patient presenting with an injury distal to the nerve being anesthetized, such as:

- Laceration
- Abscess

- Fracture
- Dislocation
- Burns

TREATMENT
Ulnar Nerve Block

The ulnar nerve supplies sensation to the medial third of the dorsal hand, small finger, and the ulnar half of the ring finger. The ulnar nerve runs along the volar aspect of the wrist, bordered medially by the ulnar artery, and laterally by the flexor carpi ulnaris. Note that the ulnar nerve lies just below this tendon flexor, making a volar approach difficult (Figures 10.1–10.3). Identification of the proximal carpi ulnaris at the proximal palmar crease is simplified by having the patient flex the wrist against resistance.

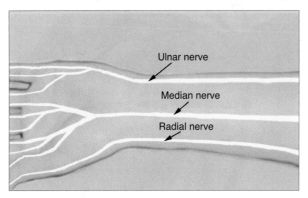

FIGURE 10.1 Ulnar, radial, and median nerves; volar wrist.

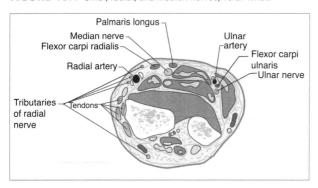

FIGURE 10.2 Cross-section of a wrist.

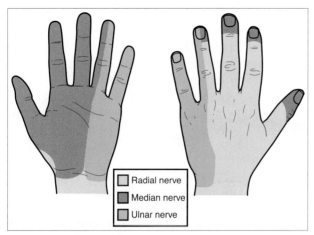

FIGURE 10.3 Dermatones of the hand.

Radial Nerve Block

Proximal to the wrist, the radial nerve is divided into tributaries that enter the radial aspect of the wrist. Sensation is provided in the lateral two thirds of the dorsal hand, the proximal dorsal thumb, the index finger, the long finger, and the radial half of the fourth finger. Note that the nail beds of the fingers are supplied by the median nerve, which makes up half of the dorsal digital nerve (Figures 10.1–10.3).

Median Nerve Block

The median nerve provides sensation to the lateral two thirds of the palm. It also supplies the distal dorsal thumb, the index and middle fingers, and the lateral half of the distal ring finger. The median nerve at the wrist is bordered medially by the palmaris longis tendon and laterally by the flexor carpi radialis at a depth just below the former tendon. Note that 20% of the population may be without the palmaris longis tendon. The palmaris longis is identified by having the patient oppose the thumb and small finger in wrist flexion with resistance. Note that the flexor carpi radialis is just lateral to this (Figures 10.1–10.3).

Posterior Tibial Nerve and Sural Nerve Blocks

The posterior tibial nerve and the sural nerve are tributaries of the tibial nerve. The posterior tibial nerve supplies the majority of the plantar surface sensation, along with the sural nerve medially and the saphenous nerve laterally. The posterior tibial nerve runs along the medial aspect of the ankle just deep and posterior to the posterior tibial artery between the medial malleolus and the Achilles tendon. It is identified by palpating the posterior tibial artery, which is located just posteriorly to the medial malleolus. The sural nerve runs subcutaneously between the lateral malleolus and the Achilles tendon. Often, these two nerves are blocked simultaneously to anesthetize the plantar surface entirely—a posterior ankle block (Figures 10.4–10.6).

Intercostal Nerve Block

This is one of the most underused nerve blocks. The fear of causing an iatrogenic pneumothorax with this procedure is unwarranted as the incidence is less than 0.1%. Rib fractures, contusions, and post–chest tube thoracostomy are ideal for its use. Although the duration of action of long-acting LAs is 8 to 12 hours, patients get continued relief for up to 3 days with this procedure. It should be noted that the intercostal nerve block has the potential for rapid vascular absorption though doses used are well below toxic levels. Care must be taken

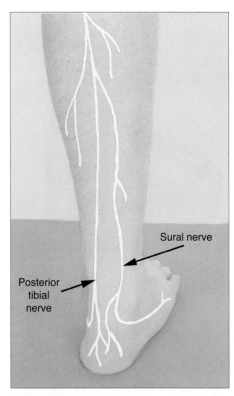

FIGURE 10.4 Posterior tibial nerves.

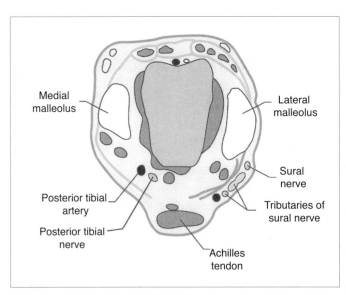

FIGURE 10.5 Cross section of the ankle.

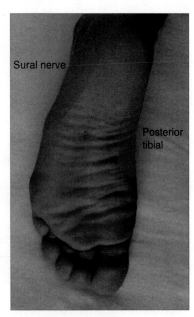

FIGURE 10.6 Dermatome of plantar foot.

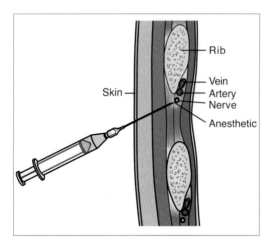

FIGURE 10.7 Intercostal groove contents of inferior rib border.

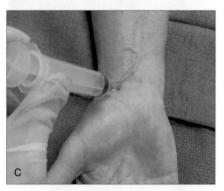

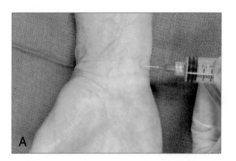

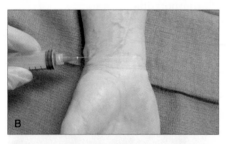

FIGURE 10.8A, 10.8B, and 10.8C Needle entry points for **A.** ulnar nerve block; **B.** radial nerve block; and **C.** median nerve block.

to correctly calculate the maximum dose of LA, though typically this is not reached. This minimizes the splinting associated with rib injuries and its sequelae of atelectasis and pneumonia.

The intercostal groove accommodates, in a superior to inferior manner, the intercostal vein, artery, and nerve. Posteriorly, it is separated from the pleural space by only a thin intercostal fascia. Laterally, it is sandwiched between the internal and external intercostal muscles. The entry point of the needle should be at the inferior border of the rib on the lateral chest wall. A post-procedure chest x-ray is not needed (Figure 10.7).

Penile Block

The two dorsal nerves of the penis each supply half of the dorsal glands and shaft. They lie just off the midline at the 10 and 2 o'clock positions at the base of the shaft. They are just deep to the fibrous buck's fascia. The anterior surface is supplied by cutaneous sacral plexus nerves. Because of this, nerve blocks can anesthetize the dorsal penis, whereas a ring block must be used to anesthetize the anterior penis.

PROCEDURE PREPARATION

- Wrist blocks are best accomplished with the patient in the supine position with the forearm/wrist resting with the volar surface.
- Posterior ankle blocks are best positioned with the patient prone and the ankle hanging off the end of the stretcher with the foot in slight dorsiflexion.

CONTRAINDICATIONS

- Allergy
- Compartment syndrome

PROCEDURE
Ulnar Nerve Block

- Insert a 25-gauge needle horizontally into the medial wrist just under the flexor carpi ulnaris at the level of the proximal palmar crease (Figure 10.8A).
- Inject 5 mL of the LA.
- Inject a subcutaneous partial ring block from the lateral border of the flexor carpi ulnaris and continue medially to the dorsal half of the wrist in order to anesthetize cutaneous fibers.

Radial Nerve Block

- Insert a 25-gauge needle horizontally into the lateral wrist until it is just lateral to the radial artery at the level of the palmar crease (Figure 10.8B).
- Inject 5 mL of the LA.
- Inject a subcutaneous partial ring block from this lateral entry point and continue laterally to the dorsal half of the wrist in order to anesthetize cutaneous fibers.

Median Nerve Block

- Insert a 27-gauge needle perpendicular to the skin between the palmaris longis and the flexor carpi radialis at the level of the proximal palmar crease (Figure 10.8C).
- Inject 5 mL of the LA.

Posterior Tibial Nerve Block

- Insert a 25-gauge needle at a 45-degree angle anteriorly just posterior to the posterior tibial artery at the level of the superior surface of the medial malleolus (Figure 10.9A).
- Inject 5 mL of the LA.
- If no paresthesia elicited, direct the needle in a more perpendicular direction.

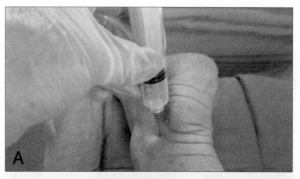
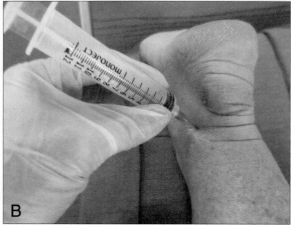

FIGURE 10.9A and 10.9B Needle entry points for ankle blocks for **A.** posterior tibial nerve and **B.** sural nerve.

Sural Nerve Block

- Insert a 25-gauge needle anteriorly between the Achilles tendon and the lateral malleolus about 1 cm superior to the lateral malleolus (Figure 10.9B).
- Inject 5 mL of the LA.
- Inject a subcutaneous partial field block between the Achilles and the lateral malleolus in order to anesthetize cutaneous fibers.

Intercostal Nerve Block

- Patient should be sitting upright with legs hanging off the side of the stretcher.
- Insert a 25-gauge needle perpendicular to the skin between the mid- and posterior axillary line directly.
- After striking the rib with the needle, retract the needle slightly (without withdrawing completely) and readvance in a slightly more inferior position in an attempt to "walk" the needle down the rib.

- At a point just below the intercostal groove, advance the needle 3 mm beyond the inferior border (Figure 10.10).
- Inject 5 mL of the LA.
- Repeat this procedure for one or two ribs above and below the site of injury in order to anesthetize cross-innervation.

Penile Block

- Insert a 25-gauge needle perpendicular to the abdominal wall, at the base of the penis at the 10 and 2 o'clock positions.
- Inject 5 mL of the LA in both sides.
- The depth of the needle should be 0.5 cm below the skin. One may feel a "pop" as buck's facia is penetrated.
- Inject a subcutaneous partial ring block around the posterior base of the penis.

COMPLICATIONS

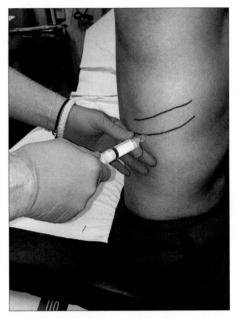

FIGURE 10.10 Intercostal nerve block.

- Infection
- Bleeding
- Peripheral nerve injury
- Compartment syndrome
- Cardiovascular toxicity
- Central nervous system toxicity
- Vasovagal syncope

PEARLS

- Allow at least 15 minutes to take effect, and more time if the injury is more distal to the block.
- Epinephrine allows the LA to remain near the nerve longer and increases the duration of action.
- Eliciting distal paresthesia with the needle before injection implies contact with the nerve.
- Keep in mind that some structures have secondary cutaneous innervation (i.e., hand and penis) and note the importance of a circumferential ring block to complement the primary target nerve.
- Dual nerves in some structures (i.e., the wrist [radial and ulnar]), may be required for a particular area to receive full anesthesia.
- Intercostal nerve blocks are safe and offer significant relief of pain.

RESOURCES

Crystal, C. S. (2007). Anesthetic and procedural sedation techniques for wound management. *Emergency Medicine Clinics of North America, 25*(1), 41–71.

Higginbothan, E., & Vissers R. J. (2004). Local and regional anesthesia. In J. Tintinalli & G. Kelen (Eds.), *Emergency medicine: A comprehensive study guide* (pp. 264–274). New York, NY: McGraw-Hill.

McCreight, A., & Stephan, M. (2008). Local and regional anesthesia. In C. King & F. Henretig (Eds.), *Textbook of pediatric emergency procedures* (pp. 439–469). Philadelphia, PA: Lippincott Williams & Wilkins.

Morgan, G. E., & Mikhail, M. S. (2002). Peripheral nerve blocks. In G. E. Morgan, M. S. Mikhail, & M. J. Murray (Eds.), *Clinical anesthesiology* (3rd ed., pp. 283–308). New York, NY: Lange Medical Books.

Simon, B., & Hern, G. (2006). Wound management principals. In J. Marx, R. Hockberger, & R. Walls (Eds.), *Rosen's emergency medicine concepts and clinical practice* (pp. 845–846). Philadelphia, PA: Mosby, Elsevier.

CHAPTER **11**

Procedures for Performing Digital Anesthesia

Keith A. Lafferty

BACKGROUND

By far, a digital nerve block is the most commonly used regional nerve block in the outpatient setting. It provides fast, effective, and simple anesthesia. Because the structure of the distal finger has fibrous septations, local infiltrative anesthesia is not only impractical but also nearly impossible.

As in most procedures, the key to a successful outcome is a fundamental understanding of the anatomy. A common digital nerve runs along the side of the metacarpals and, at the level of the metacarpal heads, bifurcates into volar and dorsal tributaries.

The end result is that there are lateral, dorsal, and medial digital nerves as well as their radial counterparts. Specifically, they lay alongside the phalanx at the 2, 10, 4, and 8 o'clock positions. Dorsal fibers are derived from the radial and ulnar nerves, whereas volar fibers stem from the median and ulnar nerves. Although both a dorsal and palmar approach can be used, the former is more desirable as it has less subcutaneous pain fibers. The innervation of the toes follows a similar pattern.

A metacarpal nerve block that is more proximal can also be used before the bifurcation at the metacarpal head. Its advantage is that it provides more proximal anesthesia; however, it is more difficult and occasionally less effective.

The thumb and hallux (great toe) have accessory nerves running over the dorsal lateral surface, much more so than the other digits. Because of this, the provider should make a circumferential subcutaneous ring pattern with the local anesthetic.

PATIENT PRESENTATION

Digital pathology of the finger/toe, including the following:

- Lacerations
- Paronychia

- Nail bed injuries
- Fracture
- Dislocation
- Ring removal
- Tendon injuries

TREATMENT

Local anesthetic injection should occur at least 10 minutes before the procedure to allow complete anesthesia. Although it is commonly stated that epinephrine should not be used, there is no evidence supporting this. In fact, according to current evidence, the use of epinephrine with lidocaine in standard commercial concentrations for digital blocks is not harmful and is likely advantageous, as epinephrine with lidocaine decreases the use of tourniquets and repeated sticks.

CONTRAINDICATIONS

- Compartment syndrome of the finger

PROCEDURE PREPARATION

- Patient should be supine with the finger well exposed and comfortably resting on the table
- Skin antiseptic solution
- Bupivacaine or lidocaine
- 25- or 27-gauge needle

PROCEDURE

- Follow skin-cleansing technique as described in Chapter 10.
- Sterile technique
- The volar surface of the hand is placed on the table.
- The needle is inserted at a 90-degree angle in the dorsal hand at the level of the web space along the proximal phalynx tenting the volar skin.
- Upon slow withdrawal of the needle, 2 mL of local anesthetic is deposited.
- Just before needle withdrawal from the skin, a 1-mL deposit is injected in the dorsal surface of the finger.
- The needle is reinserted in the other side of the finger through the anesthetized dorsal surface as described previously (Figure 11.1).

PEARLS

- Allow adequate time for onset of this peripheral nerve block—at least 10 minutes.
- Bupivacaine lasts longer than lidocaine.
- The finger tips are not amenable to the infiltrate of local anesthesia secondary to fibrous septae.

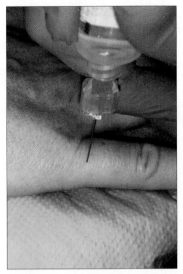 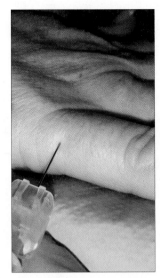 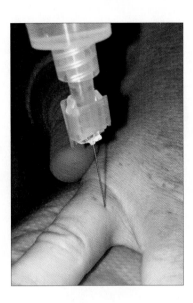

FIGURE 11.1 Digital nerve block insertion sites.

RESOURCES

Kelly, J. J., & Spektor, M. (2004). Nerve blocks of the thorax and extremities. In J. Roberts & J. Hedges (Eds.), *Clinical procedures in emergency medicine* (pp. 567–590). Philadelphia, PA: Saunders.

McCreight, A., & Stephan, M. (2008). Local and regional anesthesia. In C. King & F. Henretig (Eds.), *Textbook of pediatric emergency procedures* (pp. 439–464). Philadelphia, PA: Lippincott Williams & Wilkins.

Volfson, D. (January 27, 2010). *Anesthesia, regional, digital block*. Retrieved from http://emedicine.medscape.com/article/80887-overview

Waterbrook, A. L. (2007). Is epinephrine harmful when used with anesthetics for digital nerve blocks? *Annals of Emergency Medicine, 50*(4), 472–475.

CHAPTER 12

Procedures for Performing Beir Anesthesia

Keith A. Lafferty

BACKGROUND

The Beir anesthesia technique was first described in 1908 and has withstood the test of time, although it is much underused. This type of venous anesthesia involves intravenous (IV) infusion of a local anesthetic (LA) in the distal extremity via the proximal part constricted via a pneumatic tourniquet. The LA is forced to permeate the venous walls and capillaries and to remain in the portion of the extremity distal to the pneumatic cuff, which has a higher pressure than the systolic blood pressure. The technique allows rapid onset of limb anesthesia (paresis), provides a bloodless field, and is safe, effective, and easy to perform. Although this involves a large dose of an LA intravenously, a recent review in the literature shows no mortality and very little morbidity.

Different mechanisms of action probably contribute to its overall effect. Besides the sodium channel blockade theory, ischemia and acidosis probably contribute to the anesthesia, as prior to the discovery of LAs, surgical procedures were carried out just with pneumatic compression of nerve tunnels.

PATIENT PRESENTATION
- Large extremity lacerations (repair)
- Extremity fractures (reduction)
- Extremity dislocations (reduction)
- Extremity burns (debridement)
- Extremity abscess incision and drainage
- Extremity tendon lacerations (repair)

TREATMENT

Because the position of the pneumatic cuff overlies the proximal extremity, this procedure is best used for injuries at or below the elbow and knee. The area is exsanguinated before the procedure begins in order to maintain a bloodless field. A key feature of this procedure is that all of the LA is contained in the extremity and does not enter the systemic circulation. Two pneumatic cuffs are used—a proximal and a distal. The proximal cuff is inflated first and only after onset of anesthesia distal to this cuff is reached, then the distal cuff is inflated and the proximal cuff is deflated. This is done to decrease the pain induced by the cuff pressure.

Lidocaine is chosen over bupivacaine because it is less cardiac toxic and may remain active after cuff deflation. The concentration of lidocaine to be used is 0.5%. Although the literature states that lidocaine can be used at a dose of 3 mg/kg, a mini dose of 1.5 mg/kg can be used with similar efficacy and less potential toxicity. If needed, repeat doses of 0.5 mg/kg can be given. Expected onset is 5 to 10 minutes in a progression of paresthesia, anesthesia, to paresis in a distal to proximal manner.

CONTRAINDICATIONS
- Raynaud's disease
- Homozygous sickle cell disease
- Significant cardiac disease
- Unreliable tourniquet

PROCEDURE PREPARATION
- Patient should be supine on the stretcher.
- An IV is placed in the ipsilateral extremity for the LA.
- Another IV is placed in the contralateral extremity for the administration of resuscitation medications if needed.
- Two pneumatic tourniquets
- Elastic bandage
- Cardiac monitor with pulse oximeter
- Resuscitation cart in room
- Lidocaine 0.5% without epinephrine
- Large syringe for the lidocaine injection

PROCEDURE
- Place the patient in a supine position on cardiac monitor and pulse oximeter.
- Place IV in both extremities.

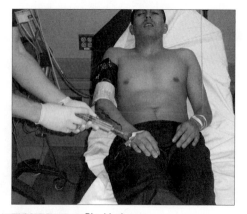

FIGURE 12.1 Bier block

- Exsanguinate the extremity via arm raising and Ace-wrap compression in a distal to proximal manner.
- Inflate the proximal pneumatic cuff to 100 mmHg above the patient's systolic blood pressure.
- Remove Ace wrap.
- Inject lidocaine at a dose of 1.5 mg/kg over 1 minute (Figure 12.1).
- At onset of effect, inflate the distal cuff and deflate the proximal cuff in order to decrease cuff-induced pain.
- Rebolus 0.5 mg/kg of lidocaine if needed.
- After completion of procedure, deflate the cuff for 10 seconds and then reinflate. Do this for three cycles.

COMPLICATIONS

Complications are rare and usually result from an improper and malfunctioning tourniquet and subsequent release of a large bolus of the LA into the systemic circulation. Treatment is with standard resuscitation techniques; however, it should be noted that benzodiazepines treat most of these signs and symptoms (see Chapter 9 for complete treatment of local anesthetic toxicity). If complications occur, observe the following signs/symptoms.

- Nausea
- Vomiting
- Dizziness
- Tinnitus
- Brady dysarhythmias
- Decreased mentation
- Seizures

PEARLS

- It is of paramount importance to repeatedly check and maintain proper cuff inflation throughout the procedure.
- Use the mini dose of lidocaine (1.5 mg/kg instead of the standard 3 mg/kg dose) as it has similar efficacy but less toxicity if systemic release occurs.
- If used on the lower extremity, the cuff should not be higher than the midcalf to prevent peroneal nerve injury.
- Confirm the absence of a radial pulse before injection of the LA.
- Skin blanching after the injection of the LA is normal and probably a result of blood extravasation from capillaries as it is being displaced by the LA.
- If 0.5% lidocaine cannot be found, it can be made from a 1% solution by creating a 50/50 solution with normal saline.

RESOURCES

Bolte, R. G., & Stevens, P. M. (1994). Mini-dose Bier block intravenous regional anesthesia in the emergency department treatment of pediatric upper-exremity injuries. *Journal of Pediatric Orthopaedics, 14*(4), 534–537.

Guay, J. (2009). Adverse events associated with intravenous regional anesthesia (Bier block): A systematic review of complications. *Journal of Clinical Anesthesia, 21*(8), 585–594.

McCreight, A., & Stephan, M. (2008). Local and regional anesthesia. In C. King & F. Henretig (Eds.), *Textbook of pediatric emergency procedures* (pp. 439–468). Philadelphia, PA: Lippincott Williams & Wilkins.

Mohr, B. (2006). Safety and effectiveness of intravenous regional anesthesia (Bier block) for outpatient management of forearm trauma. *Canadian Journal of Emergency Medicine, 8*(4), 247–250.

CHAPTER 13

Procedures for Performing Auricular Anesthesia

Theresa M. Campo

BACKGROUND

Anesthesia for the external ear, also known as auricular blocks or auricular anesthesia, can be used to treat extensive lacerations, auricular hematomas, and other painful procedures to the external ear.

The ear, also known as the auricle, is divided into three areas: external, middle, and internal structures. Discussion here will be limited to the external auricle. The external ear is innervated by four branches of nerves: (a) the greater auricular nerve (branches off from the cervical plexus), (b) lesser occipital nerve, (c) auricular branch of the vagus nerve, and (d) auriculotemporal nerve (Table 13.1 and Figure 13.1).

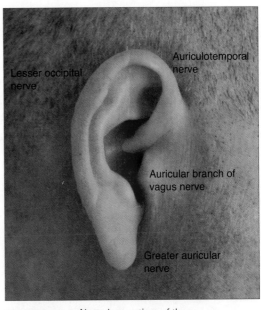

FIGURE 13.1 Nerve innervations of the ear.

CONTRAINDICATIONS AND RELATIVE CONTRAINDICATIONS

- Cellulitis
- Severe allergy to anesthetic agent

PROCEDURE PREPARATION

- Syringe (10 mL)
- Lidocaine 1% or bupivacaine 0.25% (Epinephrine should *not* be used for direct infiltration of the ear/auricle)
- Needle—25 to 30 gauge

TABLE 13.1 Auricular Nerve Branch and Innervation

Nerve Branch	Innervation
Greater auricular nerve (branch of cervical plexus)	Auricle Posteromedial Posterolateral Inferior
Lesser occipital nerve (branch of cervical plexus)	Few branches may contribute to: Auricle Posteromedial Posterolateral Inferior
Auricular branch of vagus nerve (cranial nerve [CN] X)	Concha Most of the auditory meatus tympanic membrane
Auriculotemporal nerve (mandibular branch of trigeminal nerve, CN V)	Auricle Anterosuperior Anteromedial

PROCEDURE

- Cleanse the area for infiltration with skin cleanser.
- Fill the 10-mL syringe with either lidocaine or bupivacaine.
- Attach the needle to the syringe.

Local Nerve Branch Blocks

These are for the greater auricular and lesser occipital nerve branches.

- Insert needle at the posterior sulcus pointing to the superior pole following the curve of the auricle (Figures 13.2 and 13.3).
- Gently aspirate and then inject 3 to 4 mL of anesthetic block.

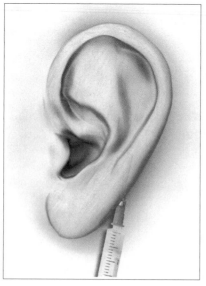

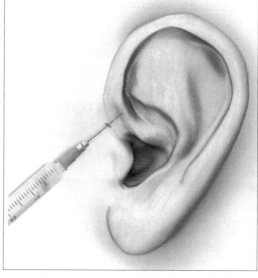

FIGURE 13.2 Local nerve block for greater auricular and lesser occipital nerve blocks.

FIGURE 13.3 Local nerve block for auriculotemporal nerve block.

Auriculotemporal Nerve Branch (Figure 13.3)

- Insert needle superior and anterior to the tragus.
- Gently aspirate and then inject 2 to 4 mL of anesthetic.

Ring Block/Regional Block (Figure 13.4)

- Insert the needle subcutaneously approximately 1-cm superior to the auricle in the direction just anterior to the tragus.
- Gently aspirate and then inject 3 to 4 mL of anesthetic.
- Remove the needle.
- Insert the needle into the same place but direct it posteriorly.
- Gently aspirate and then inject 3 to 4 mL of anesthetic.
- Remove the needle.
- Insert the needle inferior to the ear lobule.
- Repeat the aforementioned steps injecting anteriorly and posteriorly.

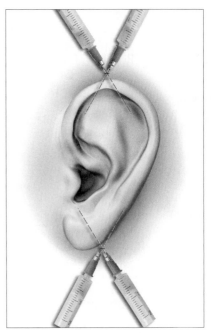

FIGURE 13.4 Ring-region nerve block of the ear.

POST-PROCEDURE CONSIDERATIONS

- Pain with injection of anesthetic
- Consult ear, nose, and throat (ENT) specialist

COMPLICATIONS

- Possible cannulation of the superficial facial artery

PEARLS

The use of lidocaine with epinephrine has generally been contraindicated for the outer ear. However, recent literature suggests that the use of epinephrine does not block the circulation to this area of the ear and, therefore, does not cause necrosis. Over 60 years ago, epinephrine was used only with the anesthetics procaine and cocaine, and necrosis was found to occur. However, it was later discovered that it was the acidity of the anesthetics (especially procaine) not the epinephrine that caused the necrosis. The decision to use epinephrine for local infiltration of the outer ear is at the clinician's discretion and should be based on the most up-to-date evidence-based practice. Epinephrine is also acceptable for regional block of the ear.

RESOURCES

Hutchens, D. J., Rosh, A. J., & Cloyd, J. (2014). *Ear anesthesia*. Retrieved from http://emedicine
    .medscape.com/article/82698-overview

Knowles, J. (2015). *Exploring the lidocaine with epinephrine myth*. Retrieved from http://www
    .clinicaladvisor.com/exploring-the-lidocaine-with-epinephrine-myth-hospital-emergency-
    medicine/article/393435/#

Riviello, R. J. (2014). Otolaryngologic procedures. In J. R. Roberts & J. R. Hedges (Eds.), *Clinical procedures in emergency medicine* (6th ed.). Philadelphia, PA: Saunders Elsevier. Retrieved from https://www.clinicalkey.com/#!/content/book/3-s2.0-B978145570606800063X

Riviello, R. J., & Brown, N. A. (2010). Otolaryngologic procedures. In J. R. Roberts & J. Hedges (Eds.), *Clinical procedures in emergency medicine* (5th ed., pp. 1195–1197). Philadelphia, PA: Saunders Elsevier.

Rosh, A. J. (2009). *Anesthesia, ear.* Retrieved from http://emedicine.medscapre.com/article/82698-overview and http://emedicine.medscapre.com/article/82698-treatment

UNIT VI

Skin and Wound Management Procedures

CHAPTER **14**

Overview of Wound Healing and Soft Tissue Ultrasound

Theresa M. Campo

SKIN ANATOMY

Skin is a component of the integumentary system and is known as the cutaneous membrane. The cutaneous membrane consists of three major areas: cutaneous, subcutaneous, and deep fascia. It is a key component of our existence as it provides protection, excretion, temperature regulation, sensory perception, and the synthesis of vitamin D. The skin also acts as a water barrier, specifically the stratum epithelial layer. Disruption of this layer can result in large water loss (i.e., burn victims).

Skin acts as a protective barrier to the external environment. It facilitates vasoconstriction and vasodilatation for temperature regulation and excretes salt and water through perspiration. Nerve endings are encompassed to provide pain reception and the sensations of touch and pressure. Finally, skin is involved in the photosynthesis of vitamin D.

The dermal and epidermal layers comprise the cutaneous layer. The epidermis is the outermost layer and is made up of stratified squamous epithelial cells. There are two layers that are important to wound healing: the stratum germinativum, which continually makes new keratinocytes as old ones are shed (basal layer), and the stratum corneum (horny or keratinized layer), which progressively moves up from the basal layer. These layers are very thin (0.2-mm thick) and difficult to differentiate from the dermal layer.

The dermis is the main component of the wound-healing process. It is thicker, lies below the epidermis, and is made up primarily of connective tissue. The main cells of the dermis are fibroblasts, which are key in the facilitation of wound healing. They deposit fibrous proteins (elastin fibers and collagen), which give the wound its intrinsic strength. Blood vessels, nerves, and sebaceous and sudoriferous glands are contained within the loose connective tissue of this layer.

The layer lying beneath the dermis is the superficial fascia or subcutaneous layer. It is primarily composed of loose connective and adipose tissues. During trauma and significant temperature changes, these tissues provide insulation and protection to major blood vessels and underlying structures. Sensory nerves and major blood vessels pass through this layer.

The deepest layer of the skin is the deep fascial layer. It is composed of fibrous, thick, and dense tissue that supports the superficial layers of skin. This layer contains sensory nerve fibers, blood vessels, and lymphatics. The functions of this layer are to provide protection from the spread of infection, as well as to support and protect the underlying muscle and soft tissue structures. See Figure 14.1 for the layers of the skin.

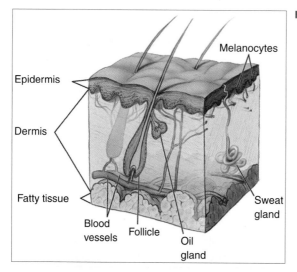

FIGURE 14.1 Layers of the skin.

PHASES OF WOUND HEALING

There are three main phases of wound healing. The components of the initial inflammatory phase are hemostasis and inflammation. The second phase is the proliferative phase; the final is the remodeling phase. During wound healing, there are many events occurring, separately and simultaneously. These phases begin at the onset of the wound and can continue for 1 to 2 years.

Hemostasis begins minutes after the injury via vasoconstriction, activation of the clotting cascade, and platelet aggregation. The platelets release thrombin and growth factors that attract fibroblasts and monocytes to the wound, activating the intrinsic clotting cascade. This helps to limit the initial damage of the wound by ceasing bleeding and sealing the wound surface through retraction of the wound edges and clot formation.

The inflammatory phase is characterized by activation of the complement system, which causes increased vascular permeability, migration of cells into the wound, and angiogenesis. Clinically, this constitutes erythema, swelling, warmth, and pain. Chemoattractant agents bring the neutrophils and monocytes to the wound within 24 to 48 hours. The neutrophils clean the area by trapping and killing bacteria. The monocytes become tissue macrophages that produce growth factors and cytokines to remove nonviable tissue and bacteria. Epidermal cells begin to migrate into the wound from surrounding tissue.

Neovascularization, fibroplasia, and epithelialization are the main components of the proliferative phase. Granulation occurs during this phase and the wound edges move closer together. A loose arrangement of collagen fibers begin to fill the wound as new capillaries begin to grow.

During the maturation phase, remodeling and wound contraction begin to occur. Wound contraction occurs as a result of myofibroblasts pulling collagen toward the cell body and epithelization is the migration of epithelial cells to resurface the wound. A more organized and stable form of collagen replaces the soft collagen. This increases the intrinsic tensile strength of the wound. This phase usually lasts about a year but can take 2 years to complete. Approximately 1 week after the wound occurs, the tensile strength is around 10% and at 1 year it can be 80%. Healed wounds never regain their original full tensile strength.

TYPES OF WOUND HEALING

Wound healing can occur in one of three ways: first intention, second intention, or third intention. First intention occurs when the wound is closed with sutures, staples, skin adhesive, or Steri-strips. Closure depends on time, contamination, and tissue devitalization. These wounds are either clean lacerations or surgical incisions.

Second intention occurs when the wound is left open to heal on its own. This is a slower process than first intention and allows the wound to heal through granulation from the inside out. These wounds can be caused by abscess, ulceration, puncture, or animal/human bites that have a high risk of infection if closed primarily. These wounds can be grafted or revised at a later date when the risk of infection is considered minimal.

The final method of healing that is widely underutilized is a delayed primary closure. This is also known as third intention. Wounds that are significantly contaminated may be closed 4 to 5 days after occurrence to help reduce the risk of infection. This time frame corresponds with the stages of wound healing when the risk of infection is significantly decreased. Delayed closures can occur weeks or months after the initial injury.

FACTORS COMPLICATING WOUND HEALING

Wound healing is a complex process that can be affected by numerous factors. Trauma, extent of the wound, patient age, type of closure, alcoholism, diabetes, connective tissue disorders, medications, vitamin deficiencies, nutritional status, and circulation are all factors that affect wound healing. Consideration of underlying factors and prevention of further damage to the wound during any interventions are key to efficient wound healing.

WOUND CARE

Wound care before and after any procedure is crucial to wound healing. All wounds require cleansing with sterile normal saline, sterile water, or tap water. This can be completed through irrigation, scrubbing, and soaking. The method used will depend on the type and extent of contamination of the wound. The use of hydrogen peroxide and povidone iodine are no longer recommended as they cause damage to viable tissue. Any time these substances are used, they should be diluted. Whenever possible, commercially prepared skin cleanser should be used (i.e., chlorhexidine). Skin cleansers should also be used before any infiltration or invasive procedure to limit contamination with normal skin flora, dirt, and debris.

SOFT TISSUE ULTRASONOGRAPHY

The use of ultrasonography to identify soft tissue infections and foreign bodies is becoming more widely utilized in the emergency, urgent, and primary care settings. Ultrasound can be useful in identifying cellulitis, necrotizing fasciitis, abscess, and retained foreign bodies. It is important to identify the normal structures of soft tissue before discussing ultrasound-guided procedures specifically. The equipment, techniques, and normal anatomy of soft tissue are discussed in this section.

Layers of Soft Tissue

The underlying makeup of the layers of soft tissue can be easily distinguished on ultrasound. Table 14.1 shows the tissue echogenicity, appearance, and an accompanying picture to demonstrate the characteristics of the tissue layers.

TABLE 14.1 Layers of Soft Tissue With Ultrasound

Tissue Layer	Tissue Echogenicity	Appearance	Picture
Cutaneous	Hyperechoic	Thin and regular	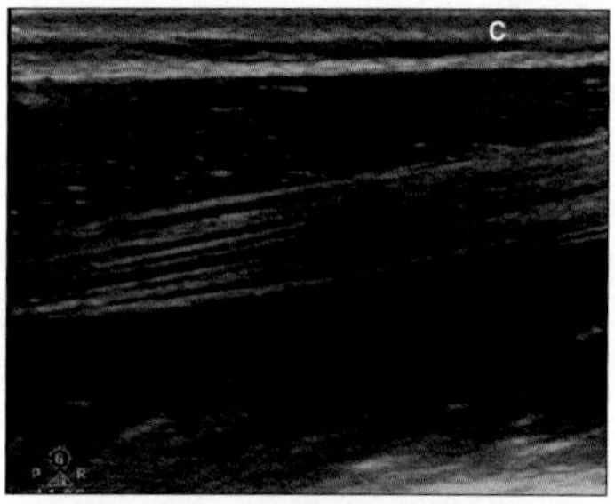
Subcutaneous	Hypoechoic	Transversed by hyperechoic connective tissue	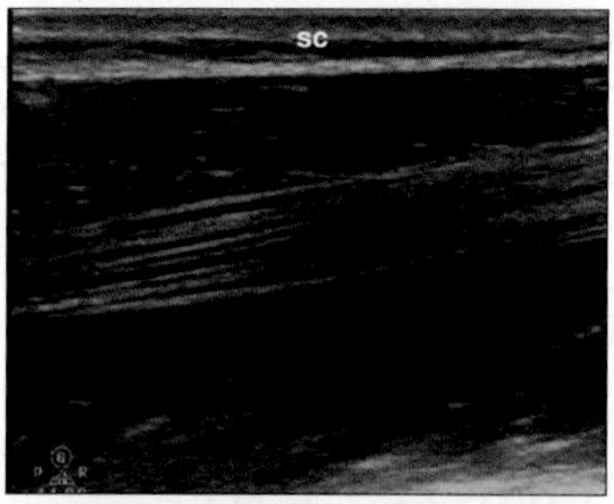
Fascia	Hyperechoic	Thin and regular	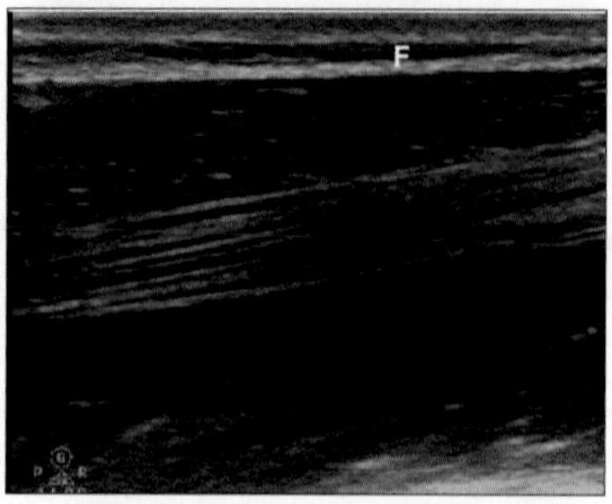

(*continued*)

TABLE 14.1 Layers of Soft Tissue With Ultrasound (*continued*)

Tissue Layer	Tissue Echogenicity	Appearance	Picture
Muscle	Hypoechoic and isoechoic with subcutaneous fat	Organized in bundles divided by fibroadipose septa Long axis: "featherlike" or "veins on a leaf" Short axis: speckled "starry night"	
Vessel	Anechoic	Long axis: rectangular Short axis: round or oval Arteries—pulsatile Veins—collapsible	
Lymph node	Echogenic center surrounded by hypoechoic rim	Irregular, circular structure	

(*continued*)

TABLE 14.1 Layers of Soft Tissue With Ultrasound (*continued*)

Tissue Layer	Tissue Echogenicity	Appearance	Picture
Bone	Bright echogenic cortex Dense acoustic shadow	Seen in the far field of the image Useful landmark and depth perspective	

Ultrasonography of Soft Tissue

When evaluating soft tissue for foreign bodies or infection, it is important to utilize the appropriate equipment and techniques. The use of a high-frequency linear array transducer (7–12 MHz) or a convex array tranducer (3.5–5 MHz) should be considered. The convex tranducer may be preferred to identify deep collections of fluid such as purulent fluid or abscess in the buttock area. When evaluating fluid collections two planes should always be used to define the shape and depth of the fluid collection. When evaluating soft tissue in the pediatric patient, consider a high-frequency (6–13 MHz) linear transducer to produce a small footprint. The gain can also be increased to visualize subtle detail of high water content of subcutaneous tissue. Visualization of superficial foreign bodies may be facilitated with the use of a water bath, a standoff gel pad, or a thick layer of acoustic gel. You should always compare the contralateral side to define normal anatomical structures and tissue layers.

PEARLS

- There are three general causes for wounds that are delayed in healing or become worse: retained foreign body, infection, and cancer.
- Pink or beefy red granulation tissue is a sign of proper wound healing and represents the proliferation phase.

TYPES OF WOUNDS

There are six categories of wounds, which include abrasion, avulsion, combination, crush, laceration, and puncture. The characteristics and extent of the wound are dependent on the causative force. See Table 14.2 for the description of wounds in each of these categories and their causative force.

WOUND MANAGMENT

All wounds presented in this book should be treated with general care. Cleaning the skin with a skin cleanser (diluted povidone iodine or chlorhexidine) should be done before any injection procedure. Remember, the solution for pollution is dilution. Open wounds should always be irrigated with normal saline before progressing with any procedure. It would be redundant to list this step for each procedure involving an open wound. If a specific method of wound cleaning is necessary, it will be noted in the respective chapters.

SPECIAL CONSIDERATIONS

Ring Removal

Background

Any injury to the upper extremity can cause swelling to the finger(s). For this reason, all rings should be removed before swelling begins. In cases in which the swelling has begun, the ring(s) can be removed using one of three techniques: lubricant, string technique, and ring cutter. Patients' rings not only have financial value but also sentimental value. For these reasons, attempts at removal with a lubricant and/or string should be made before resorting to a ring cutter. Some metals are very strong

TABLE 14.2 Description of Wounds

Force	Wounds Characteristics	Example
Skin and object in opposite directions	Rough appearance with loss of epidermis and superficial dermis	"Road rash," "skinned knee"
Shearing Tensile force	Partial or complete loss of skin layers	Skin tear Flap of skin
Crush Shear Tensile	Takes on numerous appearances depending on the force	Compression injury Explosions Motor vehicle crash
Compression of tissue against hard surface or bone	Devitalized tissue Ecchymosis surrounding wound	Rough, jagged wound edges
Shear Compression Tensile	Clean, tidy Rough, jagged	Incision Knife injury Hitting head on solid object
Tensile Compression	Depth of wound is greater than width Inability to visualize end of wound	Stepping on nail Bites

(i.e., tungsten) and difficult to cut through and may lead to further injury of the digit (i.e., lacerations, edema).

PROCEDURE PREPARATION

Lubricant
- Gloves
- Water-based lubricant (K-Y Jelly)
- Gauze or paper towel

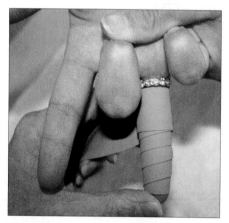

FIGURE 14.2 Ring removal via Penrose tourniquet application.

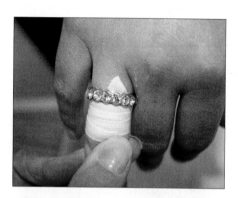

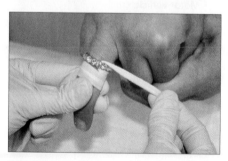

FIGURE 14.3 Ring removal via string application.

String Method
- Gloves
- Wide-width Penrose drain or tourniquet
- 20-in. length of string, umbilical tape, or 1/4-in. packing

Ring Cutter
- Gloves
- Manual or powered ring cutter

PROCEDURE

Lubricant
- Liberally apply lubricant to the finger and rub around the ring.
- Turn the ring in a circular motion (one direction only).
- Apply traction, moving the ring off the finger past the proximal interphalyngeal joint.
- Clean the finger with gauze or paper towel.

String Method

If there is significant trauma to the finger or the patient is apprehensive and anxious, a digital block can be performed before beginning this procedure (see Chapter 11).

- Take the Penrose drain, or tourniquet, and wrap it around the finger distal to proximal.
- Allow it to stay in place for a few minutes (Figure 14.2).
- Remove the Penrose drain and pass the string material between the finger and ring.
- Wrap the string as close to the ring as possible distally on the finger.
- Begin to unwrap the string from the proximal end (Figure 14.3), which will begin to move the ring off the finger.

Ring Cutter

- Place the hook end of the cutter between the ring and finger (Figure 14.4).
- Allow the wheel to rest on the ring.
- Begin turning the handle if the cutter is manual or start the power on the power cutter.
- Once through the ring, attempt to spread the metal.
- If the ends of the metal are too difficult to spread, another cut may be necessary.

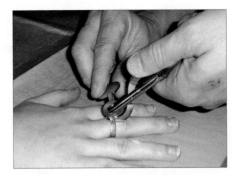

FIGURE 14.4 Ring removal via manual ring cutter.

EDUCATIONAL POINTS

- Advise the patient that the ring can be repaired by a jeweler.

PEARLS

- Give reassurance and encouragement to the patient during the procedure.
- Ask if there are any inscriptions in the ring and try to avoid that area if possible.
- Manufactured ring cutters can be either manual, electrical, or battery operated (Figure 14.5).

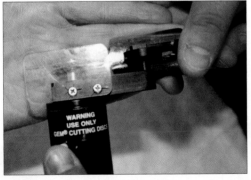
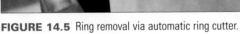
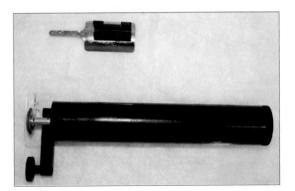

FIGURE 14.5 Ring removal via automatic ring cutter.

RESOURCES

Fishman, T. D. (2013). *Phases of wound healing.* Retrieved from http://www.medicaledu.com/phases.htm

Hollander, J. E. (2003). Patient and wound assessment: Basic concepts of the patient history and physical examination. In A. J. Singer & J. E. Hollander (Eds.), *Lacerations and acute wounds: An evidence-based guide* (pp. 9–12). Philadelphia, PA: F. A. Davis.

Lammers, R. L. (2010). Principles of wound management. In J. R. Roberts & J. R. Hedges (Eds.), *Clinical procedures in emergency medicine* (5th ed., pp. 563–575). Philadelphia, PA: Saunders Elsevier.

Lammers, R. L., & Smith, A. E. (2014). Principles of wound management. In J. R. Roberts & J. R. Hedges (Eds.), *Clinical procedures in emergency medicine* (6th ed., chap. 34). Philadelphia, PA: Saunders Elsevier. Retrieved from https://www.clinicalkey.com/#!/content/ book/3-s2.0-B9781455706068000343

Moscati, R. M., Mayrose, M., Reardon, R. F., Janicke, D. M., & Jehle, D. V. (2007). A multicenter comparison of tap water versus sterile saline for wound irrigation. *Society for Academic Emergency Medicine, 14*(5), 404–409. Retrieved from http://onlinelibrary.wiley.com/doi/10.1111/j.1553-2712.2007.tb01798.x/epdf

Pieknik, R. (2006a). Wounds. In *Suture and surgical hemostasis: A pocket guide* (pp. 1–19). Philadelphia, PA: Saunders.

Pieknik, R. (2006b). Wound healing. In *Suture and surgical hemostasis: A pocket guide* (pp. 20–41). Philadelphia, PA: Saunders Elsevier.

Simon, P. E., Moutran, H. A., & Romo, T. (2014). *Skin wound healing*. Retrieved from http://emedicine.medscape.com/article/884594-overview

Singer, A. J., & Clark, R. A. (2003). The biology of wound healing. In A. J. Singer & J. E. Hollander (Eds.), *Lacerations and acute wounds: An evidence-based guide* (pp. 1–8). Philadelphia, PA: F. A. Davis Company.

Singer, A. J., & Clark, R. A. F. (1999). Cutaneous wound healing. *The New England Journal of Medicine, 341*(10), 738–746.

Trott, A. T. (2005a). Anatomy of wound repair. In A. T. Trott (Ed.), *Wounds and lacerations: Emergency care and closure* (3rd ed., pp. 13–18). Philadelphia, PA: Mosby Elsevier.

Trott, A. T. (2005b). Surface injury and wound healing. In A. T. Trott (Ed.), *Wounds and lacerations: Emergency care and closure* (3rd ed., pp. 19–34). Philadelphia, PA: Mosby Elsevier.

Trott, A. T. (2005c). Wound care and the pediatric patient. In A. T. Trott (Ed.), *Wounds and lacerations: Emergency care and closure* (3rd ed., pp. 35–48). Philadelphia, PA: Mosby Elsevier.

CHAPTER 15

Procedures for Managing Puncture Wounds

Theresa M. Campo

BACKGROUND

Puncture wounds can have a small or large opening depending on the causative force and object (depth > width). Puncture wounds make it difficult to predict outcome because of the inability to visualize the end of the wound. The area of the body injured, level of contamination, and barriers between the offending object and the skin (e.g., shoes) can impact the interventions used and ultimately affect wound healing. Most important, the depth of penetration dictates innervation. Penetration into avascular structures, such as bursae, tendons, and joint spaces, allows organisms to proliferate. Some puncture wounds heal with minimal intervention; others become infected or have delayed healing regardless of the interventions and prophylaxis. Of note, 90% of puncture wounds to the foot involve stepping on a nail and 10% to 15% of these injuries become infected.

PATIENT PRESENTATION

- Pain
- Swelling
- Ecchymosis
- Open wound (can be as small as 1 mm)
- Bleeding

TREATMENT

The end of most puncture wounds is smaller than the entrance of the wound, making cleaning and debriding difficult for the provider. Pressure irrigation of the puncture track can cause more damage by spreading contaminants and bacteria into surrounding tissue or spaces that cannot be visualized (e.g., tendon sheath of a puncture wound to the hand). Copious irrigation is the treatment method of choice. Forcible irrigation can also increase soft tissue swelling, lead to further tissue damage, and hinder healing.

Significantly contaminated puncture wounds can be treated by either performing a coring excision or incising the wound to convert it to a linear laceration. Determination of the technique is based on the extent of the contamination, depth of the wound, presence of a foreign body (FB), and the underlying tissue and structures. Plain films should be ordered when the possibility of a radiopaque FB is suspected; ultrasonography or exploration should occur with radiolucent FBs.

SPECIAL CONSIDERATIONS

- Diabetics
- Immunocompromised patient
- Arterial or venous insufficiencies
- Anticoagulant therapy
- Steroids

PROCEDURE PREPARATION

- Absorbent pads
- Sterile normal saline solution
- Gauze
- Basin
- Splash guard or 16- to 18-gauge angio-catheter
- 35- or 65-mL syringe

If incising the area to remove contamination

- No. 11 or No. 15 scalpel
- Forceps

PROCEDURE

- Place the absorbent pad under the affected area.
  - If the wound is on the hand, soak the area in normal saline and/or scrub the area. Otherwise, the following procedure can be performed. Remember not to exert excessive pressure during irrigation.
- Adequate pressure needs to be 5 to 8 pounds per square inch (PSI) and can be achieved with either the angio-catheter or splash shield and syringe.
- Draw up the normal saline in the syringe.
- Place the splash guard on the tip of the syringe.
- Begin to irrigate the area.
  - The rate of speed and the height of the stream will affect the amount of pressure on the tissue.
- If the wound is contaminated, scrub the area to free the debris.
- Irrigate to cleanse the area.
- Apply antibiotic ointment and a dressing to the wound.
  - For grossly contaminated areas: Incise the area to remove contamination (debridement).
- Cleanse the area.
- Perform a local anesthesia (see Chapter 9).

- With the scalpel, extend the puncture wound (Figure 15.1).
- Debride the area of dirt, nonviable tissue, and FBs.
- Irrigate as described previously.
- Apply topical antibiotic and dressing.

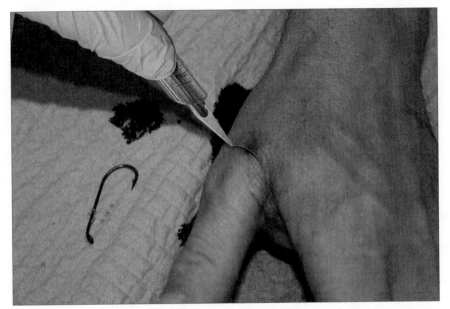

FIGURE 15.1 Incising a contaminated puncture wound.

POST-PROCEDURE CONSIDERATIONS
Antibiotic Prophylaxis

With contaminated wounds, antibiotic prophylaxis and tetanus prophylaxis should be considered. Puncture wounds occurring from stepping on a nail with a rubber-soled shoe should be treated with antibiotics that also address *Pseudomonas* infection, as this organism is harbored in rubber soled shoes (fluoroquinolone for adults and trimetoprim-sulfametoxazole for children).

Elevation

If the puncture wound is on an extremity, have the patient elevate the extremity to reduce the swelling or potential swelling resulting from the trauma. Reduction of swelling is key to promote tissue healing and to reduce pain.

Pain

Pain medication should be prescribed based on the patient's level of pain. Acetaminophen and nonsteroidal anti-inflammatory drugs (NSAIDs) are usually sufficient and well tolerated by the patient. Crutches can be used for a few days to reduce the discomfort of a puncture wound to the foot.

EDUCATIONAL POINTS

- Clean with soap and water.
- Change dressing daily and as needed.
- Advise on risk, benefits, and side effects of oral antibiotics, if prescribed.
- Follow up for wound evaluation 2 to 3 days post-injury.

COMPLICATIONS

- Infection, including cellulitis, deep-space abscess, septic arthritis, and osteomyelitis, are frequent complications of puncture wounds. Good wound hygiene at the time of injury and throughout the wound healing process and close follow-up are key to prevention of infection.
- Retained FB.

PEARLS

- A combination of light irrigation and scrubbing can minimize contamination and the risk for infection.
- Puncture wounds occurring through rubber-soled shoes should be excised via a coring method.
- Pain is the most common symptom of infection.
- The greatest failure in treating a puncture wound is the tendency to under-treat secondary to the benign appearance of the puncture wound.
- All puncture wounds have a FB until proven otherwise.

RESOURCES

Lammers, R. (2003). Plantar puncture wounds. Basic concepts of the patient history: A physical examination. In A. J. Singer & J. E. Hollander (Eds.), *Lacerations and acute wounds: An evidence-based guide* (pp. 157–160). Philadelphia, PA: F. A. Davis.

Lammers, R. L. (2010). Principles of wound management. In J. R. Roberts & J. R. Hedges (Eds.), *Clinical procedures in emergency medicine* (5th ed., pp. 565–566). Philadelphia, PA: Saunders Elsevier.

Lammers, R. L., & Smith, A. E. (2014). Principles of wound management. In J. R. Roberts & J. R. Hedges (Eds.), *Clinical procedures in emergency medicine* (6th ed., chap. 34). Philadelphia, PA: Saunders Elsevier. Retrieved from https://www.clinicalkey.com/#!/content/book/3-s2.0-B9781455706068000343

Marx, J. A., Hockberger, R. S., & Walls, R. M. (2010a). Forensic emergency medicine. In *Rosen's emergency medicine* (7th ed.). Retrieved from http://www.mdconsult.com/das/search/results/187068169-10?searchId=962524726&kw=puncture%20wound&bbSearchType=single&area=BookFast&set=1&DOCID=2084

Marx, J. A., Hockberger, R. S., & Walls, R. M. (2010b). Wound management principles. In *Rosen's emergency medicine* (7th ed.). Retrieved from http://www.mdconsult.com/book/player/book.do?method=display&type=bookPage&decorator=header&eid=4-u1.0-B978-0-323-05472-0..00056-6–s0320&uniq=187068169&isbn=978-0-323-05472-0&sid=962524726

Simon, B. C., & Hern, H. G. (2014). Wound management principles. In *Rosen's emergency medicine* (8th ed.). Retrieved from https://www.clinicalkey.com/#!/content/book/3-s2.0-B9781455706051000592

CHAPTER **16**

Procedures for Removing a Soft Tissue Foreign Body

Theresa M. Campo

BACKGROUND

Foreign bodies (FBs) in the soft tissue can be of any material—organic material, such as wood, thorns, and vegetative material, causes a rapid inflammatory response (usually infective) or inorganic material (glass, metal, plastic, and rubber), which usually does not cause a severe reaction. FBs are more common in children and occur most frequently on the extremities. The most commonly seen FBs are glass, wood, and metal. Your geographical region may influence the type and frequency of FB seen. For example, areas along the coast may see more fishhooks, wood splinters, and fish spines than the Midwest. Studies have shown more than one third of soft tissue FBs are missed on initial examination.

Fishhook removal can be a challenge to the provider. There are numerous types of hooks and the patient may not be astute as to the type and size of the hook. Always ask the patient about the type of hook (no barb, barbed with single or multiple barbs, or treble) (Figure 16.1). The technique for removal depends on the depth and type of hook that is embedded.

Ticks embed themselves in order to feed from the host. There are numerous types of ticks and they can carry bacteria, viruses, toxins, spirochetes, Rickettsiae, and protozoa. Lyme disease, ehrlichiosis, Rocky Mountain spotted fever, and other illnesses can be caused by a prolonged tick bite.

PATIENT PRESENTATION

- Puncture wound with or without visible FB
- Pain
- Bleeding
- Discoloration (bruising, object)
- Swelling
- Nonhealing wound
- Granuloma formation
- Cellulitis
- Abscess formation

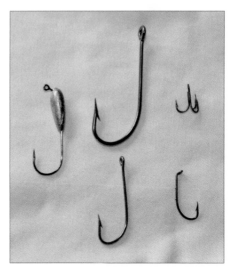

FIGURE 16.1 Types of fishhooks.

TREATMENT

Treatment is based on the location, depth, timing, and type of FB. Organic FBs do not show on plain radiographs. They are better visualized with ultrasound (US). CT scan can also be used to visualize FBs with a higher sensitivity than plain radiographs. The overall sensitivity is 95%, specifically 100% for metal, 75% for glass, and 7% for wood. CT is more expensive than plain radiographs and should be used when an FB is suspected and not found on x-ray or US. Metal and glass can be well visualized on plain radiographs except when hidden by bone or if very small (usually < 5 mm). Multiple views on plain x-ray are needed to detect FBs. Plastic materials may show on plain radiographs but are better seen with US.

Plain radiographs and US are beneficial and cost effective. Radiographs allow for visualization and estimation of depth. US can be used for guided removal of elusive and organic FBs and is mainstream for detecting radiolucent FBs (greater than 90% sensitivity), such as wood and rubber, when used properly.

There are various methods for FB removal, and they are based on the location, type, and depth of the FB. The possible positions of FBs in regard to soft tissue are superficial horizontal, vertical, subungual, and elusive. There are multiple methods used for fishhook removal, which are also discussed in this chapter.

Superficial horizontal FBs sit in the dermal and epidermal layer of the skin along the horizontal axis. You can see and palpate the FB, and it can be removed by excision. The vertical FB is perpendicular to the skin surface with only a very small surface, if any, exposed. This FB is difficult to remove and can be very deep. Incision and coring are used to remove this FB. The subungual FB is located beneath the nail plate. Cutting the nail in a "V" shape and removing the splinter is the most common method of removal. Performing a digital block and elevating the nail for removal is another option. Elusive FBs usually require referral for guided removal with either fluoroscopy or US. Plain radiographs can assist with placement and depth of the FB. However, the object may become displaced when an incision is made, making removal more complicated and causing more trauma to the tissue.

Obtaining the location, mechanism, timing, material of the FB, occupation, tetanus status, history of diabetes or immunosuppression, and hand dominance (if upper extremity is involved) are key features of the history. Assessment of contamination, location of FB, surrounding structural function (nerve, tendon, muscle, etc.) are imperative to ensure that the provider properly identifies and provides proper treatment of the patient. If the patient states that he or she feels an FB, you must exhaust all measures to confirm whether there is an FB present. A missed FB can lead to infections, including osteomyelitis, deep-space abscess, and granuloma formation.

CONTRAINDICATIONS AND RELATIVE CONTRAINDICATIONS

- Deep, elusive FBs
- Inability to obtain and maintain hemostasis for complete evaluation and removal
- Poor cosmetic outcome

SPECIAL CONSIDERATIONS

- Diabetics
- Immunocompromised patients
- Anticoagulant therapy

PROCEDURE PREPARATION

Foreign Body

Superficial Horizontal, Vertical, and Subungual

- Skin cleanser
- Absorbent pad
- Gloves
- Topical or injectable anesthetic
  - Small, superficial FBs, and/or callused skin may not require any anesthetic.
- No. 11 or No. 15 scalpel
- Splinter or fine forceps
- Small scissors
- Hemostat
- Normal saline for irrigation
- 35- to 65-mL syringe (for irrigation)
- 16- to 18-gauge angiocath or splash guard
- Skin cleanser scrub
- Dressing material
- Antibiotic ointment

Elusive

Removal should not be attempted if the object cannot be visualized. Referral is recommended for these patients.

Fishhook

Retrograde

- Gloves
- Normal saline for irrigation
- Skin cleanser

String Yank
- Gloves
- Normal saline for irrigation
- Skin cleanser
- String (thick suture material or umbilical tape)

Needle Cover
- Gloves
- Normal saline for irrigation
- Skin cleanser
- Injectable anesthetic
- Large-gauge needle (18 gauge or larger)

Advance and Cut
- Gloves
- Normal saline for irrigation
- Skin cleanser
- Injectable anesthetic
- Needle driver, hemostat, or pliers

PROCEDURE
Foreign Body
Superficial Horizontal (Figure 16.2)
- Cleanse the skin.
- Use topical or local anesthetic.
  - The type of anesthetic is determined by size, location, and depth of the FB and patient tolerance.
- Make an incision along the FB. Incise the entire length to ensure full removal.
- Apply gentle pressure to one end of the FB while lifting the opposite side.

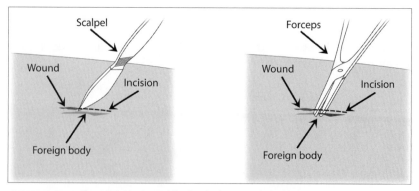

FIGURE 16.2 Superficial horizontal foreign-body removal technique.

- Grab the FB with forceps.
- Irrigate with copious amount of normal saline.
- Scrub the area to loosen debris and contamination, if necessary.
- Apply dry sterile dressing with Vaseline or antibiotic ointment.

Vertical (Figure 16.3)

- Cleanse the skin.
- Perform local anesthetic.
- Make an incision over the FB.
- Secure the FB, if possible, with the forceps.
- Incise around the FB (coring).
- Remove the entire section.
- Irrigate with a copious amount of normal saline.
- Scrub the area to loosen debris and contamination, if necessary.
- Apply dry sterile dressing with antibiotic ointment.

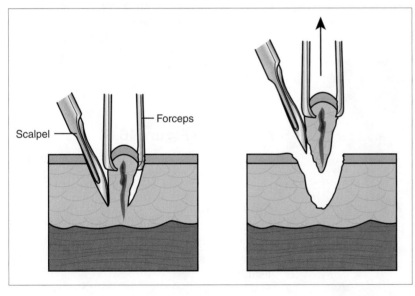

FIGURE 16.3 Vertical foreign-body removal technique.

Subungual (Figure 16.4)

- Cleanse the area.
- Perform a digital block.
- With either the scalpel or small scissors cut a "V" shape from the distal nail.
  - The point of the "V" should go to the proximal end of the FB.
  - Be careful not to cut or cause undue trauma to the nail bed.
- Remove the piece of nail with either the forceps or hemostat.
- Grasp the FB with the splinter forceps and remove by gently pulling.
- Irrigate with a copious amount of normal saline.
- Scrub the area to loosen debris and contamination if necessary.
- Apply dry sterile dressing with antibiotic ointment.

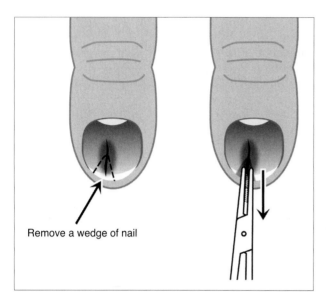

FIGURE 16.4 Removal of a subungual foreign body.

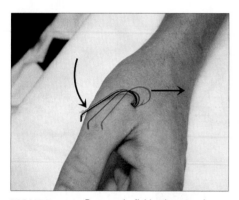

FIGURE 16.5 Retrograde fishhook removal technique.

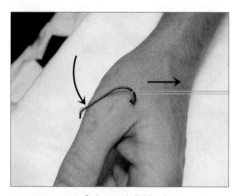

FIGURE 16.6 String-yank fishhook removal technique.

Fishhook

Key to successful removal of fishhooks is disengaging the barb from the tissue.

Retrograde (Figure 16.5)

This technique should be used for hooks that are barbless and superficially positioned. It can be attempted if the hook is small and barbed.

- Apply downward pressure to the base or shank of the hook.
- Gently rotate to disengage the barb.
- Begin to back the hook out.
  - If any resistance, stop the procedure and use another method.
- Irrigate with a copious amount of normal saline.
- Scrub the area to loosen debris and contamination, if necessary.
- Apply dry sterile dressing with antibiotic ointment.

String Yank (Figure 16.6)

This technique is best for small to medium fishhooks. Successful removal is best on fixed body parts.

- Cleanse the area.
- Topical or local anesthetic may be needed based on the patient's tolerance.
- Wrap the string around the center of the fishhook.
- Hold the ends tight.
- Rest the affected area on the table.
- Apply downward pressure to the base or shank of the hook.
- Push the distal end of the hook (the eye) against the skin while pulling on the string.
- Irrigate with a copious amount of normal saline.
- Scrub the area to loosen debris and contamination, if necessary.
- Apply dry sterile dressing with antibiotic ointment.

Needle Cover (Figure 16.7)

This technique can be used for any size fishhook with a single barb.

- Cleanse the area.
- Perform local anesthesia through the wound to reduce trauma to the area.
- Line up the large-gauge needle with the bevel facing the hook.
- Advance the needle through the opening and follow the hook.
- Push the hook forward and down slightly.
    - You may have to slightly rotate the fishhook to help disengage the tissue.
- Then begin to pull the hook out with the bevel of the needle over the barb.
- Irrigate with copious amount of normal saline.
- Scrub the area to loosen debris and contamination, if necessary.
- Apply dry sterile dressing with antibiotic ointment.

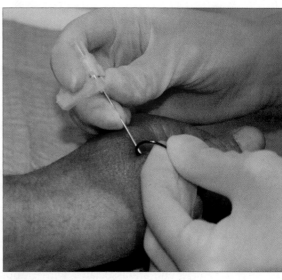

FIGURE 16.7 Needle cover fishhook removal technique.

Advance and Cut (Figure 16.8)

This technique can be used for any size hook with a single or multiple barbs.

Single Barb

- Cleanse the area.
- Perform local anesthetic.
- Push the point of the fishhook through the skin where it was tenting.
    - If unable to push through the skin, make a small incision.

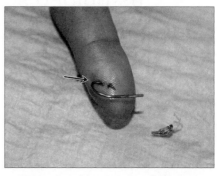

FIGURE 16.8 Advance and cut fishhook removal technique.

- Grab and secure the point of the hook with a needle driver or hemostat.
- Cut the point of the hook below the barb with wire cutters or other available cutting tools.
- Grasp the proximal end of the hook (the eye) and back the hook out.
- Irrigate with a copious amount of normal saline.
- Scrub the area to loosen debris and contamination, if necessary.
- Apply dry sterile dressing with antibiotic ointment.

Multiple Barbs

- Follow the aforementioned procedure, but cut the eye of the hook and pull the hook by the point (barb end).

Tick Removal

There are over-the-counter tick-removal devices (TRIX, Tick key, Sawyer tick pliers, etc.). Do not apply any products to the tick to attempt to kill or"stun"the tick. This may cause the tick to regurgitate and spread infection.

- Wear gloves. Ticks can pass infection with direct contact, not just bites.
- With fine-tipped forceps, grasp the tick as close to the skin as possible.
- Apply even traction while pulling upward until the tick is removed.
  - Do not twist, crush, or jerk when removing.
  - Inspect for and remove any retained mouth or body parts.
- Cleanse the area with soap and water.

POST-PROCEDURE CONSIDERATIONS

- Copious irrigation is needed after the FB is removed.
- Marine spines (stingray, lionfish, and sea urchin) carry slime and calcareous material and are associated with granuloma formation—coverage for *Vibrio* infection should be considered.
- A nail through a rubber-soled shoe should be covered for *Pseudomonas* infection with ciprofloxacin or another fluoroquinolone. Children should receive trimethoprim–sulfamethoxazole.

US-GUIDED SOFT TISSUE FB REMOVAL

Ultrasonography can be very helpful in not only identifying a radiolucent FB but also in the removal of the FB. Difficulty in identification and removal of soft tissue FBs can lead to infection, necrosis, and malpractice claims. US can be beneficial in detecting an FB that is not easily visualized or palpated, can indicate the size and shape of the FB, identify surrounding structures, and facilitate removal. US of an FB in the hand or foot can be difficult due to the complexity and sensitivity of the structures.

The most common FBs are glass, wood, and metal, which are hyperechoic with varying degrees of acoustic shadowing or reverberation artifact. Table 16.1 outlines the type of FB and its appearance with ultrasonography.

TABLE 16.1 Foreign-Body Appearance With Ultrasound

Foreign Body	Appearance
Gravel and wood	Acoustic shadow
Large wood	Brightly echogenic anterior surface
Metallic	Comet tail Reverberation artifact Bright parallel regularly spaced lines distal to the object
Glass	Acoustic shadow Comet tail Diffuse beam scatter
Retained FB (24–48 hours)	Echolucent halo

Superficial FB

A near-field acoustic dead space can occur immediately adjacent to the transducer surface and impede visualization of the superficial FB. There are three methods used to help avoid this from occurring. The use of either an US standoff pad, liberal use of the gel, and water-bath technique. The standoff pad is made of a low acoustic impedance material that elevates the transducer eliminating the near-field acoustic dead space. These are commercially prepared pads, for example, the "Aquaflex ultrasound gel pad"

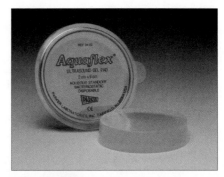

FIGURE 16.9 Standoff pad.
Permission granted by Parker Laboratories.

(Figure 16.9). The water-bath technique allows the provider to submerge the area in water and is useful for the very sensitive or tender areas with palpation and use of the transducer against the affected area.

- High-frequency linear array transducer for superficial FB or low-frequency transducer for deeper tissue penetration.
- Apply a probe cover if an open wound is present.
- Use slow, methodical scanning in multiple planes to identify the FB.
- Once FB is identified, place the center of the probe over the FB and mark with a pen.
- Note the location and depth of the FB.
- Incise at the most superficial point of the FB.
- Advance splinter forcep toward the object while maintaining the image.
- Gently grasp the object and remove.
- Evaluate the area with the transducer to ascertain any retained pieces.

For deeper, irregularly shaped FBs, the needle localization method may be considered but is less suitable for sensitive structures of the hands and feet.

- High-frequency linear array transducer for superficial FB or low-frequency transducer for deeper tissue penetration.
- Apply a probe cover if an open wound is present.
- Use slow, methodical scanning in multiple planes to identify the FB.
- Once FB is identified, place the center of the probe over the FB.
- Insert one needle at a 45-degree angle to the FB.
- Inject lidocaine.
- Insert another needle at a 45-degree angle on the other side of the FB, making a 90-degree angle between the two needles.
- Make an incision and dissect down to the tip of the needle intersection.
- Grasp the FB and remove.
- Remove the needles.
- Scan the area to ascertain any retained pieces.

EDUCATIONAL POINTS

- Complete removal of the FB and irrigation are essential.
- Antibiotic prophylaxis and close follow-up for grossly contaminated wounds and for patients with comorbidity are recommended.
- Have the patient regularly clean the wound with soap and water and apply antibiotic ointment.

COMPLICATIONS

- Infection
- Retained FB
- Further injury
  - Surrounding tissue affected during removal
- Neurovacular damage/compromise

PEARLS

- Education and counseling go a long way with patients with tick bites as most patients and/or parents are very anxious about the risk of Lyme disease and other illnesses. There are limited studies regarding antibiotic prophylaxis and the use of a one-time dose of doxycycline. The studies that have been done have shown that the incidence of transmission is low and the use of antibiotic prophylaxis inconclusive. Testing for Lyme disease should not be done immediately after the tick bite and/or after tick removal due to the high incidence of false results.
- Always use the proper type and amount of anesthesia before FB exploration.
- The use of a tourniquet for hemostasis will aid in visualization and removal of FBs.
- A glove filled with US gel can be used in place of a commercial standoff pad.

RESOURCES

Bannerman, C. C., & Ojike, N. I. (2014). *Wound foreign body removal*. Retrieved from http://emedicine.medscape.com/article/1508207-overview

Bass, A. M., & Levis, J.T. (2010). *Foreign body removal, wound*. Retrieved from http://emedicine.medscape.com/article/1508207-overview & http://emedicine.medscape.com/article/1508207-treatment

Chan, C., & Salam, G. A. (2003). Splinter removal. *American Family Physician, 67*(12), 2557–2562.

Consoli, R. J. (2007). Emergency medicine. In R. E. Rakel (Ed.), *Textbook of family medicine* (7th ed.). Philadelphia, PA: Saunders Elsevier. Retrieved from http://www.mdconsult.com/das/book/body/187280795-6/963092363/1481/466.html#4-u1.0-B978-1-4160-2467-5..50042-7–cesec45_2366

Edlow, J. A. (2009). *Tick-borne diseases, Lyme*. Retrieved from http://emedicine.medscape.com/article/1413603-overview & http://emedicine.medscape.com/article/1413603-treatment

Geria, R. (n.d.). *Ultrasound guided procedures – V. foreign body localization*. Retrieved from http://www.sonoguide.com/foreign_bodies.html

Halaas, G.W. (2007). Management of foreign bodies in the skin. *American Family Physician, 76*(5), 683–690. Retrieved from http://www.mdconsult.com/das/article/body/187280795-4/jorg=journal&source=MI&sp=19952104&sid=963088564/N/607270/1.html?issn=0002-838X

Lammers, R. (2003). Foreign bodies in wounds. In A. J. Singer & J. E. Hollander (Eds.), *Lacerations and acute wounds: An evidence-based guide* (pp. 147–156). Philadelphia, PA: F. A. Davis.

Levine, M. R., & Cheema, N. (2013). Soft tissue injury. In *Emergency medicine: Clinical essentials* (2nd ed.). Retrieved from https://www.clinicalkey.com/#!/content/book/3-s2.0-B9781437735482001877

Otten, E. J., & Mohler, D. G. (2007). Hunting and other weapon injuries. In P. S. Auerbach (Ed.), *Wilderness medicine* (5th ed.). Philadelphia, PA: Mosby Elsevier. Retrieved from

http://www.mdconsult.com/das/book/body/187280795-6/963092363/1483/198.html#4-u1
.0-B978-0-323-03228-5..50027-6–cesec16_1268

Shiels, W. E. (2007). Soft tissue foreign bodies: Sonographic diagnosis and therapeutic management. *Ultrasound Clinics, 2*(4), 669–681. Retrieved from http://www.mdconsult.com/
das/article/body/187280795-4/jorg=journal&source=&sp=20606707&sid=96308856
4/N/638044/1.html?issn=1556-858X

Stone, D. B., & Levine, M. R. (2010). Foreign body removal. In J. R. Roberts & J. R. Hedges (Eds.),
Clinical procedures in emergency medicine (5th ed., pp. 634–648). Philadelphia, PA: Saunders
Elsevier.

Stone, D. B., & Scordino, D. J. (2014). Foreign body removal. In J. R. Roberts & J. R. Hedges (Eds.),
Clinicalproceduresinemergencymedicine(6thed.).Philadelphia,PA:SaundersElsevier.Retrieved
from https://www.clinicalkey.com/#!/content/book/3-s2.0-B9781455706068000367

Thommasen, H. V. (2005). The occasional removal of an embedded fish hook. *Canadian Journal
of Rural Medicine, 10*(4), 254–259.

Winland-Brown, J. E., & Allen, S. (2010). Wound care: Foreign bodies in the skin. *The Nurse
Practitioner: American Journal of Primary Health Care, 35*(6), 42–47. Retrieved from http://
www.nursingcenter.com/lnc/static?pageid=1037067

CHAPTER **17**

Managing Animal and Human Bites

Theresa M. Campo

BACKGROUND

Animal bites can occur at any age and for many reasons. Animal bites in children usually occur from "roughhousing" with a pet or bothering an animal when it does not want to be disturbed. Bites in adults usually occur while attempting to break up fighting dogs or attempting to assist a distressed animal. Any unprovoked attack should be considered suspicious for rabies. Patients should be considered for rabies in any suspicious bite when the offending animal cannot be located and quarantined/tested. The patient's tetanus immunization status should be assessed and vaccination with either tetanus toxoid or tetanus with diphtheria and pertussis should be administered. The administration of tetanus with diphtheria and pertussis is based on the patient's age. Please refer to the new guidelines.

Dog bites most frequently occur in children 10 years old or younger and occur on the face, neck, and/or head and represent 80% to 90% of bites presenting to the emergency department. Bites to adults usually occur on the hands or arms from attempting to break up dogs that are fighting. Dog bites become infected less than 15% of the time. The teeth of dogs are round and large and tend to cause more crushing injuries than cats and can generate pressure of 200 to 450 pounds per square inch (PSI) and can crush sheet metal. Wound care, as well as the possibility of soft tissue injury, bone fracture, and foreign bodies, should always be considered.

Cat bites are less frequent and are at greater risk of becoming infected. The bite of a cat tends to leave a deeper puncture wounds, but are smaller in size than that of a dog. The teeth of cats are sharp and pointed and tend to "inoculate" bacteria deep into the tissue. When infection occurs, it usually advances more rapidly than in a dog bite and can include muscle, bone, and, most frequently, tendons (especially in the hands).

Human bites occur the least frequently but have a high rate of infection due to the polymicrobial nature of the human mouth. There are numerous organisms that can be found in our mouths at any given time. These bites can occur from altercations, assaults, sexual activity, seizures, and during medical and dental procedures (Figure 17.1A and 17.1B). Bites can be either intentional (true bite) or unintentional (closed fist).

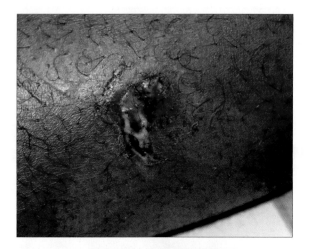

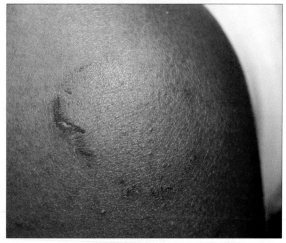

FIGURE 17.1 Human bite wound

A true bite can occur from the action of being bitten unintentionally when two people collide and the tooth of one person is pushed into the skin of another. Any open wound on the dorsal aspect of the hand, especially over the fourth or fifth metacarpalphalyngeal (MCP) joint, is considered to be a bite when it occurs with a closed hand or fist. Most patients will deny this mechanism to avoid "getting into trouble." However, it is important to discuss the increased risk of infection with these injuries and to reassure patients that they will not be penalized for their honesty. It is also very important to document the discussion on the patient's chart. It is of extreme importance to evaluate the joints for range of motion (ROM) in order to uncover a tendon and/or joint injury. Furthermore, these wounds may need to be extended in order to properly visualize the extent of the wound.

Another important consideration with human bites is the risk of transmission of hepatitis, HIV, syphilis, and other communicable diseases. Whenever possible, the patient and the person causing the bite, regardless of method, should be tested.

PATIENT PRESENTATION

Patients with either human or animal bites can present with varying degrees of severity and injuries.

- Pain
- Swelling
- Abrasion
- Ecchymosis
- Laceration
- Puncture wound
- Avulsion or partial avulsion
- Crushing injury
- Redness
- Drainage

TREATMENT

The goals of treatment are hemostasis, minimizing the risk of infection, reducing swelling, debridement of devitalized tissue, and improving cosmetic outcome. The history should include the time of the injury, circumstances leading up to the attack, and any past medical history of diabetes, immunosuppression, chemotherapeutics, and the immunization status of the patient and animal or human attacker. Radiographs should be ordered to rule out fracture and/or the presence of a foreign body. Injuries to the hand, involving a punch injury, should always be assessed for full ROM, tendon and joint function, and strength in all digits. Copious irrigation and debridement should also be performed and referred to a hand specialist for close follow-up.

Minor injuries can be treated with direct pressure, irrigation/washing, topical antibiotic, ice, and elevation for swelling. Major bites can be deep, extensive, and involve the head, face, hands, and extremities. The severity and type of injury stipulates the treatment required. Facial wounds should be closed by primary intention, and should be given antibiotics and close follow-up. Recommended antibiotics and common organisms from dog, cat, and human bites can be viewed in Table 17.1.

CONTRAINDICATIONS AND RELATIVE CONTRAINDICATIONS

Age of the Wound
- Wounds that are older than 8 hours should be left open to heal by second intention. The older the wound, the higher the risk for developing infection.
- Dog bites to the face can be sutured up to 12 hours after the bite. Some literature even recommends suturing up to 24 hours as long as antibiotic prophylaxis and close follow-up are done.
- Delay in evaluation and treatment leads to increased rates of infection.

Cause of the Wound
- Human and cat bites should not be closed unless they are very large due to the risk of infection. Cat bites should not be closed when they involve the hand.

History of Diabetes, Immunosuppression, and HIV
- Patients with diabetes, immunosuppression, and HIV should have close follow-up. The wounds should remain open and heal by second intent unless it is gaping.

PROCEDURE PREPARATION
- Absorbent pad
- Normal saline for irrigation
- 35- to 65-mL syringe

- Splash shield or 16- to 18-gauge angiocatheter
- Surgical scrub
- 4 × 4 gauze
- Topical antibiotic

Any bite to the hand or any human or cat bite should not be closed by first intention. Bites to the hand tend to have a higher infection rate (up to 28%) due to the number of enclosed compartments, nerves, tendons, joints, and fascial planes. Closure by second intention may be the best option due to the higher infection rate. Refer to Chapter 18 for closure techniques.

TABLE 17.1 Common Organisms and Antibiotic Treatment for Dog, Cat, and Human Bites

Bite	Organism(s)	First-Line Antibiotic	Alternative
Dog	**Aerobic** • *Pasteurella multocida* • *Staphylococcus aureus* • *Streptococcus* species **Anaerobic** • *Cornebacterium* species • *Eikenella corrodans* • *Capnocytphaga canimorsus*	Prophylaxis—3–5 days Infection—10 days • Amoxicillin-clavulonate	Doxycycline can be used in the following: • Children older than 8 years of age • Penicillin allergy **Adults** • Clindamycin and fluoroquinolone **Children** • Clindamycin and trimethoprim-sulfamethoxazole
Cat	**Aerobic** • *Pasteurella multocida* • *Streptococcus* species (inc. *S. pyogenes*) • *Staphylococcus aureus* • *Moraxella cataralis* **Anaerobic** • Fusobacterium • *Bacteroids fragilis* • Porphyromonas • *Capnocytophaga canimorsus*	Prophylaxis—3 to 5 days Infection—10 days • Amoxicillin-clavulonate • Do not use cephalexin	Doxycycline can be used in the following: • Children older than 8 years of age • Penicillin allergy **Adults** • Clindamycin and fluoroquinolone **Children** • Clindamycin and trimethoprim-sulfamethoxazole
Human	**Aerobic** • *Eikenella corrodans* • Alpha and beta hemolytic streptococcus • *Staphylococcus aureus* and *S. epidermidis* • *Corynebacterium* species **Anaerobic** • *Peptostreptylococcus* species • *Bacteroid fragilis* and nonfragilis • Fusobacterium • Veillonella	Prophylaxis—3 to 5 days Infection—10 days • Amoxicillin-clavulonate • Ampicillin/sulbactam	Clindamycin and trimethoprim-sulfamethoxazole • Penicillin allergy • Children • Pregnancy

- Place the absorbent pad under the affected area.
- Pour the normal saline into the basin.
- Draw up the saline with the syringe.
- Place the splash shield or catheter on the end of the syringe. (Do not use high-pressure irrigation with bites to the hands.).
- Irrigate the area.
- Use a surgical scrub to free any debris.
- Dry completely.
- Apply topical antibiotic.
- Dress the wound.

POST-PROCEDURE CONSIDERATIONS

Infection

If the wounds are 8 hours and older; contaminated; involve bone, joint, or tendon; or the patient has diabetes or immunosuppression, then it is best to leave them open for secondary healing. Broad spectrum antibiotics can be prescribed for approximately 5 days to help prevent infection. Groin injuries should also be considered for antibiotic prophylaxis.

Pain

Pain medication should be prescribed based on the severity of the injury and pain tolerance. Elevation and ice can help reduce the swelling and pain.

Rabies Prophylaxis

Rabies prophylaxis should be initiated with any suspicious animal bite (i.e., strays). The patient should receive rabies immunoglobin 20 IU/kg. Inject up to 50% around the wound(s) and the remainder via intramuscular (IM) injection. The patient will need to receive the rabies vaccine (Imovax, RabAvert) on the day of the injury, day 0, and on days 3, 7, and 14. The dose is standard at 1-mL IM in the deltoid.

EDUCATIONAL POINTS

- Dressings should remain in place for 24 hours.
- Clean with soap and water.
- Antibiotic ointment should be applied.
- Apply topical antibiotics to facial wounds frequently (every couple of hours) to avoid crusting and scar.

COMPLICATIONS

- Infection is always a consideration with bite wounds.
- Dogs have the lowest incidence of infection.
  - Parallel nonbite wound infection rates
- Cat bites have the highest infection rate of 60% to 80% due to the shape and structure of a cat's teeth.
- Facial wounds have:
  - Excellent blood supply
  - A low risk for infection, even if closed primarily

- Risk of superinfection must be discussed with the patient prior to closure.
- Generally, the better the vascular supply and the easier the wound is to clean (i.e., laceration vs. puncture), the lower the risk of infection.
- Early intervention, cleaning of the wounds, and close follow-up can help prevent these infections.

PEARLS

- If the wound is gaping, you can loosely close it so that it can drain and easily be opened if needed.
- Rapid onset of infection, usually within 12 to 24 hours, tends to be caused by *Pasteurella multocida*, whereas most other infections present 48 to 72 hours after the injury.
- Bites to the hands, from any source, demands the use of antibiotics and no closure.
- First-generation antibiotics are not as effective as amoxicillin-clavulanate due to resistance by *Eikenella corrodans* and anaerobic organisms.

RESOURCES

Barrett, J., & McNamara, R. M. (2010, April 8). *Bites, human*. Retrieved from http://emedicine .medscape.com/article/768978-overview

Barrett, J., & Revis, D. R. (2014). *Human bites*. Retrieved from http://emedicine.medscape.com/ article/218901-overview

Booth Norse, A. (2013). Mammalian bites. In *Emergency medicine: Clinical essentials* (2nd ed.). Retrieved from https://www.clinicalkey.com/#!/content/book/3-s2.0-B9781437735482001385

Dire, D. J. (2003). Animal bites. In A. J. Singer & J. E. Hollander (Eds.), *Lacerations and acute wounds: An evidence-based guide* (pp. 133–146). Philadelphia, PA: F. A. Davis.

Freer, L. (2007). Bites and injuries inflicted by wild and domestic animals. In P. S. Auerbach (Ed.), *Wilderness medicine* (5th ed.). Philadelphia, PA: Mosby Elsevier. Retrieved from http://www .mdconsult.com/das/book/body/187280795-8/0/1483/457.html?tocnode=54236968&- fromURL=457.html#4-u1.0-B978-0-323-03228-5..50056-2_2767

Habif, T. P. (2009). Animal and human bites. In *Clinical dermatology: A color guide to diagnosis and treatment* (5th ed.). Retrieved from http://www.mdconsult.com/book/player/ book.do?method=display&type=bookPage&decorator=header&eid=4-u1.0-B978-0- 7234-3541-9..00024-9-s0735&uniq=187280795&isbn=978-0-7234-3541-9&sid= 963112235#lpState=open&lpTab=contentsTab&content=4-u1.0-B978-0-7234-3541-9..0002 4-9-s0735%3Bfrom%3Dtoc%3Btype%3DbookPage%3Bisbn%3D978-0-7234-3541-9

Lee, C. K., & Hansen, S. L. (2009). Management of acute wounds. *Surgical Clinics of North America*, *89*(3), 659–676.

Nelson, S. W., & Gibbs, M. A. (2013). Hand and wrist injuries. In *Emergency medicine: Clinical essentials* (4th ed.). Philadelphia, PA: Elsevier. Retrieved from https://www.clinicalkey. com/#!/content/book/3-s2.0-B9781437735482000896

Oehler, R. L., Velez, A. P., Mizrachi, M., Lamarche, J., & Gompf, S. (2009). Bite related and septic syndromes caused by dogs and cats. *Lancet*, *9*, 439–447.

Perkins, A., & Harris, N. S. (2009, June 25). *Bites, animal.* Retrieved from http:// emedicine.medscape.com/article/768875-overview

Perkins Garth, A., Salas, R. N., Harris, N. S., & Spanierman, C. S. (2014). *Animal bites in emergency medicine.* Retrieved from http://emedicine.medscape.com/article/768875-overview

Prescutti, R. J. (2001). Prevention and treatment of dog bites. *American Family Physicians, 63,* 1567–1574.

Rhoads, J. (2009). Managing bites and stings. *Nurse Practitioner, 34*(8), 37–43.

Shoemaker, D. M., Jiang, P. P., Williamson, H., & Roland, W. E. (2007). Infectious disease: Bite infections. In R. E. Rakel (Ed.), *Textbook of family medicine* (7th ed.). Philadelphia, PA: Saunders Elsevier. Retrieved from http://www.mdconsult.com/das/book/body/187280795-12/0/1481/241.html#4-u1.0-B978-1-4160-2467-5..50024-5–cesec111

Weber, E. J., & West, H. H. (2010). Mammalian bites. In *Rosen's emergency medicine* (7th ed.). Philadelphia, PA: Elsevier. Retrieved from http://www.mdconsult.com/book/player/book. do?method=display&type=bookPage&decorator=header&eid=4-u1.0-B978-0-323-05472-0..00058-X&displayedEid=4-u1.0-B978-0-323-05472-0..00058-X–s0010&uniq=187280795&isbn=978-0-323-05472-0&sid=963109534

West, H. H., & Weber, E. J. (2014). Mammalian bites. In *Rosen's emergency medicine* (8th ed.). Philadelphia, PA: Elsevier. Retrieved from https://www.clinicalkey.com/#!/content/ book/3-s2.0-B9781455706051000610

CHAPTER 18

Procedures for Wound Closure

Theresa M. Campo

BACKGROUND

The goal of a wound healing through primary intent is to facilitate decreased healing time, reduce infection, and minimize scarring. This can be achieved through rapid assessment and interventions that minimize contamination, which includes debriding devitalized tissue, obtaining hemostasis, removal of any foreign body, and approximating tissue edges. It is imperative to make an accurate and thorough assessment, not only of the wound, but also of the circumstances that led to the wound (mechanism and time). It is also important to assess for past medical history, allergies to anesthetics, neurological and motor function, presence or suspicion of foreign body, and underlying structural damage (tendon, vessel, joint capsule, and nerve).

Delay in wound healing can have multifaceted consequences. The mechanism of the injury alone can put the patient at risk for infection and complication (i.e., crush, foreign body). Medical conditions and medications also play a role in wound healing. Patients with diabetes, immunosuppression, obesity, malnutrition, tobacco use, older age, and steroid usage are at greater risk for infections and delayed wound healing. It is important to help the patient to manage these risk factors whenever possible.

PATIENT PRESENTATION

- Pain
- Bleeding
- Open wound(s)
- Decreased or loss of sensation or function
- Anxiety

TREATMENT

Treatment begins with a thorough history, including mechanism, time of incident, medications, medication allergies, and immunization status (tetanus). Once the history is complete, do a careful examination of the wound and surrounding areas to ensure that there are no hidden foreign bodies or other injuries. If a foreign body is suspected, further studies should be ordered (plain radiograph, ultrasound, etc.). Regardless of the size of the wound, the patient will experience pain and should be anesthetized before wound cleansing and exploration.

The skin should first be cleansed. The area should then be anesthetized and irrigated with moderate pressure (5–8 pounds per square inch [PSI] with normal saline irrigation), and/or gently scrubbed. Once this has been completed, the wound should be probed for debris, foreign body, and devitalized tissue. The type of closure will depend on the type of wound, location, time since injury, contamination, and depth. Suture, staple, skin adhesive, and tape closures will be discussed in this chapter. Each method has its advantages and disadvantages, which will be discussed at the beginning of each procedure. Because of wound contraction during the healing phase, eversion is of paramount importance in all closures.

CONTRAINDICATIONS AND RELATIVE CONTRAINDICATIONS

- Grossly contaminated wounds
- Cause of the wound(s)
    - Puncture wound
    - Human and animal bite (depending on source and location)
- Delay in seeking treatment
    - Face and scalp—up to 24 hours
    - Hands and feet—less than 6 hours

SPECIAL CONSIDERATIONS

- Diabetes
- Immunosuppression
- Tobacco use
- Steroids
- Chemo and radiation therapies
- Malnutrition

PROCEDURE PREPARATION

- Nonsterile gloves
- Absorbent pad
- 4 × 4 gauze
- Skin cleanser
- Topical anesthetic
- Injectable anesthetic
- Normal saline for irrigation
- 20- to 30-mL syringe
- Splash guard
- Surgical scrub
- Nonadherent gauze
- Topical antibiotic

Suture

- Sterile gloves
- Suture kit (needle holder, toothed forceps, suture scissors, sterile drapes, basin and cups for cleanser, and normal saline)
- Suture material
    - Subcuticular and subcutaneous—absorbable (vicryl, chromic)

- Percutaneous—nonabsorbable (nylon, polypropylene)
- Face—thinner material (6-0)
- Extremities, torso, and scalp (3-0 to 5-0)

Staple
- Sterile gloves
- Suture kit (needle holder, toothed forceps, suture scissors, sterile drapes, basin and cups for cleanser, and normal saline)
- Staple gun

Skin Adhesive
- Sterile pack 4 × 4 gauze
- Skin adhesive (Cyanoacrylate glue–Dermabond, Indermill)
- Skin tape (Steri-Strips, butterflies)

Tape
- Benzoin
- Cotton-tipped applicators
- Skin tape (1/4 in., 1/2 in.)

PROCEDURE

Suture

Suturing is a great method of wound closure that offers, precision-wound edge approximation, and tensile strength. The disadvantages of sutures are the need for injectable anesthetic, removal of the sutures, tissue reactivity (especially with absorbable sutures), increased cost, and increased time to perform the procedure. There is also a great expectation by the patient or parents for a "perfect closure" and no scar formation (**Video 18.1**).

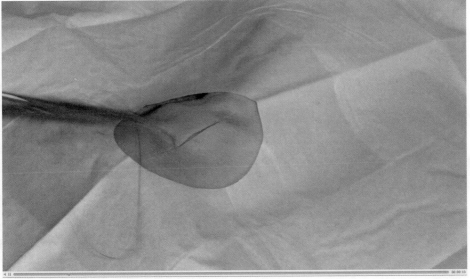

▶ **VIDEO 18.1** Simple interrupted suture.
springerpub.com/campo

- Put on nonsterile gloves.
- Cleanse the skin.
- Apply topical anesthetic.
  - Children, especially on faces
- Perform local, digital, or regional block based on the location and size of the wound (see Chapters 9 and 10).
- While the anesthetic is taking effect, open the suture kit and place the equipment needed onto your sterile field.
- Put on sterile gloves.
- Draw up the normal saline for irrigation in the large syringe.
- Attach the splash guard.
- Irrigate the wound with moderate pressure: 5 to 8 PSI, which can be achieved using a 35- to 65-mL syringe and either a splash shield or 16- to 18-gauge angiocatheter.
  - Use a gentle scrub for the eyebrow and around the eye as pressure irrigation can cause further damage to this sensitive area.
- Gently scrub the area if there is debris and contamination that was not removed with irrigation.
- Place the fenestrated sterile drape over the wound.
- Probe and visualize the wound for debris, contamination, and devitalized tissue, and remove.
- Open the suture material.
- Hold the needle holder in your dominant hand with the thumb in one hole and the ring finger in the other (Figure 18.1).
- Using your index finger to support the needle holder, open the locking mechanism.
- Grab the suture needle at the 1/3 junction of the proximal and midsection.
  - The needle holder should be perpendicular to the needle (Figure 18.2).
- Secure the locking mechanism.
- Remove the fingers from the holes and hold the needle holder in the palm of your hand.
- Put the forceps in your nondominant hand between the thumb and index fingers (Figure 18.3).
- Use the forceps to gently evert the wound edge.
- Insert the needle at 90 degrees to the skin (Figure 18.4) and press the needle through the skin and out the center of the wound. This angle ensures proper skin-edge eversion.

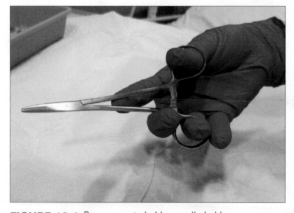

FIGURE 18.1 Proper way to hold a needle holder.

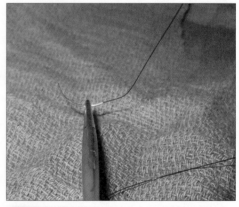

FIGURE 18.2 Proper way to hold a suture needle with the needle holder.

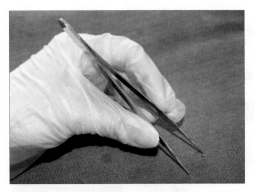

FIGURE 18.3 Holding the forceps.

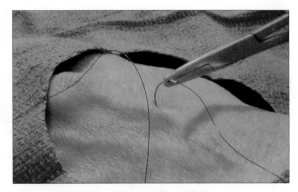

FIGURE 18.4 Inserting the needle at 90 degrees.

- Supinate your hand to give the proper motion and direction through the skin.
- Release the needle.
- Grab the needle with either the forceps or needle holder, pull through the wound, and reposition the needle holder on the needle as described previously.
- Use the forceps to evert the opposite side of the wound.
- Push the needle through the inside of the wound adjacent to the first insertion and push through the skin at the same distance from the wound on the opposite side entering the tissue at a 90-degree angle (Figure 18.5).
- Grab the needle with either the forceps or needle holder.
- Pull the material through the tissue leaving a 1- to 2-cm tail.
- Place your needle holder parallel to the wound (Figure 18.6A).
- Loop the needle end of the material two times and then grasp the tail with the needle holder and pull across, keeping the twist flat (Figure 18.6B).
- Place the needle holder parallel over the wound and loop one time in the opposite direction.
- Grasp the tail and pull across—again, the twist should be flat.
  - Approximate the wound edges, being careful not to "strangulate" the wound edges (Figure 18.6C).
- Repeat the aforementioned two steps.
- Knot(s) should be to the side of the wound and not directly over the wound itself.

Simple Interrupted Suture

- Snip both ends of the material approximately 1 cm above the knot.
- Repeat these steps as many times as needed.
- Appropriate spacing (Figure 18.7).
  - Allow equal space from the entry point to the wound and the wound to the exit.
  - Allow equal space between the sutures.
- Where to start:
  - Start in the center and work your way out the edges on each side, or start at one end and finish on the oppo-site side.

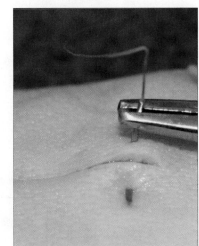

FIGURE 18.5 Needle through the other side.

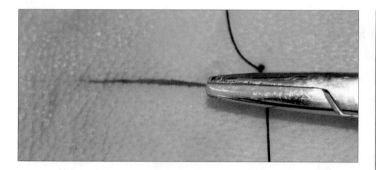

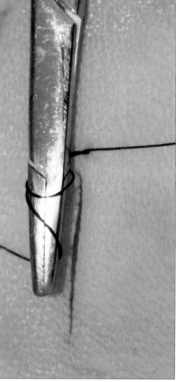

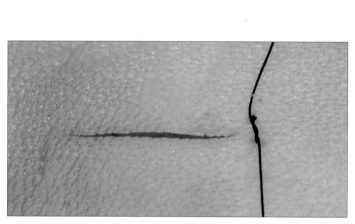

FIGURE 18.6 Tying a suture knot.

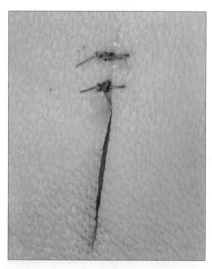

FIGURE 18.7 Appropriate spacing of a suture.

Continuous Suture (also Known as a Running Suture) (Video 18.2)

- Snip only the tail end to approximately 1 cm.
- Insert the needle beside the first insertion and come out on the other side of the wound.
- Continue the entire length of the wound.
- When you have made your last pass through the wound, do not pull the material all the way through; leave a loop.
- Make a knot as described previously, grabbing the loop in place of the free tail. Continuously check the alignment of the unsutured wound edges for potential misalignment, which is known as "dog-ears" (Figure 18.8).
- Continuous sutures take less time but if one area breaks, then they all break. Intermittently locking with a knot can help prevent this from occurring.

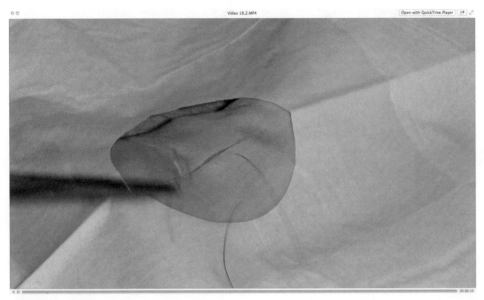

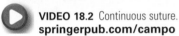

VIDEO 18.2 Continuous suture.
springerpub.com/campo

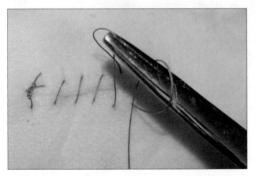

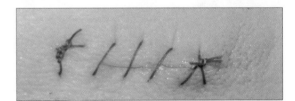

FIGURE 18.8 Making a knot at the end of a continuous suture.

Vertical Mattress Suture

Best method for everting the wound edges for healing and best used in areas where inversion easily occurs (i.e., palmer surface of hand). This method has two components. The first component is used for wound tension and is deep into the dermis, and the second component is superficial and everts the wound edges. These components allow for a meticulous wound-edge approximation (**Video 18.3**).

- Insert the needle slightly farther away than you would for a simple or continuous stitch.
- Push through the skin and wound as described previously, keeping the exit the same distance from the wound as the insertion.
- Turn the needle around and insert it between the exit and the wound, and come out the other side between the wound edge and the insertion (Figure 18.9).
- Tie a knot as described previously (Figure 18.10).
- Repeat as necessary.

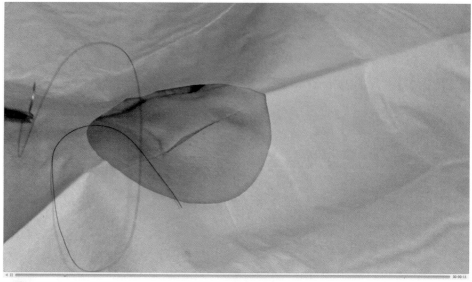

▶ **VIDEO 18.3** Vertical mattress suture.
springerpub.com/campo

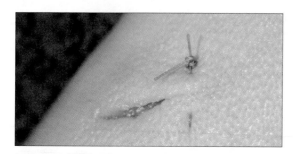

FIGURE 18.9 Performing a vertical mattress suture.

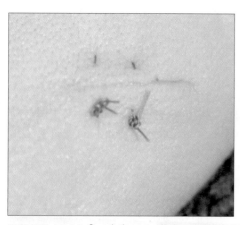

FIGURE 18.10 Completing a vertical mattress suture.

Subcutaneous Suture (Video 18.4)

- Insert the needle into the dermal layer at one end of the wound and exit toward the center of the wound (Figure 18.11).
- Insert the needle adjacent to the exit and push through adjacent to the first entrance (making a circle).
- Tie a knot as previously described.
- Repeat as necessary to close the dermal layer of the wound.

Subcuticular Suture (Figure 18.12)

- Insert the needle at the base of the subcutaneous tissue and exit just above it.

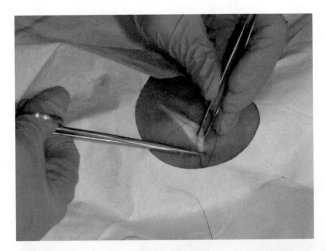

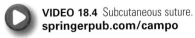

VIDEO 18.4 Subcutaneous suture.
springerpub.com/campo

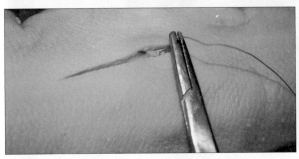

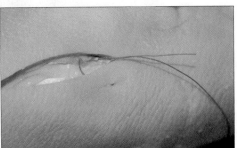

FIGURE 18.11 Performing a subcutaneous suture.

FIGURE 18.12 Performing a subcuticular suture.

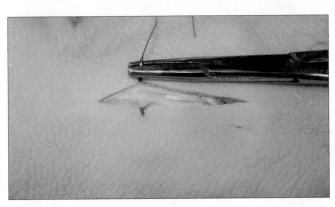

- Insert the needle adjacent to the exit and push through to the base of the subcutaneous layer (adjacent from the first insertion).
- Tie a knot as previously described.
- Repeat as necessary to close the deep space.

Skin adhesive can be applied or fine percutaneous sutures can be added to close the percutaneous layer.

Staple

The benefits of a staple closure include minimal time required for the procedure, decreased tissue reactivity, and decreased cost compared to suture closure. However, the provider does not have the same control with this method of closure and the staples can interfere with some radiological studies (i.e., CT scan and MRI). Staples should not be used on the face.

- Have an assistant hold the wound edges everted with forceps.
- Place the stapler perpendicular to the wound.
- Press down as you squeeze the trigger and place the staple.
- Repeat as necessary.
- Spacing should be equal as with sutures (Figure 18.13).

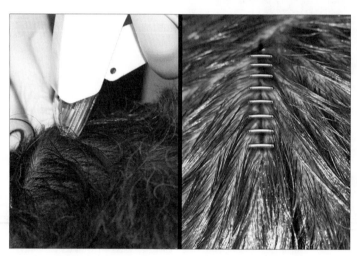

FIGURE 18.13 Performing a staple closure (note the equal spacing).

Skin Adhesive

Skin adhesives are easy to use, painless, and are a cost-effective method of closure. However, if you work in an area where water sports and water activities are an everyday or seasonal occurrence, then this method may not be your first choice. Skin adhesives should not get wet, be placed over joints or mobile areas, or be placed on wounds with high tension or skin-edge distance that have a greater chance of dehiscence than suture or staple closures. Studies have shown that skin adhesives can take 24 hours to gain full maximum strength and last 5 to 7 days before tensile strength decreases rapidly secondary to breakdown. They are ideal for superficial and small lacerations. Topical or injectable anesthetics are not required for this method of closure. Studies have shown cosmetic outcomes similar to sutured wounds, making this an advantageous closure technique.

- Irrigate and cleanse the area.
- Dry completely.
  - Any moisture, including blood, will hinder the skin adhesive from working.
- Approximate the wound edges.
- Apply the adhesive to the wound. Do *not* place skin adhesive inside the wound as this may cause a foreign-body reaction.
- Never place antibiotic ointment or cream over the skin adhesive as it will hasten breakdown.
- Skin adhesive cannot be used in high-tension wounds unless subcuticular/subcutaneous sutures are placed first.
- Allow to dry.
- Applying skin tape to the area is optional.

Skin Tape

Skin tape is ideal for superficial wounds as well as a re-enforcement of suture, staple, and glue closures. It tends to fall off prematurely and causes the highest rate of wound dehiscence compared to other methods of wound closer when used alone.

- Irrigate and cleanse the wound as described previously.
- Dry the area thoroughly.
- Dip the cotton-tipped applicator into the benzoin.
- Apply to the wound edges.
- Allow to dry.
- Cut the tape to fit the wounds, allowing approximately 1 cm on each side of the wound.
- Approximate the wound edges.
- Stick the tape to one side of the wound and gently pull to the other side (this will aid in the approximation).
- Repeat as necessary the entire length of the wound.

POST-PROCEDURE CONSIDERATIONS

Bleeding

- Bleeding and "oozing" from a sutured or stapled wound can be common.
- Elevate the wound and apply direct pressure.
- Light-pressure dressings can be applied to the wound.

Antibiotic Prophylaxis

- If the wound is older than 8 hours or grossly contaminated, antibiotics should be prescribed unless the wound is on the face or if edges will be excised before closure.
- Antibiotics should be given to patients with diabetes, immunosuppression, or on steroids.

Pain

- Closure, dressings, elevation, and immobilization of joints with wounds will help decrease pain.
- Pain medication can be prescribed, if necessary, based on the patient's pain tolerance and extent of the wound.
- Nonsteroidal anti-inflammatory medications should be avoided as they have been linked to delayed healing.

EDUCATIONAL POINTS

Wound Care

- Avoid dressing changes for 24 hours to help the healing process and the laying down of granulation tissue.
- Instruct the patient to clean with soap and water, and to avoid antiseptics (betadine, alcohol, and hydrogen peroxide) as these can hinder the healing process.

Follow-Up

- Wound re-evaluation is recommended in 48 hours.
- Follow up with a specialist is needed for any wounds with tendon, nerve, or deep-structure involvement.

COMPLICATIONS

- Infection is always a risk, even with timely irrigation, closure, and dressing of the wound.
- Educating the patient of the possibility of infection and instructing him or her to return if any signs of infection develop is always prudent.

PEARLS

- When considering the type of closure, always treat the patient as though he or she is a close family member.
- When dealing with children and parents, remember that this is an anxiety-producing event. Frequent reassurance and a confident attitude go a long way. Even if you do not feel confident, give the performance of your life and it will be better for all involved.
- When performing a procedure on a child or on a complex wound, try to focus only on the wound. Focusing your concentration takes the pressure off and allows you to treat the wound as any other you have encountered.
- With jagged, uneven wounds, strategically place sutures. Remember that if you do not like the way it is closing or the tension is not what you expected, there is nothing wrong with removing the suture and replacing it.
- Open communication with the patient, even when the patient is a child, is very important. Do not ever lie to a patient or parent or try to "candy coat" what you are going to do. They will never trust you again.
- You can place skin adhesive over sutures to help keep children from pulling knots out.
- In general, secondary wound infection occurs 24 to 72 hours after the initial injury. Hence, schedule a 48-hour wound check follow-up.
- All wounds contain a foreign body until proven otherwise with proper exploration.
- Wound anesthesia should precede wound cleansing.

SPECIAL CONSIDERATIONS/CLOSURES

Lip Laceration Involving the Vermilion Border or Intraoral Cavity

Lip lacerations occur frequently from falls, assaults, animal bites, and motor vehicle crashes. The goal of treatment is a good cosmetic outcome and hemostasis. The lips are composed of three layers: skin, muscle, and oral mucosa. The vermilion border is the area that separates the lip and skin. Unlike facial skin, its stratified squamous epithelium does not contain keratin and has fewer melanocytes. For this reason, underlying blood vessels are more apparent; hence the red color. Improper closure can lead to disfigurement. Wounds that extensively involve large pieces of the vermilion border and/or where the commissure is missing (junction where the upper and lower lips join) should always have plastic surgery repair.

Procedure Preparation

- Nonsterile gloves
- Absorbent pad

- 4 × 4 gauze
- Skin cleanser
- Topical anesthetic
- Local anesthetic or nerve block (based on location and extent of injury)
- Normal saline for irrigation
- 35- to 50-mL syringe
- Splash guard or 16- to 18-gauge angiocatheter
- Surgical scrub
- Suture kit
- Suture material
- Skin tape
- Topical antibiotic

Procedure Laceration Involving the Vermilion Border (Figure 18.14)

- Place the absorbable pad under the patient's chin
- Cleanse the area
- Apply topical anesthetic
- Perform anesthesia/block
- While the anesthetic takes effect, prepare the other equipment
- Cleanse the area and cover with a fenestrated sterile drape.
- Place deep suture as necessary.
- Approximate the vermilion border with the first suture using 6-0 nonabsorbable suture material.
    - You can also approximate the vermilion border and place a mark with a pen of where you will put the first suture.
    - Misalignment of as little as 1 mm can cause disfigurement.
- Once the border is aligned, continue closure using simple interrupted sutures.
- Apply topical antibiotic.

Procedure Intraoral Laceration

Any laceration that is gaping, > 1.0 cm, or has the potential for food particles to become entrapped, should be sutured. The size and depth of the wound will determine how many layers of sutures will be required for closure. If there is a deep space, then internal suture(s) should be performed. Simple interrupted or continuous sutures can be used to close the surface layer with absorbable material.

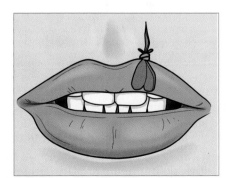
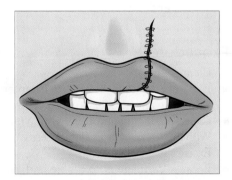

FIGURE 18.14 Closure of a lip laceration involving the vermillion border.

Ear Laceration

The ear is unique in that it contains vascular skin tissue covering avascular cartilage tissue. Proper repair of the injury most often results in a good outcome with regard

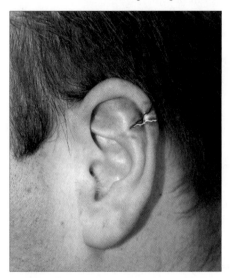

to healing and cosmetic result. Any large avulsions or cartilage involvement should be referred immediately to a plastic surgeon for repair. When small areas of cartilage are involved, the area must be debrided and covered with skin for proper healing and outcome. This will decrease the chance of developing chondritis. The auricular cartilage is avascular and depends on the perichondrium and surrounding tissue for nutrients. A laceration involving the cartilage is seen in Figure 18.15. Most lacerations of the ear that involve only the skin layers should be closed using the aforementioned methods of closures based on the extent of the laceration. All avascular cartilage must be covered to prevent hematoma formation and promote healing. Local anesthesia must be avoided as it can distort important landmarks. Regional nerve blocks should be used as discussed in Chapter 13. Closing a laceration to the pinna with exposed cartilage is discussed here.

FIGURE 18.15 Wound to the pinna.

Procedure Preparation

- Nonsterile gloves
- Absorbent pad
- 4 × 4 gauze
- Skin cleanser
- Topical anesthetic
- Local anesthetic or auricular block
- Normal saline for irrigation
- 35- to 65-mL syringe
- Splash guard or 16- to 18-gauge angiocatheter
- Surgical scrub
- Suture kit
- No. 15 scalpel
- Suture material
- Topical antibiotic

Procedure

- Cleanse the area.
- Perform anesthetic block (see Chapter 13).
- While the anesthetic takes effect, prepare the other equipment.
- Cleanse the area and cover with a fenestrated sterile drape.
- With the scalpel, cut a full thickness wedge (triangle) from the antihelix (Figure 18.16A).
- Excise the cartilage.
- Because cartilage is so friable and avascular, either do not suture or place sutures through the perichondrium only.
- Leave 1 mm of overhanging skin to ensure eversion during closure.

- With 6-0 nonabsorbable suture material, perform closure (Figure 18.16 B and C).
- Apply a pressure dressing to prevent auricular hematoma.
- Close follow-up is required.

When closing percutaneous lacerations of the ear not involving the cartilage, close as you would other lacerations but begin posteriorly and end anteriorly. Vertical mattress sutures may be needed when repairing the helix of the ear to ensure eversion.

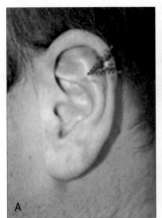 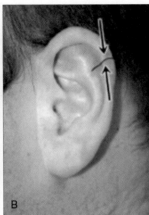 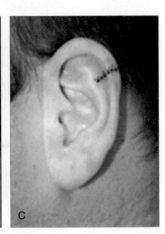

FIGURE 18.16 (A, B, and C) Wedge excision and repair of an ear laceration.

Nail Bed Laceration

The goal of treatment is to preserve as much tissue as possible, minimize debridement, and prevent further damage/trauma to the nail bed. Educating the patient that the nail may not grow in properly or may never grow is imperative. It can take 6 months to 1 year before you know the outcome. The eponychium (cuticle) is the proximal portion of skin at the base of the nail that folds over on itself and supplies the layer of dead skin over the nail plate. If the nail plate is removed during repair, this tissue must not be allowed to come into contact with the nail bed as it will cause scarring and future nail growth disfigurement. Plain radiographs may be necessary to evaluate for underlying tuft or distal phalanx fracture. Children may require conscious sedation to repair the nail bed.

Procedure Preparation

- Nonsterile gloves
- Absorbent pad
- 4 × 4 gauze
- Skin cleanser
- Digital block
- Normal saline for irrigation
- 35- to 65-mL syringe
- Splash guard or 16- to 18-gauge angiocatheter
- Surgical scrub
- Suture kit
- Suture material
- No. 11 scalpel
- Nonadherent gauze
- Topical antibiotic

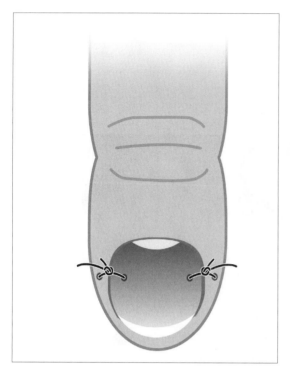

FIGURE 18.17 Securing the nail after repair of a nail bed laceration.

Procedure

- Cleanse the area to prepare for a digital block.
- Perform a digital block.
- While the anesthetic takes effect, prepare the other equipment.
- Cleanse the area and cover with a fenestrated sterile drape.
- Cut off the tip from a finger of a glove and then cut again.
- Place at the base of the finger to aid with hemostasis.
- Elevate the nail with either the scalpel or scissors and remove the remainder of the nail.
- Make sure you keep the scissors or scalpel horizontal to the nail bed, being careful not to cause further damage/trauma to the nail bed.
- Once the nail is lifted, remove with a hemostat/needle holder.
- Irrigate the nail bed with normal saline and debride any devitalized tissue.
- Place the sutures using 6-0 absorbable suture material.
- Once you have finished with the sutures, reapply the nail by placing a 4-0 nonabsorbable suture through the nail on each side of the base of the nail and securing it to the surrounding skin (Figure 18.17).
- Apply a dry sterile dressing and splint as necessary.

Tendon Lacerations

Flexor tendon lacerations usually involve the synovial membrane and should always be handled by a hand specialist immediately. Repair of the tendon should not be attempted due to the risk of tenosynovitis. Debridement with copious irrigation should be performed. Extensor tendons do not possess the synovial membrane and can be either repaired or closed over after debridement and copious irrigation and referred for follow-up with a hand specialist. Flexor tendons possess a synovial membrane and repair should be done by a specialist.

RESOURCES

Brown, D. J., Jaffe, J. E., & Henson, J. K. (2007). Advanced laceration management. *Emergency Medical Clinics of North America, 25*, 83–99.

Bruns, T. B., & Worthington, J. M. (2000). Using tissue adhesive for wound repair: A practical guide to dermabond. *American Family Physician, 61*(5), 1383–1388. Retrieved from http://www.aafp.org/afp/20000301/1383.html

DeSouza, B. A., Shibu, M., Moir, G., Carver, N., Dunn, R., & Watson, S. (2002). Suturing versus conservative management of hand lacerations. *British Medical Journal, 325*, 1113–1117.

Doud Galli, S. K., & Constantinides, M. (2013). *Wound closure technique*. Retrieved from https://www.clinicalkey.com/#!/content/book/3-s2.0-B9780323074186000125

Fansler, J. L., & Schreibner, D. (2010, January 14). *Complex laceration, lip*. Retrieved from http://emedicine.medscape.com/article/83256-overview

Hollander, J. E. (2003). Selecting sutures and needles for wound closure. In A. J. Singer & J. E. Hollander (Eds.), *Lacerations and acute wounds: An evidence-based guide* (pp. 98–107). Philadelphia, PA: F. A. Davis.

Hollander, J. E. (2003). Wound closure options. In A. J. Singer & J. E. Hollander (Eds.), *Lacerations and acute wounds: An evidence-based guide* (pp. 56–63). Philadelphia, PA: F. A. Davis.

Hollander, J. E., & Singer, A. J. (1999). Laceration management. *Annals of Emergency Medicine*, *34*, 356–367.

Jolly, J. (2009). Surgical staples for scalp laceration repair: A quick and easy solution. *Advance for Nurse Practitioners*, *17*(7), 37–38.

Kumar, K. (2009, October 13). *Complex laceration, ear*. Retrieved from http://emedicine.medscape.com/article/83294-overview

Lammers, R. L. (2010). Principles of wound management. In J. R. Roberts & J. R. Hedges (Eds.), *Clinical procedures in emergency medicine* (5th ed.). Philadelphia, PA: Saunders Elsevier.

Lammers, R. L., & Smith, Z. E. (2014). Principles of wound management. In J. R. Roberts & J. R. Hedges (Eds.), *Clinical procedures in emergency medicine* (6th ed.). Philadelphia, PA: Saunders Elsevier. Retrieved from https://www.clinicalkey.com/#!/content/book/3-s2.0-B9781455706068000343

Lent, G. S., Fansler, J. L., & Schreiber, D. (2014). *Complex lip laceration*. Retrieved from http://emedicine.medscape.com/article/83256-overview

Lockwood, R. (2013). Wound repair. In Adams et al. (Eds.), *Emergency medicine: Clinical essentials* (2nd ed.). Philadelphia, PA: Elsevier. Retrieved from https://www.clinicalkey.com/#!/content/book/3-s2.0-B9781437735482001865

Patel, L. (2014). Management of simple nail bed lacerations and subungual hematomas in the emergency department. *Pediatric Emergency Care*, *30*(10), 742–745.

Quinn, J., Cummings, S., Callaham, M., & Sellers, K. (2002). Suturing versus conservative management of lacerations of the hand: Randomized controlled trial. *British Medical Journal*, *325*, 299. Retrieved from http://bmj.com/cgi/content/full/325/7359/299?view=long&pmid=12169503

Singer, A. J. (2003a). Adhesive tapes. In A. J. Singer & J. E. Hollander (Eds.), *Lacerations and acute wounds: An evidence-based guide* (pp. 64–72). Philadelphia, PA: F. A. Davis.

Singer, A. J. (2003b). Surgical staples. In A. J. Singer & J. E. Hollander (Eds.), *Lacerations and acute wounds: An evidence-based guide* (pp. 73–82). Philadelphia, PA: F. A. Davis.

Singer, A. J., & Hollander, J. E. (2003). Wound preparation. In A. J. Singer & J. E. Hollander (Eds.), *Lacerations and acute wounds: An evidence-based guide* (pp. 13–22). Philadelphia, PA: F. A. Davis.

Singer, A. J., & Quinn, J. V. (2003). Tissue adhesive. In A. J. Singer & J. E. Hollander (Eds.), *Lacerations and acute wounds: An evidence-based guide* (pp. 83–97). Philadelphia, PA: F. A. Davis.

Sodovsky, R. (2000). *Management of lacerations to avoid infection and scarring*. Retrieved from http://www.aafp.org/afp/2000/0301/p1501.html

Sutijono, D., & Silverberg, M. A. (2009, May 7). *Nailbed injuries*. Retrieved from http://emedicine.medscape.com/article/827104-overview

Thomsen, T. W., Barclay, D. A., & Setnik, G. S. (2006). Basic laceration repair. *New England Journal of Medicine*, *355*(17), e18.

Trott, A. T. (2005a). Basic laceration repair: Principles and techniques. In Trott A. T. (Ed.), *Wounds and lacerations: Emergency care and closure* (3rd ed., pp. 119–134). Philadelphia, PA: Mosby Elsevier.

Trott, A. T. (2005b). Instruments and suture material. In A. T. Trott (Ed.), *Wounds and lacerations: Emergency care and closure* (3rd ed., pp. 93–106). Philadelphia, PA: Mosby Elsevier.

Trott, A. T. (2005c). Special anatomical sites. In Trott A. T. (Ed.), *Wounds and lacerations: Emergency care and closure* (3rd ed., pp. 153–176). Philadelphia, PA: Mosby Elsevier.

Trott, A. T. (2005d). Wound cleansing and irrigation. In A. T. Trott (Ed.), *Wounds and lacerations: Emergency care and closure* (3rd ed., pp. 83–92). Philadelphia, PA: Mosby Elsevier.

Trott, A. T. (2012a). Basic laceration repair: Principles and techniques. In A. T. Trott (Ed.), *Wounds and lacerations: Emergency care and closure* (4th ed.). Philadelphia, PA: Mosby Elsevier. Retrieved from https://www.clinicalkey.com/#!/content/book/3-s2.0-B9780323074186000101

Trott, A. T. (2012b). Instruments, suture materials, and closure choices. In A. T. Trott (Ed.), *Wounds and lacerations: Emergency care and closure* (4th ed.). Philadelphia, PA: Mosby Elsevier. Retrieved from https://www.clinicalkey.com/#!/content/book/3-s2.0-B9780323074186000083

Trott, A. T. (2012c). Special anatomical sites. In A. T. Trott (Ed.), *Wounds and lacerations: Emergency care and closure* (4th ed.). Philadelphia, PA: Mosby Elsevier. Retrieved from https://www.clinicalkey.com/#!/content/book/3-s2.0-B9780323074186000125

Trott, A. T. (2012d). Wound cleansing and irrigation. In A. T. Trott (Ed.), *Wounds and lacerations: Emergency care and closure* (4th ed.). Philadelphia, PA: Mosby Elsevier. Retrieved from https://www.clinicalkey.com/#!/content/book/3-s2.0-B9780323074186000071

Wang, Q. C., & Johnson, B. A. (2001). Fingertip injuries. *American Family Physicians, 63*(10), 1961–1966.

CHAPTER 19

Managing Minor Burns

Theresa M. Campo

BACKGROUND

Burns can cause devastation and even death. This chapter outlines the type, degree, and treatment of minor burns, including sunburn. Acute management of any burn is to immediately stop the burn from causing further damage, initiate prompt treatment, and arrange referral as necessary. Always assess for the potential of severe associated injury. For instance, a patient who presents after a fire should be evaluated for smoke inhalation (burned or singed nasal hairs, hoarse voice, cough, etc.). Follow-up is imperative with burns to reduce the risk of infection, scarring, and loss of function.

Traditionally, burns were classified as first-, second-, and third-degree burns. Today, burns are classified by the depth and extent of the burn. The current classifications are epidermal, partial thickness (superficial or deep), and full thickness. The current classifications correspond with the traditional categorization.

Epidermal burns, or first-degree burns, are painful, red, and moist. Blistering does not occur and the damage is mostly to the epidermal layer of skin. Healing usually occurs in 5 to 7 days with no scarring. The most common epidermal burn is sunburn. Partial-thickness burns can be either superficial or deep. Superficial partial-thickness burns involve the epidermal layer and several dermal layers of the skin. They are painful but heal, usually with minimal scarring, in 2 to 3 weeks. Deep partial-thickness burns involve the epidermal and dermal layers and may involve some of the dermal appendages. They are not as painful as epidermal or superficial partial-thickness burns because of the loss of sensory nerves. Sensation to pinpricks is intact. Healing can be more than 3 weeks with increased scarring. Full-thickness burns involve the entire epidermal and dermal layers of the skin. They are dry, leathery, and insensitive. Patients present with little or no pain. The color of the burn can be white, brown, or black. These burns cause significant scarring, loss of function, and usually require skin grafting. Deep partial-thickness and full-thickness burns may be difficult to distinguish during the initial evaluation.

The depth and body surface area (BSA) have a direct impact on healing and mortality of burns. The rating of burns can be done using the "rule of nines," which designates a percentage to certain anatomical locations. The head and each arm account for 9% each; the genitals equal 1%; and the anterior, posterior trunk, and each leg account for 18% each. The percentages for children using the rule of nines are more specific (Figure 19.1).

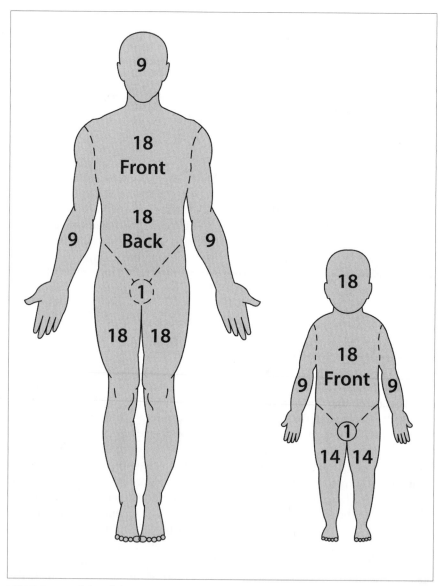

FIGURE 19.1 Rules of nines.

A more practical way to ascertain the percentage of BSA burned is to take the palm of the patient's hand, which equals 1%. This is a practical and accurate way to estimate the BSA without using calculations and diagrams (Figure 19.2).

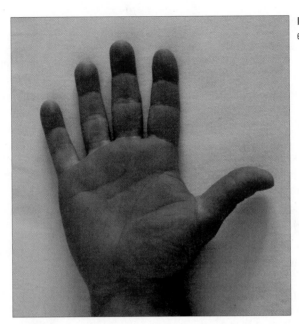

FIGURE 19.2 The palm of the hand equals 1% body surface area.

PATIENT PRESENTATION

Epidermal

- Painful
- Red
- No blisters

Superficial Partial Thickness

- Very painful
- Red
- Blanches with pressure
- Moist
- Weeping
- Blister may or may not be present (usually intact if present)

Deep Partial Thickness

- Pain
- Perception of pressure
- Waxy appearance

Full Thickness

- Not painful
- Perception of deep pressure
- Waxy white or gray color

TREATMENT

Treatment is based on depth, cause, and BSA affected. The goal of treatment is to quickly stop the burn, identify the extent of the burn, and administer pain medication immediately. Many patients will present with "home remedies" for treating burns. These can include butter, ketchup, petroleum jelly, and submersion in a bucket of ice. Although you want to cool the burn, ice cubes can attach to and tear off blistered skin. Always be careful with removal of anything that is touching the skin, including clothing, towels, and gauze. Cooling a burn can be effective for up to 3 hours after the initial injury. Applying a moist, cool towel can minimize tissue damage.

Burns that require hospitalization and/or referral to a burn center are described in the following text.

Partial and Full-Thickness Burns

- Partial thickness
  - Burns covering 15% BSA—adults
  - 10% BSA—children
- Full thickness
  - Burns of greater than 3% BSA
  - Partial or full-thickness burns of the face, genitals, hands, or feet
- Any partial or full-thickness burn to the face, genitals, hands, and feet (especially if circumferential)
- Electrical burns
- Smoke inhalation
- Suspected child abuse
- Age either older than 65 years or younger than 2 years
- Patients who are immunocompromised or have diabetes, or those patients taking chemotherapeutics or immunosuppressive medications should also be considered for hospitalization or referral to a burn center.

Any burns involving the face, hands, feet, and genitalia should be referred to a burn center. Burns that are circumferential on the hands, feet, or penis should be transferred to a burn center immediately.

SPECIAL CONSIDERATIONS

- Diabetes
- Immunosuppression
- Chemotherapeutics
- Anticoagulation
- History of electrolyte imbalance

PROCEDURE PREPARATION

- Sterile water or normal saline for irrigating
- Silver sulfadiazine (Silvadene)
  - Do not use on the face
- Topical antibiotic ointment (polymixin, bacitracin)
  - Use on the face

- Use mupirocin (Bactroban) if sulfa allergic. Both silver sulfadiazine and other topical antibiotics contain sulfa
- Nonadherent gauze
- 2 × 2 or 4 × 4 gauze (depending on area)
- Loose roll gauze (Kerlix)
- Tape

PROCEDURE

- Medicate for pain
    - Partial and full-thickness burns usually require narcotic pain medication either oral or parenteral
- Cleanse the area to remove any products applied by the patient or other persons prior to arrival
- Dry completely
- Debride the area of any loose tissue and open blisters
- Apply silver sulfadiazine
- Cover with nonadherent gauze
- Place 2 × 2 or 4 × 4 gauze over the nonadherent gauze
- Loosely wrap the rolled gauze over the area
- Do not apply dressings tightly. This can cause further damage

POST-PROCEDURE CONSIDERATIONS

- Pain medication should be prescribed.
- Close follow-up with the burn center, plastic surgeon, or primary care provider.

Educational Points

- Dressings should be changed at least once daily and optimally twice daily with application of silver sulfadiazine.
- Elevation will assist with reducing swelling.

Complications

- Infection
- Contracture
- Scarring

PEARLS

- Educate the patient to completely wash off the silver sulfadiazine before the next application. This medication has the potential to pigment the skin. This is why it is not recommended for use on the face.
- Circumferential burns of the hands, feet, or body in children should be suspected for child abuse.

RESOURCES

Bethel, C. A., & Mazzeo, A. S. (2009). Burn care procedures. In J. R. Roberts & J. R. Hedges (Eds.), *Clinical procedures in emergency medicine* (5th ed., pp. 692–714). Philadelphia, PA: Saunders Elsevier.

Caron, A., & McStay, C. M. (2009, May 18). *Sunburn.* Retrieved from http://emedicine.medscape .com/article/773203-overview & http://emedicine.medscape.com/article/773203-treatment

Druck, J. (2013). Thermal burns. In Adams et al. (Eds.), *Emergency medicine: Clinical essentials* (2nd ed.). Philadelphia, PA: Elsevier. Retrieved from https://www.clinicalkey.com/#!/ content/book/3-s2.0-B9781437735482001890

Goodis, J., & Schraga, E. D. (2009, June 28). *Burns, thermal.* Retrieved from http://emedicinemed-scape.com/article/769193-overview

Lafferty, K. A. (2009, December 9). *Smoke inhalation.* Retrieved from http://emedicine.medscape .com/article/771194-overview

Lafferty, K. A., Bonhomme, K., & Martinex, C.V. (2014). *Smoke inhalation injury.* Retrieved from http://emedicine.medscape.com/article/771194-overview

Morgan, E. D., Bledsoe, S. C., & Barker, J. (2000). Ambulatory management of burns. *American Family Physician, 62*(9), 2015–2026. Retrieved from http://www.aafp.org/afp/20001101/2015 .html

Sheridan, R. L. (2013). *Initial evaluation and management of the burn patient.* Retrieved from http:// emedicine.medscape.com/article/435402-overview

Soroff, H. S., & Brebbia, J. S. (2003). Burns. In A. J. Singer & J. E. Hollander (Eds). *Lacerations and acute wounds: An evidence-based guide* (pp. 173–187). Philadelphia, PA: F. A. Davis.

Trott, A. T. (2005). Minor burns. In A. T. Trott (Ed.), *Wounds and lacerations: Emergency care and closure* (3rd ed., pp. 253–262). Philadelphia, PA: Mosby Elsevier.

Trott, A. T. (2012). Minor burns. In A. T. Trott (Ed.), *Wounds and lacerations: Emergency care and closure* (4th ed.). Philadelphia, PA: Mosby Elsevier. Retrieed from https://www.clinicalkey .com/#!/content/book/3-s2.0-B9780323074186000174

UNIT VII

Procedures for the Management of Nail and Nail Bed Injuries

CHAPTER 20

Procedures for Managing Ingrown Toenails

Theresa M. Campo

BACKGROUND

Toenails mainly consist of the proximal nail fold, cuticle, nail plate, hyponychium, and nail bed. The proximal nail fold covers one fifth of the base of the nail and protects the nail matrix, which lies underneath. The cuticle or eponychium is formed from the proximal nail fold and attaches to the nail plate; the cuticle acts as a protector against microorganisms. The nail plate extends to the hyponychium (thick skin just underneath the distal nail plate). The nail bed facilitates the smooth movement of the nail plate distally, but does not participate in the actual nail development. It supports the nail and contains blood vessels and nerves. The nail matrix (root) is solely responsible for the formation and growth of the nail plate (Figures 20.1 and 20.2). Nails grow 1 mm in a month.

Normal nail growth is distal from the proximal nail fold and should be smooth. However, lateral growth of the nail plate into the soft tissue causes an inflammatory response. Ingrown toenails are most commonly the result of improperly fitting shoes and improper nail cutting. An ingrown toenail can also be the result of increased age, pregnancy, repetitive trauma, hyperhidrosis, poor hygiene, improper nail grooming, or underlying disorders (i.e., diabetes, immunosuppression, obesity, thyroid

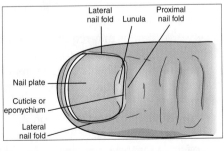

FIGURE 20.1 Anatomy of a toenail.

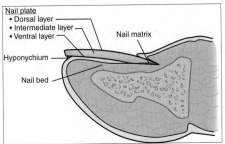

FIGURE 20.2 Lateral view of anatomy of a toenail.

disease, cardiac disease, and renal disorders). The shape of nail growth can place a person at risk of developing infected ingrown nails. The most common site is the great toe.

The severity of the ingrown nail and reaction to this form of growth can range from mild to severe. A mild presentation may consist of swelling, edema, and hyperkeratosis, whereas a moderate presentation consists of increased edema, drainage, pain, infection, and ulceration of the nail fold. Severe cases progress to increased production of granulation tissue with layering over the nail plate. This may be accompanied by infection and severe pain.

A study by De Berker et al. (2008) described a retronychia, which is the proximal ingrowing of the nail plate and is associated with multiple generations of nail plates. The most common cause is distal nail trauma from footwear pushing the nail back and upward. This pushes the proximal nail above the new growth. As the new nail grows, it displaces the previous nail growth upward rather than advancing it forward. The nail becomes thickened and discolored from the layering of nails. Granulation is common with retronychia.

PATIENT PRESENTATION

- Throbbing pain
- Edema
- Erythema
- Purulent drainage
- Granulation tissue
- Foul smell

TREATMENT

Treatment is based on the severity of the ingrown toenail. The goal of treatment is to decrease pain and inflammation as well as promote normal nail growth. Mild cases are treated with warm or cold soaks, steroids, 20% to 40% topical urea cream (Keralac, Carmol), cotton wisps under the lateral nail plate, and gutter splinting. Cases not responsive to conservative therapy may require removal of the nail spicule with or without a portion of the nail. Lateral matrixectomy may also be necessary. Matrixectomy is the removal of the nail matrix. This is done by manually removing the nail matrix with or without silver nitrate, electrocautery, or a chemical solution such as phenol or 10% sodium hydroxide solution.

Infected ingrown toenails are most commonly caused by *Staphylococcus aureus*, streptococcus, and gram-negative bacteria (i.e., *pseudomonas*). If antibiotic treatment is necessary, then coverage for these organisms should be considered.

CONTRAINDICATIONS AND RELATIVE CONTRAINDICATIONS

- Allergy to local anesthetics
- Bleeding dyscrasia
- Diabetic patients with neuropathic disease should not have matrixectomy performed

SPECIAL CONSIDERATIONS
- Diabetics
- Immunocompromised patients

PROCEDURE PREPARATION
Minor Ingrown Toenail
- Gloves (nonsterile)
- Skin tape strips (Steri-Strips)
- Small gauze angiocatheter

Moderate to Severe Ingrown Toenail
- Absorbent pads
- Skin cleanser
- 3-mL syringe with small-gauge needle (25–30 gauge) filled with lidocaine or bupivacaine
- Sterile gauze
- Bone curette
  - Tissue nipper if unavailable
- English anvil nail splitter
  - Small pointed scissors
- Forceps or hemostat
- Penrose drain
- Silver nitrate sticks
  - Aqueous phenol solution (1%) or sodium hydroxide solution (10%) if available
- Cotton-tipped applicator
  - Some of the cotton can be removed to fit the small area of the excised wound
- Topical antibiotic ointment
  - Topical antibiotic cream (i.e., silver sulfadiazine [Silvadene]) should be used if chemical solution or silver nitrate used
- Nonadherent gauze dressing
- Roll gauze

PROCEDURE
Minor Ingrown Toenail
Minimal Inflammation and No Granulation Tissue
- Warm soaks
- Place a skin-tape strip (Steri-Strip) under the affected section of the nail and secure to the toe (Figure 20.3)
  - You can also place a small piece of tubing (small-gauge angiocatheter cut to fit the area) around the lateral nail on the nail spicule and tape into place with a skin-tape strip.

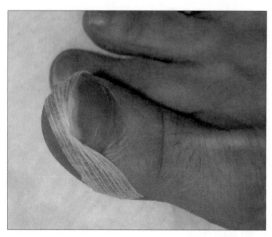

FIGURE 20.3 Skin closure (Steri-Strip) under nail.

Moderate Ingrown Toenail
Inflammation Accompanied by Granulation Tissue

Oblique section of nail removal for nails with inflammation and little to no granulation tissue.

- Cleanse the skin using a circular motion to free debris and bacteria.
- Place an absorbent protective pad under the treatment area.
- Digital block (see Chapter 11).
- Clean the area of granulation tissue with a bone curette to expose the offending nail border.
- Remove an oblique section from the distal corner of the nail using the English anvil nail splitters (Figure 20.4).
  - Small pointed scissors can be used with upward pressure and a controlled push method to minimize nail bed trauma.
  - One third to one half distal to proximal nail fold.
- Grab the cut portion of nail with forceps or hemostats and remove.
- Gently debride the area with either the forceps or hemostat.
- Silver nitrate can be applied if there is any residual bleeding.
- Dress the wound with antibiotic ointment and nonadherent gauze.
  - Topical antibiotic cream (i.e., silver sulfadiazine [Silvadene]) should be used if chemical solution or silver nitrate used.

Moderate to Severe Ingrown Toenail
Inflammation With Granulation Tissue

Nail removal can be either partial or complete. Complete nail removal is rarely needed unless both lateral nail folds are involved. Such a case should be referred to a podiatric specialist.

- Cleanse the skin using a circular motion to free debris and bacteria.
- Place an absorbent protective pad under the treatment area.
- Perform a digital block (see Chapter 11).
- Apply Penrose drain to the base of the toe.
- Mark the lateral quarter to one third of the nail on the affected side (Figure 20.5).
- Lift the nail with either forceps or hemostat.
- Using the English anvil nail splitter, cut the nail distal to proximal just past the proximal cuticle.
  - The cut should not be farther than two thirds of the nail distal to proximal to prevent nail bed damage.
- With small sharp scissors cut the final one third of the nail to just beneath the cuticle (a few millimeters).

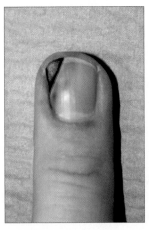

FIGURE 20.4 Oblique section removal.

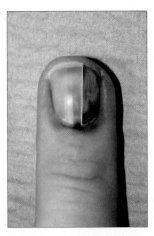

FIGURE 20.5 Partial nail removal.

- Grab the cut nail with forceps or hemostat.
- Pull the loose piece while rotating away from the lateral edge and toward the intact nail removing it from its attachment.
- Inspect the area for any remaining pieces of nail.
- Debride the area of any loose nail fragments or hyperkeratotic tissue with the forceps.

Matrixectomy

Debridement of the granulation tissue is usually sufficient and does not require matrixectomy. Consultation with podiatry should be considered if this procedure is necessary and/or performed.

Silver Nitrate
- Apply silver nitrate to the granulation tissue for 2 to 3 minutes.

> **NOTE** *Silver nitrate, electrocautery, or chemical solutions (phenol, 10% sodium hydroxide solution) can be used for this procedure.*

Electrocautery
- Apply to granulation tissue.

Phenol (Should Not Be Used If Infection Is Present)
- Soak a cotton-tipped applicator with phenol.
- Apply to area of nail matrix for 30 seconds.
- Use a rolling motion to avoid damage to nail edge or viable surrounding tissue.
- Repeat two times.
- Irrigate the area to remove phenol.
- It is important to keep the area clean and dry during the application of a chemical solution/agent.

10% Sodium Hydroxide Solution (Should Not Be Used If Infection Is Present)

- Soak a cotton-tipped applicator with 10% sodium hydroxide solution.
- Apply to the area of nail matrix for 30 seconds.
  - Use a rolling motion to avoid damage to nail edge.
- Repeat two times.
- Irrigate the area to remove the solution.
- Do not forget to remove the Penrose drain (tourniquet).
- Apply silver sulfadiazine (Silvadene) and a nonadherent dressing with rolled gauze (Kling).
- It is important to keep the area clean and dry during the application of a chemical solution/agent.

POST-PROCEDURE CONSIDERATIONS
Pain

- Ingrown nails may be exquisitely tender and digital block should be performed slowly and with a small-gauge needle (i.e., 25–30 gauge).
- Scissors can be used in place of the English anvil nail splitter.
- If phenol or other ablating solutions are available, they can be used in place of the silver nitrate. These substances will prevent further nail growth.

EDUCATIONAL POINTS
Minor Ingrown Toenails

- Warm-water soaks with Epsom salt two to three times daily
- Wound evaluation 48 to 72 hours after procedure
  - Diabetic or immunocompromised patients or patients with peripheral vascular disease should be followed more closely with strong consideration of prophylactic antibiotic use.
- Patients with ingrown nails caused by deformity should be referred to a podiatrist for definitive nail removal.

Moderate Ingrown Toenails

- Warm-water soaks two to three times daily
- Dry dressing
- Healing occurs within 2 to 4 weeks

PEARLS

- Cutting the finger of a latex/rubber glove can be used as a tourniquet in place of a Penrose drain.
- If English anvil nail splitters are not available, iris scissors can be used. However, be sure not to cut or damage the nail bed.
- Use the "push–pull" method of gentle, controlled use of the scissor while inserting under the nail plate.

COMPLICATIONS

- Complications are minimal but regrowth of the nail, infection or extending infection (abscess), osteomyelitis and delayed healing, and recurrence are all possibilities.

RESOURCES

Benzoni, T. E. (2010, March 15). *Toenails, ingrown.* Retrieved from http://emedicine.medscape.com/article/828072-overview & http://emedicine.medscape.com/article/828072-treatment

Chavez, M. C., & Maker, V. K. (2007). Office surgery. In R. E. Rakel (Ed.), *Textbook of family medicine* (7th ed.). Philadelphia, PA: Saunders Elsevier. Retrieved from http://www.mdconsult.com/das/book/body/187327964-5/963237221/1481/390.html#4-u1.0-B978-1-4160-2467-5..50036-1-cesec68_1821

De Berker, D. (2015). Diseases of the skin: Diseases of the nails. In *Conn's current therapy*. Philadelphia, PA: Saunders Elsevier. Retrieved from https://www.clinicalkey.com/#!/content/book/3-s2.0-B9781455702978004043?scrollTo=%23hl0008226

De Berker, D. A., Richert, B., Duhard, E., Piraccini, B. M., Andre, J., & Baran, R. (2008). Retronychia: Proximal ingrowing of the nail plate. *Journal of the American Academy of Dermatology, 58,* 978–983.

Habif, T. P. (2009). Nail diseases. In *Clinical dermatology: A color guide to diagnosis and treatment* (5th ed.). Philadelphia, PA: Elsevier. Retrieved from http://www.mdconsult.com/book/player/book.do? method=display&type=bookPage&decorator=header&eid=4-u1.0-B978-0-7234-3541-9..00034-1-s0315&displayedEid=4-u1.0-B978-0-7234-3541-9..00034-1-s0350&uniq=187327964&isbn=978-0-7234-3541-9&sid=963240480

Heidelbaugh, J. L., & Lee, H. (2009). Management of the ingrown toenail. *American Family Physician, 79*(4), 303–308, 311–312.

McGee, D. L. (2009). Podiatric procedures. In J. R. Roberts & J. R. Hedges (Eds.), *Clinical procedures in emergency medicine* (5th ed., pp. 939–943). Philadelphia, PA: Saunders Elsevier.

McGee, D. L. (2014). Podiatric procedures. In J. R. Roberts & J. R. Hedges (Eds.), *Clinical procedures in emergency medicine* (6th ed.). Philadelphia, PA: Saunders Elsevier. Retrieved from https://www.clinicalkey.com/#!/content/book/3-s2.0-B9781455706068000513

Mostaghimi, L. (2010). Diseases of the skin: Diseases of the nails. In E. T. Bope, R. E. Rakel, & R. D. Kellerman (Eds.), *Conn's current therapy 2010* (1st ed.). Philadelphia, PA: Elsevier. Retrieved from http://www.mdconsult.com/book/player/book.do?method=display&type=bookPage&decorator=header&eid=4-u1.0-B978-1-4160-6642-2..00013-2-s0845&uniq=187327964&isbn=978-1-4160-6642-2&sid=963240480

Richardson, E. G. (2008). Disorders of nails and skin. In S. T. Canale & J. H. Beaty (Eds.), *Campbell's operative orthopaedics* (11th ed.). Philadelphia, PA: Elsevier. Retrieved from http://www.mdconsult.com/das/book/body/187327964-6/963237528/1584/638.html#4-u1.0-B978-0-323-03329-9..50087-8-cesec1_4367

Schraga, E. D. (2009, November 10). *Ingrown toenail removal.* Retrieved from http://emedicine.medscape.com/article/149627-overview & http://emedicine.medscape.com/article/149627-treatment

Xuber, T. J. (2002). Ingrown toenail removal. *American Family Physician, 65*(12), 2547–2550.

CHAPTER **21**

Procedures for Treating Subungual Hematoma

Theresa M. Campo

BACKGROUND

A subungual hematoma is a collection of blood between the nail plate and nail bed. It is often caused by a crushing injury or blunt trauma to the distal aspect of a digit, causing accumulation of blood under the nail plate, in turn causing pressure and pain. The degree of the hematoma may be minimal or severe with or without coinciding distal phalanx or tuft fractures. Pain is the most common complaint and can be relieved quickly by performing trephination to the nail.

PATIENT PRESENTATION

- Throbbing, painful finger or toe
- Dark red to black coloration to nail

TREATMENT

The treatment of a subungual hematoma is dependent on the amount of the nail that is affected. If the hematoma is small (< 25%) and painless, then treatment is usually not required. However, if the hematoma covers more than 25% of the nail bed and pain is present, then decompression (trephination) should be performed. If the hematoma covers more than 50% of the nail, then removal of the nail should be considered and any laceration to the nail bed should be repaired. Approximately 50% of subungual hematomas covering 50% or more of the nail have associated nail bed laceration injuries. The incidence increases significantly when associated with a distal tuft fracture. Repair of nail bed lacerations is discussed in Chapter 18.

CONTRAINDICATIONS AND RELATIVE CONTRAINDICATIONS

There are no contraindications or relative contraindications for this procedure.

SPECIAL CONSIDERATIONS

- Associated nail bed laceration
- Associated distal phalanx and/or tuft fractures

PROCEDURE PREPARATION

Heat Method

- Cautery stick (may use a heated paper clip)
- Gauze

Drilling Method

- 18-gauge needle
- Gauze

PROCEDURE

- Cleanse the skin using a circular motion to remove debris and bacteria.
- Place an absorbent protective pad under the treatment area.
- Drape the patient to maintain a clean area as well as to protect the patient's privacy.

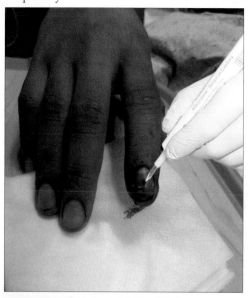

FIGURE 21.1 Trephination—heat method.

- Strict sterile technique is not required for this procedure. However, because of the era of resistance, sterile technique should be used whenever possible.

Heat Method

- Hold the cautery stick perpendicular to the nail plate.
- Once it is heated and ready, press the tip through the nail plate (Figure 21.1).
- Once it penetrates the nail plate and the hematoma, the blood will drain and cool the tip, preventing damage to the nail bed.
- Apply pressure to the nail and finger or toe to drain the hematoma.

Drilling Method

- Take the 18-gauge needle and press through the nail plate with gentle pressure while rotating the needle in a circular motion (Figure 21.2).
  - Be careful not to penetrate the nail bed as this is a common complication with this method.

POST-PROCEDURE CONSIDERATIONS

Pain

- A digital block can be performed if patient is intolerant of procedure.
- Instruct the patient to keep the finger elevated, above the level of the heart, to prevent throbbing and pain.

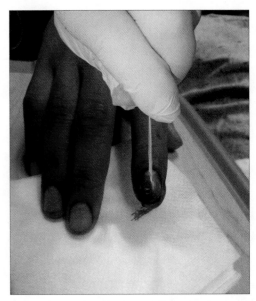

FIGURE 21.2 Trephination—drilling method.

EDUCATIONAL POINTS

- Elevation
- Clean with soap and water.
- Apply topical antibiotic.
- Systemic antibiotic therapy is not warranted but should be considered with an open tuft or phalanx fracture.
- Consideration should be given to children with a significant or recurring hematoma, and child abuse should be ruled out.
- A device approved by the Food and Drug Administration called the Path Former can decrease the amount of trauma during trephination as it offers more concise control.

COMPLICATIONS

- Infection

PEARLS

- Tube gauze may be used to give light pressure and encourage drainage.
- The heat method is preferred because of the potential nail bed trauma with the drill method.

RESOURCES

Huang, Y. H., & Ohara, K. (2005). Medical pearl: Subungual hematoma: A simple and quick method for diagnosis. *Journal of the American Academy of Dermatology, 54,* 877–878.

Lammers, R. L. (2010). Methods of wound care. In J. R. Roberts & J. R. Hedges (Eds.), *Clinical procedures in emergency medicine* (5th ed., p. 626). Philadelphia, PA: Saunders Elsevier.

Mayorga, O., & Wall, S. P. (2014). *Subungual hematoma drainage.* Retrieved from http://emedicine .medscape.com/article/82926-overview

CHAPTER **22**

Procedures for Managing Paronychia

Theresa M. Campo

BACKGROUND

Paronychia is a superficial infection of the nail fold. It is commonly caused by frequent nail biting or chewing of the periungual tissue or by aggressive manicures. Paronychia is one of the most common infections of the hand.

Paronychia can be either acute or chronic. Acute paronychia usually affects one digit and is characterized by acute onset of pulsating pain, swelling, and erythema of the periungual space, usually unilateral. Chronic paronychia is caused by frequent and increased water exposure, humidity, detergents, and irritants, which cause irritation and maceration of the proximal nail fold. This leads to inflammation, swelling of the nail fold, and cessation of cuticle production. The most common organisms found in chronic paronychia are *Candida albicans* and *Pseudomonas aeruginosa*. Acute paronychia is discussed in detail in this chapter.

Most Common Pathogens Causing Acute Paronychia

- *Streptococcus pyogenes*
- *Staphylococcus aureus*
- *Eikenella corrodens*
- Anaerobic organisms
  - *Provotella* spp.
  - *Fusobacterium nucleatum*
  - Gram-positive cocci
  - *Peptostreptococcus* spp.

> **NOTE** *Practitioners should always consider mixed oropharyngeal flora as the causative organism.*

Paronychia can be confused with a herpetic whitlow. This infection is most often seen in health care workers and immunocompromised patients. The most common presentation is localized swelling with clear vesicles. Lymphangitis, lymphadenopathy, and a dusky appearance to the nail may also be present. Viral culture should be obtained if possible and sent for Tzanck smear and serum antibody titers. Opening of the vesicles is not recommended. This infection is self-limiting and should resolve within 3 to 4 weeks.

PATIENT PRESENTATION

- Warm, erythematous, edematous, and painful unilateral or bilateral lateral nail fold.
- Frank abscess and occasional extension to the eponychia can occur.
- Lymphangitis and lymphadenopathy are usually not seen.

TREATMENT

Early paronychia is characterized by redness and mild swelling. Treatment is localized and noninvasive. Warm soaks, elevation, and antibiotic therapy with dicloxacillin or cephalexin are recommended. More extensive infection with fluctuance requires drainage of the pustulent material. This procedure will be covered in this chapter.

SPECIAL CONSIDERATIONS

- Diabetics
- Immunocompromised patients

PROCEDURE PREPARATION

- Absorbent pad
- Skin cleanser
- No. 11 or No. 15 scalpel blade with handle
- Scissors
- Culture swab
- Normal saline solution
- Large syringe (20, 30, or 35 mL)
- Gauze pads
- Kling or gauze for wrapping
- Tape

PROCEDURE

- Place an absorbent protective pad under the treatment area.
- Cleanse the skin using a circular motion to free debris and bacteria.
- Drape the patient to maintain a clean area.
- Strict sterile technique is not required for this procedure. However, because of the era of resistance, sterile technique should be used whenever possible.

> **NOTE** *Ethyl chloride or a digital block can be used based on the patient's pain tolerance and extent of the paronychia.*

Localized Pus Collection

- Position an 18-gauge needle bevel up and parallel to the nail surface.
- Insert the needle into the lateral nail fold at the point of maximum fluctuance (Figure 22.1).
- Lift the skin of the nail fold, which will release the pus.
- Use a gentle side-to-side motion and "fan out" the area allowing full expression of the contents.
- Obtain culture.
- Soak or irrigate with normal saline.
  - Irrigate with syringe and splash shield.
- Insert packing if possible.
- Apply sterile dressing.

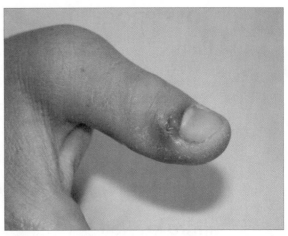

FIGURE 22.1 Releasing localized pus collection of a paronychia.

Complex

- Perform digital block technique (see Chapter 11).
- Holding the scalpel parallel to the nail surface, gently advance the scalpel under the eponychium, making sure not to invade the nail bed (Figure 22.2).
- Express the contents.
- Irrigate with normal saline.
- Insert packing.
- Apply sterile dressing.

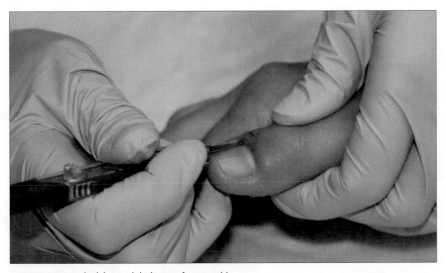

FIGURE 22.2 Incision and drainage of paronychia.

POST-PROCEDURE CONSIDERATIONS

Pain

- Digital block can be performed if patient is intolerant of the procedure.
- Instruct the patient to keep the finger elevated, above the level of the heart, to prevent throbbing and pain.

Drainage

- If the paronychia is small, you may only get a very small amount of drainage.
- Consider herpetic whitlow if pus drainage is less than expected based on the amount of swelling and presentation.

Ingrown Nail

- If an ingrown nail is present or the pus collection is under the nail, lifting the nail may be necessary or a semilunar incision proximal to the nail fold may be required.

Mobile Nail

- If the nail is mobile, removal may be necessary.

EDUCATIONAL POINTS

- Elevation
- Clean with soap and water.
- Apply topical antibiotic.
- Incision and drainage is the ideal treatment of paronychia.
- Systemic antibiotic therapy is not always warranted.
- Instruct patients not to bite or chew nails, to be careful with aggressive manicures, and not to suck on fingers.

COMPLICATIONS

- Progression of infection to surrounding tissue causing cellulitis, lymphangitis, and/or fever should be treated with antibiotic therapy.
- Recurrence of the abscess necessitates consideration of risk factors or abnormalities including foreign body, cancer, staph colonization, and immunologic disorders.

PEARL

- Ethyl chloride can be used topically to decrease the pain experienced with incision or puncture of the pustule.

RESOURCES

Billingsley, E. M., & Vidimos, A. T. (2014). *Paronychia*. Retrieved from http://emedicine .medscape.com/article/1106062-overview

Browning, J., & Levy, M., & Long, S. S. (2008). Cellulitis and superficial hand infections. In L. K. Pickering & C. G. Prober (Eds.), *Principles and practice of pediatric infectious disease* (3rd ed.).

Philadelphia, PA: Elsevier. Retrieved from http://www.mdconsult.com/das/book/body/ 187327964-17/963263349/1679/76.html#4-u1.0-B978-0-443-06687-0..50075-8- cesec12_1553

Butler, K. H. (2009). Incision and drainage. In J. R. Roberts & J. R. Hedges (Eds.), *Clinical procedures in emergency medicine* (5th ed., pp. 681–685). Philadelphia, PA: Saunders Elsevier.

Clark, D. C. (2003). Common acute hand infections. *American Family Physician, 68*(11), 2167–2176.

Habif, T. P., (2009). Nail diseases. In *Clinical dermatology: A color guide to diagnosis and treatment* (5th ed.). Philadelphia, PA: Saunders/Elsevier. Retrieved from http://www .mdconsult.com/book/player/book.do?method=display&type=bookpages&decora tor=header&eid=4u1.0-B978-0-7234-3541-9..00034-1-s0315&displayedEid=4-u1 .0-B978-0-7234-3541-9..00034-1–s0350&uniq=187327964&isbn=978-0-7234-3541- 9&sid=963240480

Holtzman, L. C., Hitti, E., & Harrow, J. (2014). Incision and drainage. In J. R. Roberts & J. R. Hedges (Eds.), *Clinical procedures in emergency medicine* (6th ed.). Philadelphia, PA: Saunders Elsevier. Retrieved from https://www.clinicalkey.com/#!/content/ book/3-s2.0-B9781455706068000379

Kellerman, R. D. (2015). Diseases of the skin: Diseases of the hand. In *Conn's current therapy*. Philadelphia, PA: Saunders Elsevier. Retrieved from https://www.clinicalkey.com/#!/ content/book/3-s2.0-B9781455702978004043

Lyn, E. T., & Mailhot, T. (2010). Hand: Infection of the hand. *Rosen's emergency medicine* (7th ed.). Philadelphia, PA: Elsevier. Retrieved from http://www.mdconsult.com/ book/player/book.do?method=display&type=bookpages&decorator=header&eid= 4u1.0-B978-0-323-05472-0..X0001-1@uniq=187327964&isbn=978-0-323-05472- 0&sid=963266130#1pstate=open&1pTab=contentsTab&content=4u1.0-B978- 0-323-05472-0..00047–st0495%3Bfrom%3Dindex%3Btype%3Dbookpage%3Bisbn %3D978-0-323-05472-0

Mailhot, T., & Lyn, E. T. (2014). Hand. In *Rosen's emergency medicine* (8th ed.). Philadelphia, PA: Elsevier. Retrieved from https://www.clinicalkey.com/#!/content/book/3-s2.0- B9781455706051000506

Mostaghimi, L. (2010). Diseases of the skin: Diseases of the nails. In E. T. Bope, R. E., Rakel, & R. D. Kellerman (Eds.), *Conn's current therapy 2010* (1st ed.). Philadelphia, PA: Elsevier. Retrieved from http://www.mdconsult.com/book/player/book.do?method=display&type= bookpages&decorator=header&eid=4u1.0-B978-1-4160-6642-2..00013-2-s0845& uniq=187327964&isbn=978-1-4160-6642-2&sid=963240480

Rockwell, P. G. (2001). Acute and chronic paronychia. *American Family Physician, 63*(6), 1113–1116.

Wright, P. E. (2008). Hand infections: Paronychia. In S. T. Canale & J. H. Beaty (Eds.), *Campbell's operative orthopaedics* (11th ed.). Philadelphia, PA: Elsevier. Retrieved from http://www .mdconsult.com/book/body/187327964-19/963269025/1584/577.html#4-u1 .0-B978-0-323-03329-9..50078-7–cesec3_4075

CHAPTER 23

Procedures for Treating Felons

Theresa M. Campo

BACKGROUND

A felon is an infection that involves the pulp of the distal finger or thumb. The finger pulp or pad is made up of numerous small compartments that are divided by fibrous septa running from the bone to the skin. The compartments contain eccrine sweat glands and fat globules, which are possible modes of bacterial invasion.

Felons are commonly caused by trauma or a foreign body, such as a splinter, thorn, and so on. An untreated paronychia can develop into a felon. *Staphylococcus aureus*, including community-acquired methicillin-resistant *S. aureus* (CA-MRSA), is the most common bacteria. However, a mixed infection with staph and strep as well as a gram-negative infection can occur.

Infection and inflammation can cause an increase in pressure within the compartments and can lead to ischemia and tissue necrosis. Bacteria can invade the periosteum and can lead to osteomyelitis and can also innervate the flexor tendon sheath.

Complications can develop if the felon is not treated or failure of therapy occurs. Possible complications include osteomyelitis, soft tissue or bone necrosis, septic arthritis of the distal interphalyngeal joint, and flexor tenosynovitis.

PATIENT PRESENTATION

- Rapid onset of pain
  - Continuous and throbbing
- Swelling to distal finger pad
  - Does not extend proximal to distal interphalyngeal joint space
- Redness
- Firmness
  - Fluctuance may be present early but is usually firm at time of patient presentation.

NOTE *Decreased pain without intervention can be a sign of extensive necrosis and nerve degeneration.*

TREATMENT

The definitive treatment for a felon is incision and drainage. Antibiotics alone can be used for minor cellulitis, but are often not curative. Treatment plans should include tetanus prophylaxis, warm compresses or soaks, and elevation. Radiographs should be considered to rule out a foreign body and osteomyelitis. Oral antibiotics should be considered and given based on current recommendations in your region.

Most felons can be effectively managed with a simple incision procedure. The techniques of a "hockey stick" or "fish mouth" incision are not advocated due to the risk of complications; no differences in healing have been found. Careful attention must be paid when incising a felon because of the potential for injury of the tendons, nerves, and vasculature. Incisions should not be performed on the radial aspects of the index finger or the ulnar surface of the thumb or little finger.

SPECIAL CONSIDERATIONS

- Diabetics
- Immunocompromised patients

PROCEDURE PREPARATION

- Absorbent pads
- Skin cleanser
- Lidocaine 1% or 2% with epinephrine (bupivacaine is another option because of its longer duration of action)
- 10-mL syringe
- 25-gauge needle for injection of lidocaine
- No. 11 or No. 15 scalpel blade with handle
- Scissors
- Culture swab
- Normal saline solution
- Large syringe (20, 30, or 35 mL)
- Gauze pads
- Kling or gauze for wrapping
- Tape

NOTE *Premade suture kits usually have the instruments and equipment used in this procedure. Check with your institution for kit contents. Please see Chapter 18 for common contents.*

PROCEDURE

- Cleanse the skin using a circular motion to free debris and bacteria.
- Place an absorbent protective pad under the treatment area.
- Drape the patient to maintain a clean area.
- Sterile technique is required for this procedure to prevent extension of the infection.
- Digital block anesthesia should be performed (see Chapter 11).
- Apply a Penrose drain to the base of the finger to give a bloodless field.

Simple Lateral Incision

- Using either the No. 11 or No. 15 blade scalpel, make an incision at the point of maximum fluctuance (Figure 23.1).
  - Incision should be lateral.
  - Avoid the center or midline finger pad as this may cause increased scarring and pain.

Transverse Incision (Most Preferred Method)

- Make an incision transversely through the point of maximum fluctuance (Figure 23.2).
  - Avoid the digital nerves.

Longitudinal Incision

- A longitudinal incision is made through the fat pad (Figure 23.3).
  - Do not extend past the distal interphalyngeal crease to avoid flexor tendon damage.
  - This technique should be avoided unless absolutely necessary because of the sensitivity of the fat pad.
- Bluntly dissect the subcutaneous tissue to break up the loculations with a hemostat.
- Investigate, evaluate, and remove foreign bodies.
- Remove any necrotic tissue.
- Irrigate the wound with sterile normal saline and a 20- to 30-mL syringe only.
  - Do not use high pressure irrigation as it may push bacteria onto the tendon sheath and extend the infection into the distal interphalyngeal joint.
- Insert packing into the wound.
  - Usually only requires a wick (small piece of packing).
- Dress the wound with gauze and Kling.

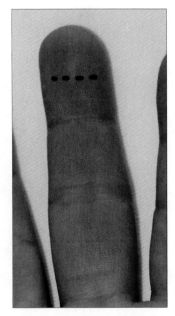

FIGURE 23.1 Felon—simple lateral incision.

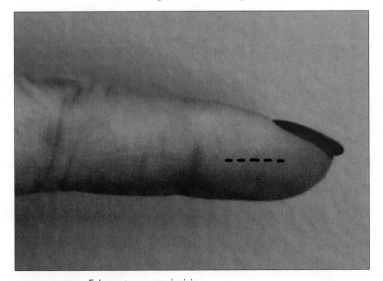

FIGURE 23.2 Felon—transverse incision.

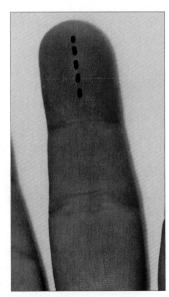

FIGURE 23.3 Felon—longitudinal incision.

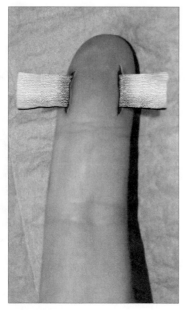

FIGURE 23.4 Felon—through-and-through technique.

Alternate Procedure— Through-and-Through Incision

- A second incision can be made similarly to the first to allow a "through-and-through" incision (Figure 23.4).
- Place gauze in the first incision.
- Grasp the gauze through the second incision and pull through.
- Trim the gauze close to the finger.
- Dress the wound with gauze and Kling.
- Finger splint may be applied.

> **NOTE** *This method is not considered a method of choice due to the increased risk of causing a flattened pad of the distal finger.*

POST-PROCEDURE CONSIDERATIONS
Pain
- Instruct the patient to keep the finger elevated, above the level of the heart, to prevent throbbing and pain.

EDUCATIONAL POINTS
- Elevate
- Warm compresses
- Packing removal 48 to 72 hours
- Narcotic analgesia with instructions not to drive or consume alcohol with medication

COMPLICATIONS
- Extension or recurrence of infection
- Osteomyelitis
- Soft tissue necrosis
- Bone necrosis
- Nerve damage
- Heightened sensitivity to the distal finger
- Scar tissue
- Flattening of the fat pads due to extensive compartment damage during procedure (through and through, simple lateral or longitudinal techniques)

PEARLS

- Premedicate with oral pain medicine if not driving home.
- Cutting the finger out of a sterile glove and placing at the base of the finger can be done in place of a Penrose drain.

RESOURCES

Browning, J., Levy, M., & Long, S. S. (2008). Cellulitis and superficial hand infections. In L. K. Pickering & C. G. Prober (Eds.), *Principles and practice of pediatric infectious disease* (3rd ed.). Philadelphia, PA: Elsevier. Retrieved from http://www.mdconsult.com/das/book/body/187327964-20/963270106/1584/578.html#4-u1.0-B978-0-323-03329-9..50078-7–cesec7_4079

Clark, D. C. (2003). Common acute hand infections. *American Family Physician, 68*(11), 2167–2176.

Holtzman, L. C., Hitti, E., & Harrow, J. (2014). Incision and drainage. In J. R. Roberts & J. R. Hedges (Eds.), *Clinical procedures in emergency medicine* (6th ed.). Philadelphia, PA: Saunders Elsevier. Retrieved from https://www.clinicalkey.com/#!/content/book/3-s2.0-B9781455706068000379

Kellerman, R. D. (2015). Diseases of the skin: Diseases of the hand. In E. T. Bope & R. D. Kellerman (Eds.), *Conn's current therapy*. Philadelphia, PA: Saunders Elsevier. Retrieved from https://www.clinicalkey.com/#!/content/book/3-s2.0-B9781455702978004043

Lyn, E. T., & Mailhot, T. (2010). Hand: Infection of the hand. In J. Marx, R. Hockenberger, & R. Walls (Eds.), *Rosen's emergency medicine* (7th ed.). Philadelphia, PA: Elsevier. Retrieved from http://www.mdconsult.com/book/player/book.do?method=display&type=bookPage&decorator=header&eid=4-u1.0-B978-0-323-05472-0..00047-5–s0705&displayedEid=4-u1.0-B978-0-323-05472-0..00047-5–s0730&uniq=187327964&isbn=978-0-323-05472-0&sid=963271883

Mailhot, T., & Lyn, E. T. (2014). Hand. In J. Marx, R. Hockenberger, & R. Walls (Eds.), *Rosen's emergency medicine* (8th ed.). Philadelphia, PA: Elsevier. Retrieved from https://www.clinicalkey.com/#!/content/book/3-s2.0-B9781455706051000506

Mostaghimi, L. (2010). Diseases of the skin: Diseases of the nails. In E. T. Bope, R. E. Rakel, & R. D. Kellerman (Eds.), *Conn's current therapy 2010* (1st ed.). Philadelphia, PA: Elsevier. Retrieved from http://www.mdconsult.com/book/player/book.do?method=display&type=bookPage&decorator=header&eid=4-u1.0-B978-1-4160-6642-2..00013-2–s0845&uniq=187327964&isbn=978-1-4160-6642-2&sid=963240480

Vaughn, G. (2010). *Felon*. Retrieved from http://emedicine.medscape.com/article/782537-overview and http://emedicine.medscape.com/article/782537-treatment

Vaughn, G., Bowman, J. G., Talavara, F., Hirshon, J. M., & Halamka, J. D. (2014). *Felon*. Retrieved from http://emedicine.medscape.com/article/782537-overview

Wright, P. E. (2008). Hand infections: Paronychia. In S. T. Canale & J. H. Beaty (Eds.), *Campbell's operative orthopaedics* (11th ed.). Philadelphia, PA: Mosby/Elsevier. Retrieved from http://www.mdconsult.com/das/book/body/187327964-19/963269025/1584/577.html#4-u1.0-B978-0-323-03329-9.50078-7–cesec3_4075

UNIT VIII

Incision and Drainage Procedures

CHAPTER 24

Abscess Overview and the Use of Sonography

Theresa M. Campo

An abscess is the formation and collection of pus that can develop in any region of the body, usually initiated by the breakdown of epidermal defense mechanisms against the normal flora. It can occur by either an inflammatory reaction to an infectious process (bacteria, parasite, or fungus) or less commonly by a foreign body or substance such as a splinter or needle. Abscesses may develop from a blocked sweat or oil gland (sebaceous), from an inflamed hair follicle, or minor break in the skin such as a puncture wound.

The most typical organism causing an abscess is *Staphylococcus aureus*; normally found on the skin, it produces an area of rapidly forming necrosis and large amounts of pus. Group A beta-hemolytic streptococcus tends to spread rapidly through the tissue, causing erythema, edema, and serous exudate with little or no necrosis. It also has a streaky appearance and is the cause of most cellulitis. In the perirectal area, enteric and/or anaerobic bacteria proliferation is typical. Necrosis and brownish, foul smelling pus are typical of abscess formation and are commonly seen with cellulitis of the surrounding tissue. Combinations of anaerobic and gram-negative organisms have been reported in the literature. Methicillin-resistant *S. aureus* has been identified as the source of many abscesses throughout the nation and the world as a result of the misuse and overuse of antibiotics.

Abscesses form when white blood cells (WBCs) move through the walls of the blood vessels into an area with organisms or foreign bodies. The WBCs collect with the damaged tissue, forming pus, which is a build up of fluid, damaged and dead tissue, and organisms, usually bacteria. A pocket forms with the pus and a wall is formed to attempt to block the bacteria from spreading to surrounding tissue or structures initiating an inflammatory response. Occasionally, bacteria escape from the walled-off area and penetrate the bloodstream and surrounding tissue or organs.

Most abscesses occur cutaneously and can be found in the extremities (especially axilla), groin and external vagina (Bartholin), tailbone (pilonidal), and areas of hair distribution causing a folliculitis, which can then form a furuncle. Abscesses can also occur in many places, including, but not limited to, the brain, liver, kidneys, lungs, teeth/periodontal region, pharynx, and tonsils. Common areas of abscess related to a patient's occupation and intravenous drug use can be viewed in Table 24.1.

TABLE 24.1 Factors Leading to Abscess Formation and Location

Factor	Body Area/Location	Cause
Occupation (manual labor)	Arms Hands	Minor trauma
Women	Axilla Groin Submammary	Shaving Constrictive clothing Overgrowth of bacteria
Intravenous drug users (may be superficial or deep)	Upper extremities Lower extremities	Penetration of skin with clean or dirty needles Skin popping

Most abscesses can be readily diagnosed based on the physical examination findings of pain, redness, swelling, and the presence of fluctuance. When the physical findings are equivocal, needle aspiration and/or ultrasonography may be performed. The use of ultrasonography is increasing in popularity and can assist in the location and diagnosis of abscess formation, especially in areas with major vessels and organs in close proximity to the affected area. Ultrasonography can easily identify surrounding arteries with the use of the Doppler color setting.

The ability to differentiate cellulitis from abscess can be accomplished with the use of ultrasonography. Findings of cellulitis with ultrasound arise from the swelling and edema produced by the response to the infective organism. Findings include increased

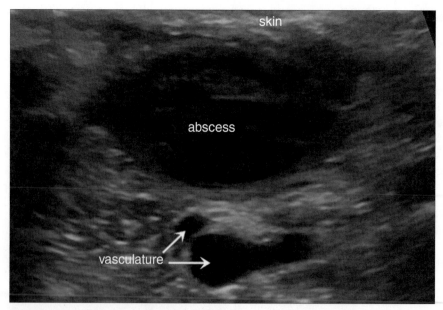

FIGURE 24.1 Ultrasound of subcutaneous abscess.

distance between the skin and underlying fascia or bone; increased echogenicity of the subcutaneous tissue accompanied with hypoechoic bands cause a cobblestone appearance. It can be difficult to differentiate edema from purulent fluid. However, the most common finding of a subcutaneous abscess is a hypoechoic roughly spherical mass. An organized collection of pus and debris in a well-formed, sharply demarcated area can be visualized. A posterior acoustic enhancement may also be present and the fluid-filled area may have motion with palpation (Figure 24.1).

RESOURCES

Abrahamian, F. M., Talan, D. A., & Moran, G. J. (2008). Management of skin and soft tissue infections in the emergency department. *Infectious Disease Clinics of North America, 22*(1), 89–116.

Anderson, D. J., & Kaye, K. S. (2007). Skin and soft tissue infections in older adults. *Clinics in Geriatric Medicine, 23*(3), 595–613.

Butler, K. H. (2010). Incision and drainage. In J. R. Roberts & J. R. Hedges (Eds.), *Clinical procedures in emergency medicine* (5th ed., pp. 657–672). Philadelphia, PA: Saunders Elsevier.

Fitch, M. T., Manthey, D. E., McGinnis, H. D., Nicks, B. A., & Pariyadath, M. (2007). Abscess incision and drainage. *New England Journal of Medicine, 357*(19), e20.

Grimm, L., & Carmody, K. A. (2009, May 20). *Bedside ultrasonography, abscess evaluation.* Retrieved from http://emedicine.medscape.com/article/1379916-overview and http://emedicine.medscape.com/article/1379916-treatment

Hammond, S. P., & Baden, L. R. (2008). Management of skin and soft-tissue infection—Polling results. *New England Journal of Medicine, 359*(19), e20.

Herchline, T. E. (2014). *Staphylococcal infections.* Retrieved from http://emedicine.medscape.com/article/228816-overview

Holtzman, L. C., Hitti, E., & Harrow, J. (2014). Incision and drainage. In J. R. Roberts & J. R. Hedges (Eds.), *Clinical procedures in emergency medicine* (6th ed.). Philadelphia, PA: Saunders Elsevier. Retrieved from http://www.clinicalkev.com/#!/content/book/3-s2.0-B9781455706080000379

Meislin, H. W., & Guisto, J. A. (2009). Soft tissue infections. In J. A. Marx, R. Hockberger, & R. Walls (Eds.), *Rosen's emergency medicine* (7th ed.). Philadelphia, PA: Elsevier. Retrieved from http://www.mdconsult.com/book/player/book.do?method=display&type=bookPage&decorator=header&eid=4-u1.0-B978-0-323-05472-0..00135-3–s0325&uniq=190201654&isbn=978-0-323-05472-0&sid=970896658

Pallin, D. J., & Nassisi, D. (2014). Skin and soft tissue infections. In J. A. Marx, R. Hockberger, & R. Walls (Eds.), *Rosen's emergency medicine* (8th ed.). Philadelphia, PA: Elsevier. Retrieved from https://www.clinicalkey.com/#!/content/book/3-s2.0-B9781455706051001378

Rogers, R. L., & Perkins, J. (2006). Skin and soft tissue infections. *Primary Care Clinical Office Practice, 33*(3), 697–710.

Singer, A. J., & Dagum, A. B. (2008). Current management of acute cutaneous wounds. *New England Journal of Medicine, 359*(10), 1037–1046.

Singhal, H., Kaur, K., & Bailey, R. (2014). *Skin and soft tissue infections: Incision, drainage, and debridement.* Retrieved from http://emedicine.medscape.com/article/1830144-overview

CHAPTER **25**

Procedures for Incision and Drainage of Subcutaneous Abscess

Theresa M. Campo

BACKGROUND

Abscesses most commonly occur in the following areas:

- Extremities (especially axilla)
- Areas of hair distribution (folliculitis, furuncle)
- Neck
- Buttocks

PATIENT PRESENTATION

- Red, raised, painful lump
- Warmth
- Firm and/or fluctuant (fluid filled, feels like a ripe piece of fruit)
- Pointing with pustule
- Lymphangitis
- Lymphadenopathy
- Localized or extensive cellulitis
- Fever

TREATMENT

Incision and drainage are considered to be the definitive treatment for cutaneous abscesses. Abscesses without cellulitis can be effectively treated with incision and drainage alone and may not require antibiotic treatment. Deep-seated abscesses or abscesses over major vessels or structures can be investigated further using ultrasonography or CT scanning. Abscesses found within or extending into the abdominal cavity, thoracic cavity, brain, and other deep tissue can be incised using guided imaging.

Abscesses that are fluctuant and draining can develop a chronic nonhealing sinus that may require surgical excision. Cultures should be obtained when incising any abscess to determine the offending organism(s), especially methicillin-resistant *Staphylococcus aureus* (MRSA). Small lesions, usually less than 5 mm, can be treated effectively with warm compresses and either topical or systemic antibiotics based on the severity and location of the infection. Larger abscesses should be incised and drained, with packing removal 24 to 48 hours after placement. Any abscess with pus formation, whether firm or fluctuant, should be incised and drained. Antibiotic treatment alone does not adequately treat loculated collections of pus and infection. Incisions should be liberal to allow for breakup of loculations and appropriate drainage of the purulent material. Accompanying cellulitis should be treated empirically based on the common organisms found in the region (i.e., MRSA). Modifications to treatment can be made once culture results are reported.

Some abscesses located at cosmetically important areas and not significant on physical examination can be evacuated by needle aspiration as long as the purulent material is not too thick for drainage. Large abscesses may require placement of a rubber drain. All abscesses should be evaluated and treated independently, with careful consideration given to the patient's past and current medical history, family history, and current trends of bacterial organism invasion in the treatment area.

CONTRAINDICATIONS AND RELATIVE CONTRAINDICATIONS

- Abscesses that lie in close proximity to major vessel.
  - Location and nature of abscess should be confirmed with needle aspiration, ultrasonography, or CT scan.
- Hand abscesses involving the palmer aspect and with passive range-of-motion pain should be referred immediately to a hand specialist for evaluation and treatment.
  - Increased severity of infection occurs because the flexor tendon has a sheath of synovial fluid and the extensor tendon does not.

SPECIAL CONSIDERATIONS

- Pediatric patient
  - Conscious sedation may be necessary for deep-seated or difficult-to-manage areas due to movement or severity.
  - Each case should be considered independently.
- General anesthesia
  - May be required for abscesses located in the perirectal, supralevator, ischiorectal areas, and those that are deep-seated or in the area of major vessels or over bony prominences.
- Abscesses located in the palmer aspect of the hand should be referred to a hand specialist to avoid tendon injury or neurovascular compromise.
- Abscesses located on the face, particularly the nasolabial fold, may drain into the sphenoid sinus, causing cavernous sinus thrombosis.
- Immunocompromised patients and those with comorbidities
  - Abscesses in organ transplant, HIV, AIDS, diabetes, and/or cancer patients should be treated more aggressively and with a lower index of suspicion for abscess and infection.

- Patients with immunosuppression may not present with classic signs and symptoms of abscess formation as they may lack the host defense and release of cytokines needed to produce the inflammatory reaction. They may only present with a low-grade fever or malaise. Atypical bacterial organisms and fungus are more common in this population
- Intravenous (IV) drug use
  - Patients with multiple abscesses or abscesses on the arms and antecubital fossa or dorsal aspect of the hand should be questioned for IV drug use, and treated more aggressively for atypical organisms and fungus.
- Pregnancy
  - Patients who are pregnant should be treated with antibiotics that are considered safe in pregnancy.
- Artificial heart valves and prosthetic joints
  - Prophylaxis based on the current American Heart Association/American College of Cardiology guidelines.
  - The timing of the procedure may need to be reconsidered to help prevent endocarditis in this group of patients.
  - Consultation with a specialist is recommended.

PROCEDURE PREPARATION

- Protective gown, gloves, and goggles—abscess contents are under pressure
- Drape
- Skin cleanser
- Lidocaine 1% or 2% with epinephrine (bupivacaine is another option because of its longer duration of action)
- 20- or 35-mL syringe for irrigation
- 10-mL syringe
- 25-gauge needle for injection of lidocaine
- No. 11 or No. 15 scalpel blade with handle
- Hemostat and scissors
- Culture swab
- Normal saline solution
- Plain or iodoform 1/4, 1/2, or 1 in. depending upon the size and depth of the abscess
- Gauze pads
- Kling or gauze for wrapping
- Tape

PROCEDURE

- Cleanse the skin using a circular motion to free debris and bacteria.
- Place an absorbent protective pad under the treatment area.
- Drape the patient to maintain a clean area as well as to protect the patient's privacy.
- Strict sterile technique is not required for this procedure. However, because of the era of resistance, sterile technique should be used whenever possible.

Infiltration

- Anesthetize the top of the wound, inserting a 25-gauge needle just under and parallel to the surface of the skin.
- Inject the anesthetic gently into the intradermal layer, until the area is large enough for incision (Figure 25.1). Field-block anesthesia can be used for larger abscesses (see Chapter 9).
- You will notice blanching of the skin.

> **NOTE** *IV pain medication and/or anxiolytics should be considered for deep-seated abscesses.*

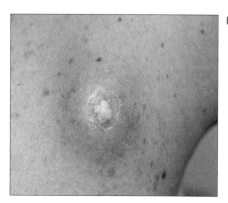

FIGURE 25.1 Abscess.

Incision

- Make a liberal incision directly over the center of the abscess with a No. 11 or No. 15 scalpel, making sure to cut through the skin and into the cavity of the abscess (Figure 25.2).
- Direct, firm pressure should be used when making the incision.
- Be careful not to puncture through the back end of the abscess wall because this can cause excessive bleeding.
- Extend the incision to allow for adequate drainage of pus and enough room for wound dissection.
- Attention should be given to the skin tension lines; these should be followed whenever possible for the best cosmetic outcome.
- Allow the pus to drain freely and apply pressure to the area to assist with expression of pus and abscess contents.
- With a culture swab, swab the *inside* of the abscess—not the drainage (Figure 25.3).
- Perform a blunt dissection with a curved hemostat in a circular motion to break up loculations (Figure 25.4).
- Never use a gloved finger, especially when a foreign body is suspected.

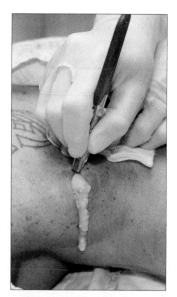

FIGURE 25.2 Incising an abscess.

- Irrigate the abscess liberally with normal saline (Figure 25.5).
- Insert iodoform or plain packing into the cavity (Figure 25.6).
- Place a sufficient amount of packing into the cavity, making certain not to overpack the wound causing pressure necrosis, which causes ischemia and death to the surrounding tissue.
- Apply a gauze dressing to help collect any drainage.
- Tetanus immunization should be up to date.
- Abscesses should not be sutured closed.

POST-PROCEDURE CONSIDERATIONS

Pain

The contents of the abscess are acidotic and can decrease the efficacy of the anesthetic. Performing a field block (see Chapter 9) and administering oral or IV pain medicine can help reduce the pain.

Drainage

- If there is little or no drainage from the abscess, consider a deeper and/or wider incision.
- If sebaceous material is extracted from the site and there is little or no pus, proceed with the procedure as described previously.

Antibiotic Therapy

Successful incision and drainage of abscesses do not require antibiotic therapy in healthy individuals unless the abscess is accompanied by cellulitis. However, patients who are immunocompromised, diabetic, or IV drug users should be considered for antibiotic treatment. It has been speculated that abscesses caused by community-acquired MRSA do not need antibiotic therapy. However, there is little data to support this at this time.

EDUCATIONAL POINTS

- Packing should be changed if persistent drainage is present; otherwise, removal within 48 hours of placement is recommended during follow-up with a provider.
- Stress the importance of follow-up.
- Risks and benefits of antibiotics and pain medicine
- Area should not get wet until packing is removed.

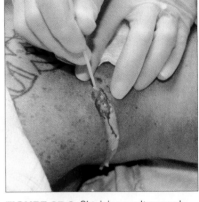
FIGURE 25.3 Obtaining a culture swab.

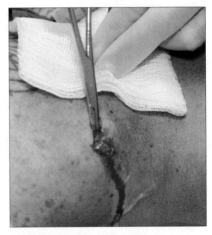
FIGURE 25.4 Blunt dissection

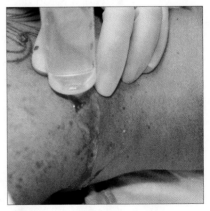
FIGURE 25.5 Irrigation of an abscess cavity.

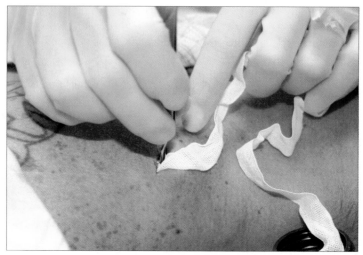

FIGURE 25.6
Insertion of packing.

- Healing occurs through tissue granulation from the base of the wound.
- Proper hygiene and handwashing are effective against recurrence and spread of infection.

COMPLICATIONS

- Progression of infection to surrounding tissue causing cellulitis, lymphangitis, and/ or fever should be treated with antibiotic therapy.
- Recurrence of the abscess necessitates consideration of risk factors or abnormalities, including foreign body, cancer, staph colonization, and immunologic disorders.

PEARLS

- Fluctuance can be described to patients as a piece of ripe or overripe fruit such as a peach.
- Premedicating with oral analgesia helps to make the procedure more tolerable.
- Peripads can be used for abscesses in the groin or buttocks or areas that are difficult to dress with tape or wrapping gauze.
- Patients presenting with pus should not leave with pus.

RESOURCES

Abrahamian, F. M., Talan, D. A., & Moran, G. J. (2008). Management of skin and soft tissue infections in the emergency department. *Infectious Disease Clinics of North America, 22*(1), 89–116.

Anderson, D. J., & Kaye, K. S. (2007). Skin and soft tissue infections in older adults. *Clinics in Geriatric Medicine, 23*(3), 595–613.

Butler, K. H. (2010). Incision and drainage. In J. R. Roberts & J. R. Hedges (Eds.), *Clinical procedures in emergency medicine* (5th ed., pp. 657–672). Philadelphia, PA: Saunders Elsevier.

Fitch, M. T., Manthey, D. E., McGinnis, H. D., Nicks, B. A., & Pariyadath, M. (2007). Abscess incision and drainage. *New England Journal of Medicine, 357*(19), e20.

Grimm, L., & Carmody, K. A. (2009, May 20). *Bedside ultrasonography, abscess evaluation.* Retrieved from http://emedicine.medscape.com/article/1379916-overview. and http://emedicine.medscape.com/article/1379916-treatment

Hammond, S. P., & Baden, L. R. (2008). Management of skin and soft-tissue infection—Polling results. *New England Journal of Medicine, 359*(19), e20.

Herchline, T. E. (2014). *Staphylococcal infections.* Retrieved from http://emedicine.medscape.com/article/228816-overview

Holtzman, L. C., Hitti, E., & Harrow, J. (2014). Incision and drainage. In J. R. Roberts & J. R. Hedges (Eds.), *Clinical procedures in emergency medicine* (6th ed.). Philadelphia, PA: Saunders Elsevier. Retrieved from http://www.clinicalkey.com/#!/content/book/3-s2.0-B9781455706068000379

Meislin, H. W., & Guisto, J. A. (2009). Soft tissue infections. In J. A. Marx, R. Hockberger, & R. Walls (Eds.), *Rosen's emergency medicine* (7th ed.). Philadelphia, PA: Elsevier. Retrieved from http://www.mdconsult.com/book/player/book.do?method=display&type=bookPage&decorator=header&eid=4-u1.0-B978-0-323-05472-0..00135-3–s0325&uniq=190201654&isbn=978-0-323-05472-0&sid=970896658

Pallin, D. J., & Nassisi, D. (2014). Skin and soft tissue infections. In J. A. Marx, R. Hockberger, & R. Walls (Eds.), *Rosen's emergency medicine* (8th ed.). Philadelphia, PA: Elsevier. Retrieved from https://www.clinicalkey.com/#!/content/book/3-s2.0-B9781455706051001378

Rogers, R. L., & Perkins, J. (2006). Skin and soft tissue infections. *Primary Care Clinical Office Practice, 33*(3), 697–710.

Singer, A. J., & Dagum, A. B. (2008). Current management of acute cutaneous wounds. *New England Journal of Medicine, 359*(10), 1037–1046.

Singhal, H., Kaur, K., & Bailey, R. A. (2014). *Skin and soft tissue infections: Incision, drainage, and debridement.* Retrieved from http://emedicine.medscape.com/article/1830144-overview

CHAPTER 26

Procedures for Managing Pilonidal Cyst/Abscess

Theresa M. Campo

BACKGROUND

The term *pilonidal* has its origins from the Latin terms *pilus* meaning hair and *nidus* meaning nest. Pilonidal abscesses were originally thought to be congenital and caused by remnants of caudal segments, hair, and other dermal debris. However, during World War II, there was an insurgence of soldiers who were jeep drivers who suffered from pilonidal abscesses. It was postulated that the cysts could be caused by repetitive trauma. The most recent theory on the development of pilonidal abscesses is that a foreign-body reaction occurs. Microtrauma causes the epithelium to line the cavity, which in turn causes an occlusion that prevents drainage. Hair follicle enlargement then causes an inflammatory response and edema. The increased pressure causes the spreading of purulent material to the surrounding subcutaneous tissue, thus promoting abscess formation. These abscesses can be quite large and are found in the gluteal fold overlying the coccyx (see Figure 26.1 to visualize a pilonidal abscess).

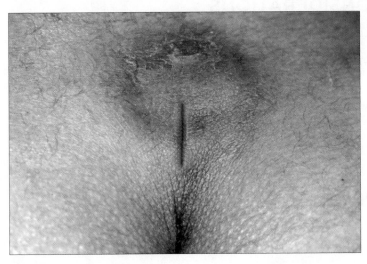

FIGURE 26.1 Pilonidal abscess.

Staphylococcus aureus, anaerobic cocci, aerobic, and anaerobic organisms cause abscess formation. Abscesses are more prevalent in men than in women. They tend to be familial and occur in persons with sitting occupations and obesity.

PATIENT PRESENTATION
- Sinus tract or "pit" sacrococcygeal region
- Tenderness to palpation
- Back pain
- Fluctuance
- Warmth
- Purulent discharge
- Localized or extensive cellulitis
- Fever

TREATMENT
The goal of treatment for pilonidal abscess is to fully remove the internalized material (i.e., hair, keratin, and cellular debris). Simple incision and drainage can be performed to treat the acute fluctuant abscess until surgical excision of the internalized material can be done. Pilonidal abscesses have a varied recurrence rate that can be as high as 90%. Even with surgical excision, 20% to 40% may recur. A flared-end de Pezzer catheter may be used for an extended period of time to allow for granulation and closure of chronic sinus. Simple incision and drainage of pilonidal abscess will be the focus of this chapter.

CONTRAINDICATIONS AND RELATIVE CONTRAINDICATIONS
- Immunocompromised patients

SPECIAL CONSIDERATIONS
- Immunocompromised patients
- Diabetes
- Cancer
- HIV-positive patient
- Pregnancy
- Pediatric and elderly patients
- Co-morbidities
- Prosthetic heart valves
- Prosthetic joints

PROCEDURE PREPARATION
- Protective gown, gloves, and goggles—abscess contents are under pressure
- Drape
- Skin cleanser

- Lidocaine 1% or 2% with epinephrine (bupivacaine is another option because of its longer duration of action)
- 20- or 35-mL syringe for irrigation
- 10-mL syringe
- 25-gauge needle for injection of lidocaine
- No. 11 or No. 15 scalpel blade with handle
- Hemostat and scissors
- Culture swab
- Normal saline solution
- Suture kit
- Plain or iodoform 1/4, 1/2, or 1 in. depending upon the size and depth of the abscess
- Gauze pads
- Kling or gauze for wrapping
- Tape

PROCEDURE

- Cleanse the skin using a circular motion to free debris and bacteria.
- Place an absorbent protective pad under the treatment area.
- Drape the patient to maintain a clean area as well as to protect the patient's privacy.
- Strict sterile technique is not required for this procedure. However, because of the increasing prevalence of bacterial resistance, sterile technique should be used whenever possible.

NOTE *Figures illustrating the following procedural steps appear in Chapter 25.*

Infiltration

- Anesthetize the top of the wound by inserting a 25-gauge needle just under and parallel to the surface of the skin.
- Inject the anesthetic gently into the intradermal layer, until the area is large enough for incision.
- You will notice blanching of the skin.

Incision

- Make a liberal incision directly over the center of the abscess with a No. 11 or No. 15 scalpel, making sure to cut through the skin and into the cavity of the abscess.
  - Direct, firm pressure should be used when making the incision.
- Be careful not to puncture through the back end of the abscess wall because this can cause excessive bleeding.
- Extend the incision to allow for adequate drainage of pus and enough room for wound dissection.
- Attention should be given to the skin tension lines; these should be followed whenever possible for the best cosmetic outcome.
- Allow the pus to drain freely and apply pressure to the area to assist with expression of pus and abscess contents.
- With a culture swab, swab the inside of the abscess—not the drainage (see Figure 25.3).

- Perform a blunt dissection with a curved hemostat using a circular motion to break up loculations.
- Never use a gloved finger, especially when a foreign body is suspected.
- Irrigate the abscess liberally with normal saline.
- Insert iodoform or plain packing into the cavity.
- Place a sufficient amount of packing into the cavity, making certain not to over-pack the wound thereby causing pressure necrosis, which causes ischemia and death to the surrounding tissue.
- Apply a gauze dressing to help collect any drainage.
- Tetanus immunization should be up to date.
- Abscesses should not be sutured closed.

POST-PROCEDURE CONSIDERATIONS

Pain

- The contents of the abscess are acidotic and can decrease the efficacy of the anesthetic.
- Performing a field block and administering oral pain medicine can help reduce the pain.

Drainage

- If there is little or no drainage from the abscess, consider a deeper and/or wider incision.
- If sebaceous material is extracted from the site and there is little or no pus, proceed with the procedure as described previously.

Antibiotic Therapy

- Successful incision and drainage of abscesses do not require antibiotic therapy in healthy individuals unless the abscess is accompanied by cellulitis.
- Patients who are immunocompromised, diabetic, or intravenous drug users should be considered for antibiotic treatment.
- It has been speculated that abscesses caused by community-acquired methicillin-resistant *Staphylococcus aureus* (MRSA) do not need antibiotic therapy. However, there is a paucity of data to support this at this time.

EDUCATIONAL POINTS

- Packing should be changed if persistent drainage is present, otherwise removal within 48 hours of placement is recommended during follow-up with a provider.
- Stress the importance of follow-up.
- Weigh the risks and benefits of antibiotics and pain medicine.
- Area should not get wet until the packing is removed.
- Healing occurs through tissue granulation from the base of the wound.
- Proper hygiene and handwashing are effective against recurrence and spread of infection.
- The use of a donut pillow will help to reduce the pressure on the affected area.

COMPLICATIONS

- Progression of infection to surrounding tissue causing cellulitis, lymphangitis, and/or fever should be treated with antibiotic therapy.
- Recurrence of the abscess necessitates consideration of risk factors or abnormalities, including foreign body, cancer, staph colonization, and immunologic disorders.

PEARLS

- Instruct patients who have sitting occupations to take frequent breaks or use donut pillows to reduce the pressure on the coccyx area.
- Do not forget to medicate for pain, as this can be a painful experience.

RESOURCES

Butler, K. H. (2010). Incision and drainage. In J. R. Roberts & J. R. Hedges (Eds.), *Clinical procedures in emergency medicine* (5th ed., pp. 677–679). Philadelphia, PA: Saunders Elsevier.

Coates, W. C. (2009). Disorders of the anorectum. In J. A. Marx, R. Hockberger, & R. Walls (Eds.), *Rosen's emergency medicine* (7th ed.). Philadelphia, PA: Elsevier. Retrieved from http://www.mdconsult.com/book/player/book.do?method=display&type=bookPage&decorator=header&eid=4-u1.0-B978-0-323-05472-0..00094-3–s0180&uniq=190201654&isbn=978-0-323-05472-0&sid=970898882

Fazeli, M. S., Ghavami, M., & Lebaschi, A. H. (2006). Comparison of outcomes in z plasty and delayed healing by secondary intention of the wound after excision of the sacral pilonidal sinus: Results of a randomized, clinical trial. *Diseases of the Colon and Rectum, 49*(12), 1831–1836.

Holtzman, L. C., Hitti, E., & Harrow, J. (2014). Incision and drainage. In J. R. Roberts & J. R. Hedges (Eds.), *Clinical procedures in emergency medicine* (6th ed.). Philadelphia, PA: Saunders Elsevier. Retrieved from https://www.clinicalkey.com/#!/content/book/3-s2.0-B9781455706068000379

Lanigan, M. D. (2009, August 6). *Pilonidal cyst and sinus*. Retrieved from http://emedicine.medscape.com/article/788127-overview & http://emedicine.medscape.com/article/788127-treatment

Lanigan, M. D. (2014). *Pilonidal cyst and sinus*. Retrieved from http://emedicine.medscape.com/article/788127-overview

Lee, P. J., Raniga, S., Biyani, D. K., Watson, A. J., Faragher, I. G., & Frizelli, F. A. (2008). Sacrococcygeal pilonidal disease. *Colorectal Disease, 10*(7), 639–650.

Pallin, D. J., & Nassisi, D. (2014). Skin and soft tissue infections. In J. A. Marx, R. Hockberger, & R. Walls (Eds.), *Rosen's emergency medicine* (8th ed.). Philadelphia, PA: Elsevier. Retrieved from https://www.clinicalkey.com/#!/content/book/3-s2.0-B9781455706051001378

Tajirian, T., Lee, J. L., & Abbas, M. A. (2007). Is wide local excision for pilonidal disease still justified? *The American Surgeon, 73*(10), 1075–1078.

CHAPTER **27**

Procedures for Managing
Bartholin Abscess

Theresa M. Campo

BACKGROUND

The Bartholin gland is a secretory organ approximately the size of a pea. It is located at the posterior introitus bilaterally at 5 and 7 o'clock on each side of the vestibule of the vagina. This gland drains through ducts that empty into the vestibule. It maintains the moisture of the vaginal mucosa. Obstruction of the duct may result in the formation of a cyst or abscess when there is retention of secretions, which causes the duct to dilate. A Bartholin abscess can be a common problem in women of reproductive age. It is distinguishable from a cyst in that an abscess produces a rapid onset of swelling and pain in the vulvar area. Cysts are often asymptomatic in nature. Figure 27.1 shows a Bartholin gland abscess.

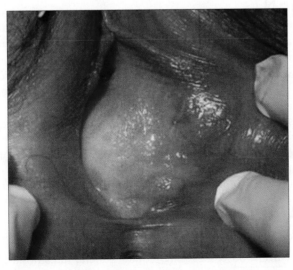

FIGURE 27.1
Bartholin abscess.

MOST COMMON ORGANISMS

Aerobic

- *Neisseria gonorrhoeae*
- *Staphylococcus aureus*
- *Streptococcus faecalis*
- *Escherichia coli*
- *Pseudomonas aeruginosa*
- *Chlamydia trachomatis*

Anaerobic

- *Bacteroides fragilis*
- *Clostridium perfringens*
- *Peptostreptococcus* species
- *Fusobacterium* species

PATIENT PRESENTATION

- Acute unilateral swelling of labia minora
- Pain with walking and sitting
- Exquisitely tender mass—grape size
- Dyspareunia—painful intercourse
- Fluctuant
- Erythema
- Spontaneous rupture with purulent drainage
- Localized cellulitis
- Systemic infection is not common with this type of abscess

TREATMENT

Simple incision and drainage with or without insertion of a word catheter is the initial treatment for a Bartholin abscess. Removal of the gland or marsupalization may be performed if recurrence is an issue but is not often considered for initial treatment. The goal of treatment is drainage of the abscess contents, prevention of fluid reaccumulation, and pain relief. Bartholin abscesses are painful, and patient comfort during the incision and drainage should be a priority.

Simple incision and drainage with and without insertion of a word catheter will be covered in this chapter. Whenever a word catheter is available, it should be used for both initial and long-term treatment, as it may obviate the need for marsupalization. The word catheter allows for epithelialization to occur.

CONTRAINDICATIONS AND RELATIVE CONTRAINDICATIONS

Complex or recurrent abscesses may require general anesthesia for removal of the Bartholin gland.

Special Considerations

- Immunocompromised patients
- Diabetics
- Cancer
- HIV-positive patients
- Pregnancy

PROCEDURE PREPARATION

- Protective gown, gloves, and goggles—abscess contents are under pressure
- Absorbent pad
- Drape
- Skin cleanser
- Lidocaine 1% (bupivacaine is another option because of its longer duration of action)
- 20- or 35-mL syringe for irrigation
- 10-mL syringe
- 25-gauge needle for injection of lidocaine
- No. 11 or No. 15 scalpel blade with handle
- Hemostat, scissors
- Culture swab
- Normal saline solution
- Plain or iodoform 1/4, 1/2, or 1 in. depending on size and depth of abscess
- Peri-pad
- Word catheter, if available or plain packing

PROCEDURE

- Cleanse the skin using a circular motion to free debris and bacteria.
- Place an absorbent protective pad under the treatment area.
- Place the patient in the lithotomy position.
- Drape the patient to maintain a clean area as well as to protect the patient's privacy.
- Strict sterile technique is not required for this procedure. However, because of the era of resistance, sterile technique should be used whenever possible.

Infiltration

- Insert a 25-gauge needle into the subcutaneous layer of the labia minora just under the mucosa.
- Infiltrate the area with lidocaine 1% (1–3 mL).

Incision

- Make a small incision along the medial mucosa at or behind the hymenal ring, not the skin, with a No. 11 scalpel.
- Use the tip of the scalpel or a hemostat to puncture the abscess cavity.
- Make an incision that is large enough to allow for proper drainage of fluid contents (Figure 27.2).

- Be careful not to puncture through the back end of the abscess wall, as this can cause excessive bleeding.
- Allow the pus to drain freely; apply pressure to the area to assist with expression of pus and abscess contents.
- With a culture swab, swab the inside of the abscess, not the drainage.
- Never use a gloved finger especially when a foreign body is suspected.
- Perform a blunt dissection with a curved hemostat in a circular motion to break up loculations.
- Irrigate the abscess liberally with normal saline.
- Insert iodoform or plain packing into the cavity.
- Place a sufficient amount of packing into the cavity making certain not to over-pack the wound causing pressure necrosis, which causes ischemia and death to the surrounding tissue.

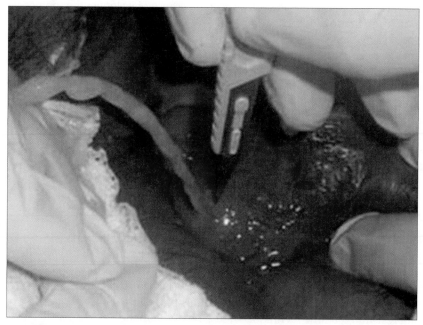

FIGURE 27.2 Incising a Batholin abscess.

Insertion of a Word Catheter

- Make the incision large enough to fit the deflated word catheter but small enough to hold the inflated balloon of the catheter in place.
- Place the deflated catheter inside the cavity (Figure 27.3).
- Using a 25-gauge needle, instill 2- to 4-mL of water into the stopper.
- Place the free end of the catheter into the vagina.
- The catheter should remain in place for 2 to 4 weeks.
- Apply a gauze dressing to help collect any drainage.
- Tetanus immunization should be up to date.
- Abscesses should not be sutured closed.

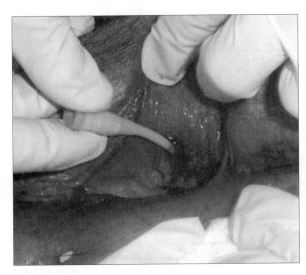

FIGURE 27.3 Insertion of Word catheter.

POST-PROCEDURE CONSIDERATIONS

Incising the Abscess
■ Failure to obtain pus or to feel a "pop" after the small incision is made in the mucosa and the cavity has been punctured may indicate a failed procedure.
■ "Skewer" the abscess onto a hemostat by stabilizing the abscess between the thumb and index finger first.

Persistent Pain
■ Can occur if too much fluid accumulation after packing or Word catheter insertion
■ Make a larger incision to facilitate proper drainage, then reinsert packing.
■ Consider the marsupalization procedure.

Word Catheter Falls Out
■ Incision too big to hold catheter in place—consider using packing
■ Word catheter reinsertion can be done if it falls out before the 2- to 4-week time period.

EDUCATIONAL POINTS
■ Packing should be changed if persistent drainage is present, otherwise removal within 48 hours of placement is recommended during follow-up with a provider.
■ Stress the importance of follow-up.
■ Risks and benefits of antibiotics and pain medicine.
■ Area should not get wet until the packing is removed.
■ Area can get wet if word catheter inserted.

- Word catheter should ideally remain in place for 2 to 4 weeks but may fall out within 1 week.
- Sexual intercourse is not contraindicated with a Word catheter insertion.

COMPLICATIONS

- Bleeding
- Progressive infection, cellulitis, and sepsis
- Recurrence

PEARLS

- Do not forget to medicate for pain, as this can be a painful experience.
- Use a peri-pad to protect clothing from drainage.
- Alert patients of the foul odor that may emanate from the abscess once it is incised. Use peppermint oil or air freshener before the procedure.
- Placing a fracture bedpan under the patient's buttocks will assist in drainage accumulation. Some abscess drain a lot of fluid and patients would not want to lie in it.

RESOURCES

Birnbauer, D. M., & Anderegg, C. (2009). Sexually transmitted diseases. In J. A. Marx, R. Hockberger & R. Walls (Eds.), *Rosen's emergency medicine* (7th ed.). Philadelphia, PA: Elsevier. Retrieved from http://www.mdconsult.com/book/player/book.do?method= display&type=bookPage&decorator=header&eid=4-u1.0-B978-0-323-05472-0..00096-7– s0035&uniq=190201654&isbn=978-0-323-05472-0&sid=970896658#lpState= open&lpTab=contentsTab&content=4-u1.0-B978-0-323-05472-0..00096-7– s0035%3Bfrom%3Dtoc%3Btype%3DbookPage%3Bisbn%3D978-0-323- 05472-0

Butler, K. H. (2010). Incision and drainage. In J. R. Roberts & J. R. Hedges (Eds.), *Clinical procedures in emergency medicine* (5th ed., pp. 674–677). Philadelphia, PA: Saunders Elsevier.

Hill, D. A., & Lense, J. J. (1998). Office management of Bartholin gland cysts and abscesses. *American Family Physician, 57*(7), 1611–1616. Retrieved from http://www.aafp.org/afp/ 980401ap/hill.html

Holtzman, L. C., Hitti, E., & Harrow, J. (2014). Incision and drainage. In J. R. Roberts & J. R. Hedges (Eds.), *Clinical procedures in emergency medicine* (6th ed.). Philadelphia, PA: Saunders Elsevier. Retrieved from https://www.clinicalkey.com/#!/content/book/3-s2.0- B9781455706068000379

Meislin, H. W., & Guisto, J. A. (2009). Soft tissue infections. In J. A. Marx, R. Hockberger, & R. Walls (Eds.), *Rosen's emergency medicine* (7th ed.). Philadelphia, PA: Elsevier. Retrieved from http://www.mdconsult.com/book/player/book.do?method=display&type=bookPage& decorator=header&eid=4-u1.0-B978-0-323-05472-0..00135-3–s0325&uniq =190201654&isbn=978-0-323-05472-0&sid=970896658

Omole, F., Simmons, B. J., & Hacker, Y. (2003). Management of Bartholin duct cyst and gland abscess. *American Family Physician, 68*(1), 135–140.

Pallin, D. J., & Nassisi, D. (2014). Skin and soft tissue infections. In J. A. Marx, R. Hockberger, & R. Walls (Eds.), *Rosen's emergency medicine* (8th ed.). Philadelphia, PA: Elsevier. Retrieved from https://www.clinicalkey.com/#!/content/book/3-s2.0-B9781455706051001378

Patil, S., Sultan, A. H., & Thaker, R. (2007). Bartholin's cysts and abscesses. *Journal of Obstetrics and Gynaecology, 27*(3), 241–245.

Peibert, J. F. (2003). Genital chlamydial infections. *New England Journal of Medicine, 349*(25), 2424–2430.

Schecter, J. C., & Quinn, A. (2009). *Bartholin gland disease.* Retrieved from http://emedicine.medscape.com/article/777112-overview & http://emedicine.medscape.com/article/777112-treatment

Schlamovitz, G. Z. (2009). *Drainage, Bartholin abscess.* Retrieved from http://emedicine.medscape.com/article/80260-overview & http://emedicine.medscape.com/article/80260-treatment

Schlamovitz, G. Z. (2014). *Bartholin abscess.* Retrieved from http://emedicine.medscape.com/article/80260-overview

Singhal, H., Kaur, K., & Bailey, R. (2014). *Skin and soft tissue infections: Incision, drainage, and debridement.* Retrieved from http://emedicine.medscape.com/article/1830144-overview

UNIT **IX**

Procedures for Examination and
Management of Common
Eye Injuries

CHAPTER **28**

Eye Examination

Larry Isaacs

BACKGROUND

Before the eye examination, taking a history and getting the timing of the complaint are important. Obtain pertinent ophthalmologic history such as surgeries, prescription drop use, or corrective glasses/contact lens use. If a chemical injury to the eye has occurred, any detailed examination should be performed after copious irrigation with water or saline of the affected eye(s).

GENERAL EYE EXAMINATION

Visual Acuity

Corrected visual acuity should be documented. If vision is severely affected, counting fingers and light perception are two measures for documenting severely impaired vision. One can use an index card with a pinhole if the patient does not have his or her glasses.

External Exam

Begin with lids/lashes, looking for swelling, discharge (matted lashes), and lacerations. Notice any proptosis, ptosis, or asymmetry. Any lid laceration on the medial third of the lid gives risk of lacrimal duct injury and should be considered for repair by an ophthalmologist.

Extraocular Movements

Cranial nerves III, IV, and VI control eye movements; cranial nerve III also controls pupillary constriction and lid elevation. Have the patient move his or her eyes in all directions, including diagonally. Globe rupture is the only contraindication in evaluating the extraocular muscles.

Pupils

Note the size, shape, and reactivity of the pupils. A teardrop-shaped pupil often indicates a globe rupture. Some patients will have 1 to 2 mm of anisocoria (pupillary size difference); this can be normal. Afferent pupillary defect (APD) is determined by the swinging flashlight test. This test should be performed under slightly dim lighting conditions. Normally, both pupils will constrict when a light is shone into one eye. In normal eyes, swinging the light back and forth will keep both pupils constricted. If the eye has a process that blocks light to the optic nerve, that eye will dilate. Optic nerve dysfunction and large hemorrhages are two causes of an APD.

Sclera and Conjunctiva

The surface of the globe is composed of the conjunctiva, sclera, and cornea. The sclera is the white, tough collagenous part of the eye that anteriorly becomes the cornea. The conjunctiva is a thin vascular membrane that covers the sclera and inner eyelids.

Cornea

The cornea is a thin, clear extension of the sclera. It is 500- to 600-μm thick, is very sensitive, and is innervated by the fifth cranial nerve. Please see the section titled "To Use Fluorescein Stain," which follows.

Anterior Chamber

This is the space between the iris and the cornea. It is filled with a clear fluid (the aqueous humor), which provides oxygen and nutrients to the cornea and lens. The slit lamp (see the following) is the best way to examine the anterior chamber.

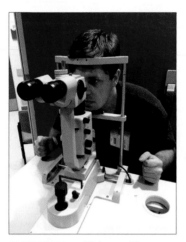

FIGURE 28.1 Slit lamp with person in proper position. Note the chin is positioned in the chin rest and the forehead remains leaning forward on the headrest.

SLIT LAMP

Patient Positioning

Have the patient sit facing the examiner, with his or her chin in the chinrest and forehead against the forehead strap (Figure 28.1). This will keep the patient's eyes within the focal range of the slit lamp.

Using the Slit Lamp

Although each slit lamp model is slightly different, the controls are generally similar (Figure 28.2). Most lamps use a joystick to focus the eyepiece. Elevation (getting the patient's eye in the center of your field) is first accomplished by grossly adjusting the chinrest up or down. The patient's eyes should be aligned with the black indicator marks on the slit lamp vertical bars. Fine tuning of elevation is then performed by spinning the joystick.

Once the eye is in focus, examine the lids/lashes for foreign bodies, debris, or lacerations. If a foreign body is suspected, be sure to evert (flip) the lids to examine behind each lid and deep into the corners.

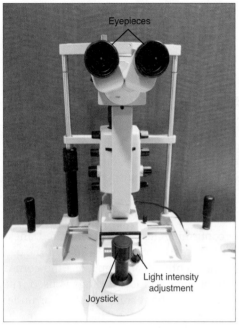 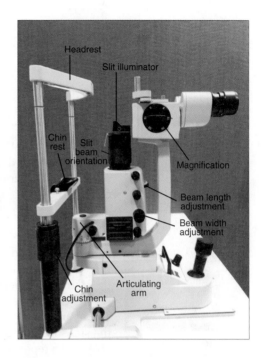

FIGURE 28.2 Two views of a slit lamp.

To View the Anterior Chamber

Swing the light source on the slit lamp toward the temporal side of the patient's head and have it project at a sharp angle across the cornea. The area between the iris and cornea should be free of cells and debris. White blood cells floating in the anterior chamber are a result of inflammation. These often look like white dust particles. "Flare" makes the anterior chamber look smoky and is a result of inflammatory proteins (note the term cells in flare). Here is where both hyphemas (blood) and hypopion (pus) are found.

Corneal Foreign Bodies and Abrasions

Shift the focus of the slit lamp to the superficial cornea. Frequently, corneal foreign bodies can be seen without the use of fluorescein stain. Fluorescein is usually needed for the detection of abrasions.

To Use Fluorescein Stain

First instill a few drops of anesthetic (i.e., proparacaine or tetracaine). The easiest way to instill drops is to pull down the lower lid, creating a well. With the patient tilting his or her head back, drop several drops into the well created by the lid. Have the patient blink several times. Once the eye is anesthetized, place one or two drops of the anesthetic onto the fluorescein strip, then touch the moistened strip to the same area where the anesthetic drops were placed—such as, into the well created by pulling down on the lower lid. Have the patient blink to distribute the stain.

Have the patient return to the slit lamp. Change the light source to cobalt blue. Again, focus on the superficial part of the cornea and look for any uptake. Corneal abrasions are usually linear; corneal ulcers are usually rounded and crater-like. Often seen with cloudy edges (edema), foreign bodies are also highlighted with the stain.

Multiple, linear, vertical abrasions suggest a foreign body under a lid. Be sure to examine under the lid.

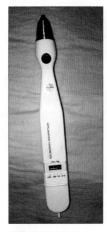

FIGURE 28.3
Commercial digital tonometer.

INTRAOCULAR PRESSURE MEASUREMENT

Most emergency departments use an electronic intraocular pressure (IOP) measuring device (i.e., Tono-Pen, Figure 28.3). The one contraindication to measuring the IOP is suspected globe rupture.

To Measure the IOP Using a Tono-Pen

Turn the device on. After confirming the device is calibrated, anesthetize the eye using drops. Place a cover (Ocu-Film) over the pen tip. With the patient supine, gently tap the tip onto the cornea several times; the average of three to four readings is used. The Tono-Pen will give the average of the readings with a bar under the statistical reliability of the readings. More than 20% is unreliable, and a repeat examination should proceed.

A reading less than 20 mmHg is normal; between 21 and 30 mmHg should be referred for urgent ophthalmologic evaluation. Readings above 30 mmHg require initiation of treatment to lower the IOP and emergent referral.

The Schiotz tonometer was historically used to measure IOP. However, other modalities, such as the Tono-Pen and applanation tonometry, have replaced this technique.

PEARLS

- Be sure the tonometer is moving freely—test on the small plate that usually is attached to the box.
- Be sure to rest your hand(s) on the orbital rim while opening the lids, not on the globe, as this will cause an increase in IOP.
- Corneal ulcer can easily be missed and must be looked for during every eye exam.

RESOURCE

Varma, R. (1997). *Essentials of eye care: The Johns Hopkins Wilmer handbook* (pp. 26–38). Philadelphia, PA: Lippincott Raven.

CHAPTER **29**

Managing Eye Injuries

Larry Isaacs

FOREIGN-BODY REMOVAL

Background

Although ocular trauma accounts for a small percentage of emergency department (ED) visits, its potential for life-changing consequences for the patient are high. During the initial assessment, there are questions to ask the patient that are important, both for documentation and to provide clues to the nature of the injury. However, do not delay irrigation, if indicated, to ask these questions. The following is a partial list of questions to ask the patient: What was the patient doing? Does the patient wear contact lens or glasses? Was the patient wearing protective glasses? Is there a foreign-body sensation? Was there a potential for a high-speed projectile?

Patient Presentation

- Pain
- Blurry vision
- Tearing
- Foreign body
- Foreign-body sensation

Treatment

First, one must determine if the foreign body is superficial or penetrating. Foreign-body removal can be accomplished with a cotton-tipped applicator or needle, and/or irrigation. The suspected object and the location and depth of the object determine the type of removal. Prior to any assessment and intervention of the eye(s), a visual acuity should always be performed.

Contraindications and Relative Contraindications

- Open globe, intraocular foreign body

Special Considerations

- Some deep corneal foreign bodies may not be amenable to ED removal—referral to ophthalmology is appropriate.
- A cooperative patient is necessary.

Procedure Preparation

- Fluorescein stain
- Ophthalmic anesthetic
- Cotton-tipped applicator
- Insulin syringe or small-gauge (27–30 gauge) needle with syringe
- Slit lamp
- Ophthalmoscope

Procedure

- Instill two drops of anesthetic.
- With the patient in the slit lamp, use an insulin syringe and a cotton swab wetted with anesthetic.
- Have the patient fix his or her gaze.
- Hold the syringe with your thumb and index fingers, resting your fifth digit and medial (ulnar) side of your hand on the patient's face (around the inferior orbital rim) for support (Figure 29.1A).
- While looking through the slit lamp, move the syringe slowly toward the patient's eye, following the syringe needle as it comes into focus.
  - Once in focus with the bevel of the needle facing you, slowly and gently attempt to flick the foreign body out of the cornea.
  - Do not dig deeply into the cornea.
  - If the foreign body sticks superficially to the cornea, take the wetted cotton swab and touch it to the now-freed foreign body and it will often stick to the swab (Figure 29.1B).

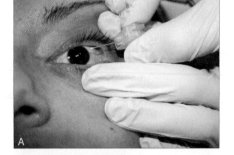
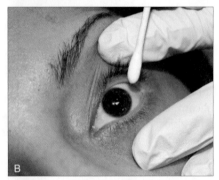

FIGURE 29.1A and 29.1B Foreign-body removal from the eye: **A.** using a small gauge needle first, followed by **B.** a wet cotton swab. Note this is generally accomplished using a slit lamp and is pictured here without a slit lamp for clarity.

RUST RING REMOVAL

Metallic foreign bodies will often leave a "rust ring"—a rust colored stain of the cornea. These patients will need follow-up with an ophthalmologist for removal of the rust ring. Topical antibiotics are indicated here, drops being more convenient for adults (i.e., polytrim) and ointment (erythromycin) for young children. If the patient wears contact lenses, then the antibiotic choice should cover *Pseudomonas* (i.e., ciprofloxacin, tobramycin, or gentamycin).

Cyanoacrylate Glue

These glues can cause a chemical keratitis upon corneal contact. They also may attach to the lid margins. Do not force the lids open if glued shut. Applying petroleum-based products (erythromycin ointment, over-the-counter antibiotic ointment, or petroleum jelly) to the lids or placing on the cornea will degrade the glue in a short time. Gentle rubbing may be required.

Post-Procedure Considerations

Rust rings should be addressed by an ophthalmologist. Cyanoacrylate glues on the cornea can leave a large, painful defect.

Educational Points

- Do not rub the eye.
- Advise the patient that irritation may return when the anesthetic wears off, but it should resolve on its own.
- Nonsteroidal anti-inflammatory medications can be taken for discomfort.
- Antibiotic ointment is often prescribed though supporting literature is scant.
- Do not use an eye patch.

Complications

- Corneal abrasion
- Infection

PEARLS

- Do not cause more damage when attempting to remove a corneal foreign body; if it is deeply embedded, an ophthalmologist may be required.
- Removal of a rust ring is not an emergency; here again, ophthalmology follow-up is all that is required.
- Corneal abrasions present similarly to foreign bodies
- High-speed metal (welding, grinding of metal) in the presentation of a foreign-body sensation demands ocular imaging (ultrasound and or CT scan) in order to rule out an intraocular foreign body.
- Multiple linear corneal abrasions, the "ice-rink sign," may result from an embedded foreign body adhered to the upper lid. The lid should always be everted fully and inspected.

CHEMICAL SUBSTANCE REMOVAL

Background

For both liquid and solid ocular injuries, the key is dilution with saline. Even before a complete ocular examination, irrigation should begin. Use of either normal saline or lactated Ringer's solution is appropriate. Alkaline substances cause a liquefactive necrosis; therefore, increased morbidity than with acidic substances, which induce a coagulative and more superficial necrosis.

Patient Presentation

- Pain
- Burning
- Tearing
- Photophobia
- Blurry vision

Treatment

- Immediate irrigation with normal saline or tap water if saline is not readily available.

Contraindications and Relative Contraindications

- Open globe

Special Considerations

- Alkaline versus acidic substance

Procedure Preparation

- Ophthalmic anesthetic
- Absorbent pads
- Large basin
- Normal saline or Ringer's lactate (liter bags intravenous [IV] solution)
- IV tubing or commercial device (Morgan lens)
- pH paper (litmus)

Procedure

IV Tubing

- Connect the normal saline or Ringer's lactate to the IV tubing and run it through.
- Instill several drops of anesthetic.
- Place an absorbent pad under the patient's head.
- Place the patient in Trendelenburg position.
- Place a large basin beneath the patient's head.
- Retract the eyelid.
- Instill several liters of fluid into the eye until a pH of 7.0 is achieved.

Morgan Lens

- Retract the eyelids.
- Place an absorbent pad under the patient's head.
- Place the patient in Trendelenburg position.
- Place a large basin beneath the patient's head.
- Place the lens under both the upper and lower lid directly onto eye.
- Connect the normal saline or Ringer's lactate to the IV tubing and run it through.
- Instill several liters of fluid into the eye until a pH of 7.0 is achieved.

Post-Procedure Considerations

- Check for corneal abrasions.

Educational Points

- Do not rub the eye.
- Advise the patient that irritation may return when the anesthetic wears off, but it should resolve on its own.
- Nonsteroidal anti-inflammatory medications can be taken for discomfort.

> ### PEARL
>
> - You can connect the end of the intravenous tubing to the end of a nasal cannula if irrigation of both eyes is required.

CONTACT LENS REMOVAL

Background

Most contact lens wearers can remove their own lenses. If they cannot find the lenses on their eyes, you may need to assist with removal. Contact lenses may need to be removed for a full eye examination by the provider. Even lenses that are manufactured to be worn for long periods of time place the person at risk for *Pseudomonas* infection and corneal ulceration. Some contact lenses "fall out" of a person's eye without his or her knowledge. A full examination should be completed to ensure that the lens is not caught in the fornices.

Patient Presentation

- Foreign-body sensation
- Pain
- Redness
- Irritation

Treatment

- Removal of the contact lens is required

Procedure Preparation

- Ophthalmic anesthetic drops
- Fluorescein stain (may permanently discolor lens)
- Cotton-tipped applicator
- Normal saline and IV tubing
- Commercially available suction cups

Procedure

- First ask whether the patient wears hard or soft lens. If the wearer cannot find the lens, it is usually up in the fornices (the deep corners behind the lids). Everting the lid may help find it.
- You can use fluorescein, but remember that this will permanently discolor the lens.
- While placing traction on the lid, have the patient look to all four quadrants and often you will find the lens stuck to the globe.
- Sometimes anesthetic drops are necessary.
- A wet cotton-tipped applicator can also be used to move the lens.
- Once found, move it to the center of the cornea, where it can be removed.
- If the lens is adherent, irrigating with saline and a soft catheter will often loosen it.

- Soft contacts, once found, can be gently squeezed between the thumb and forefinger (this will break the suction).
- Irrigation will not break the seal when removing a hard lens. Commercially available suction cups will adhere to the lens for removal.
- Always do a fluorescein examination after removal.

Post-Procedure Considerations
Fluorescein Stain Uptake

- If there is uptake, remember to prescribe an antipseudomonal antibiotic drop.

Educational Points

- Do not wear contact lenses until symptom free.
- Follow up with an optometrist/ophthalmologist.

Complications

- Corneal abrasion

PEARL
■ Once you locate the lens, you can sometimes let the patient attempt removal.

RESOURCES

http://emedicine.medscape.com/article/799316-overview
http://www.ncbi.nlm.nih.gov/pubmed/12085075
http://www.ncbi.nlm.nih.gov/pmc/articles/PMC2579545
http://www.ncbi.nlm.nih.gov/pmc/articles/PMC3779420
http://www.ncbi.nlm.nih.gov/pmc/articles/PMC3484698

CHAPTER **30**

Ocular Ultrasound

Keith A. Lafferty

BACKROUND

Ultrasound technology has become integral in clinical arenas and its use in imaging ocular pathology underlines its many proven uses. The direct (standard) ophthalmoscope is currently still in clinical practice and has not changed much since its inception in the medical world in 1915 (see Figure 30.1). Its use is far inferior to indirect ophthalmoscopy using mirrors and curved lenses. Fortunately, the eye is somewhat the perfect organ for bedside sonography as it is anteriorly positioned and, for the most part, it is fluid filled, allowing minimally inhibited conduction throughout all parts. Also, with ultrasound, dilatation is unnecessary.

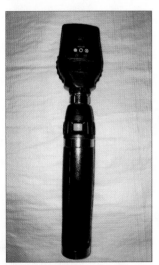

FIGURE 30.1 Direct ophthalmoscope

Vision-threatening pathology of this vital organ can be insidious and delayed diagnosis can lead to the depletion and/or loss of one of our greatest sense organs. As challenging as it is for the nonspecialist to diagnose posterior eye pathology using an antiquated ophthalmoscope, the opposite is true when the nonspecialist uses bedside ultrasonography. The focus of this chapter is on posterior pathology.

RETINAL DETACHMENT

The retina is normally tightly bound and "tacked down" to the posterior/lateral wall of the eye and is attached in two places: posteriorly at its origin, the *optic nerve*, and anterior laterally, at the *ora serrata* (serrated junction between the retina and the cilliary body where the anterior lateral non-photosensitive area of the retina is tethered down). All retina detachments will be easily sonographically visualized somewhere between these two anchored areas of fixation. This photosensitive tissue has no pain fibers and therefor this condition is painless. Retinal detachment is any separation of the retina with the choroid and occurs at a rate of in 1 in 300 over a lifetime. It will appear to be free floating, but will not continue to undulate or tumble when the patient stops moving the eye (in contrast to posterior vitreous detachment). Acute retinal detachments are attached in two places, whereas chronic detachments may be attached in one location. Next to central retinal artery occlusion, chemical burns to the eye, and endophthalmitis, it is one of the most time-critical eye emergencies encountered in the emergency setting.

Treatment in all cases generally involves "tacking down" the retina in order to halt its ongoing retinal detachment progression. In smaller tears, this usually is accomplished via laser photocoagulation or cryopexy. Larger and "mac on" (macula not involved) tears are treated more aggressively in order to preserve this vital area. With prompt diagnosis, 90% of tears can be successfully treated, although sometimes a second treatment is needed. There are three types of detachments:

- Rhegmatogenous
  - Most common type
  - Results when a tear/break in the neuronal inner retinal layer allows fluid from the vitreous to seep in-between the retina and the choroid
- Traction
  - Results from adhesions between the vitreous gel and the retina
- Exudative
  - Results from exudation of material into the subretinal space from retinal vessels
    - Hypertension
    - Central retinal venous occlusion
    - Vasculitis
    - Papilledema

Risks include:

- Age 40 years or older
- History of retinal detachment
- Family history
- Recent cataract/eye surgery
- Recent eye trauma
- Myopia

Symptoms include:

- Visual field defect (localizes detachment area)
  - May be described as a curtain closing from the side
- Photopsia—flashing lights, or a "curtain" over the field of vision
  - Not pathognomonic as can be seen in:
    - Posterior vitreous detachment
    - Migraine aura
    - Occipital lobe cerebral vascular accident (CVA)
- Floaters—vitreous blood
  - Note that floaters are not pathognomonic for blood as they can also be from aging vitreous gel strand formation.

POSTERIOR VITREOUS DETACHMENT

This is a common disorder found in 23% of autopsy cases, increasing throughout the life span to more than 50% in those older than 80 years. Many detachments are asymptomatic and usually occur spontaneously but may occur secondary to trauma or irritation secondary to recent ocular surgery or disease. Aging induces degeneration and break down of the vitreous gel causing it to liquefy in some areas and shrink in others.

The fluid collects in pockets/cavities, and thick strands of the gel form and drift through the eye and appear as floaters. When these changes occur suddenly, the vitreous membrane separates from the retina and a posterior vitreous detachment arises. Usually of little sequelae and the floaters resolve over time, the biggest fear is the formation of a traction-induced rhegmatogenous retinal tear. Risks include:

- Age 60 years or older
- Myopia
- Status after cataract surgery
- Facial trauma

Symptoms include:

- Floaters
  - May be prominent
- Photopsia

Posterior vitreous detachments will look similar to a retinal detachment, except:

- In contrast to a retinal detachment, a posterior vitreous detachment is only attached to the choroid in one place.
- A posterior vitreous detachment will be thinner and more difficult to see without the ultrasound gain set very high.
- There will be "after-movements"—having the patient move his or her eye will create undulations of the structure that continue after the eye has stopped moving.

VITREOUS HEMORRHAGE

Diabetic retinopathy is the leading cause of vitreous hemorrhage in adults, as fragile blood vessels spontaneously hemorrhage. Blood in vitreous hemorrhage can be solid, liquefied, or both. The solid blood is often found in the middle of the posterior chamber, liquefied blood will layer more posteriorly. Risks include:

- Trauma
  - Leading cause of hemorrhage in the young
- Retinal detachment
- Posterior vitreous detachment
- Sickle cell retinopathy
- Macular degeneration
- Central retinal vein occlusion

Symptoms include:

- Floaters
- Blurry vision
- Reddish tint to vision

GLOBE RUPTURE/INTRAOCULAR FOREIGN BODY

Any complete violation to the cornea or sclera is defined as an open globe injury. This is an ophthalmologic emergency and mandates immediate ophthalmology consultation. Globe rupture may occur when a blunt object impacts the orbit, compressing the globe, and inducing a sudden and transient elevation in intraocular pressure, resulting in a scleral tear. Ruptures from blunt trauma are most common at the sites where the sclera is thinnest, at the insertions of the extraocular muscles, limbus, and at the site of previous intraocular surgery. Sharp or small missile bodies traveling at high velocity may directly pierce the globe directly. The possibility of globe rupture should be considered and ruled out during the evaluation of all blunt and penetrating orbital/facial traumas as well as in all cases involving high-speed projectiles with potential for ocular penetration. One third of all cases of childhood blindness are secondary to ocular trauma.

> **NOTE** *The clinician must maintain a high clinical suspicion, as most cases are occult and the detection of very small scleral wounds are challenging to visualize, even for the astute provider.*

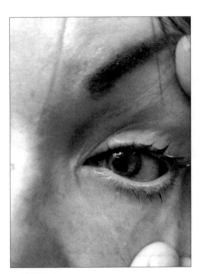

FIGURE 30.2 Tear-shaped pupil secondary to a corneal violation. Note irregular pupil and scleral injection.

On examination:

- Eccentric/teardrop pupil (Figure 30.2)
- Projecting foreign body in eye
- Diminished visual acuity
  - Afferent pupillary defect (APD)
- Extrusion of vitreous
- External prolapse of the iris, ciliary body, or choroid (black tissue)
- Tenting of the sclera or cornea at the site of globe puncture
- Volume loss of eye/misshapen globe
- Hyphemia
- Flat anterior surface

Risks for permanent visual impairment include:

- Initial poor visual
- Wounds extending posterior to rectus muscle insertion plane
- Wound length greater than 10 mm
- Blunt or missile injury

Symptoms include:

- Pain
  - May not be severe in sharp injuries with or without an intraocular foreign body.
    - Vitreous humor and retina have no pain fibers
- Diplopia
  - Usually caused by entrapment and dysfunction of extraocular muscles with associated orbital floor blowout fractures.
    - May be caused by traumatic cranial nerve palsy from associated head injury.

LENS DISLOCATION

Most common secondary to cases of blunt trauma. Hereditary presentations are usually bilateral and associated with other disorders such as Marfan's syndrome. The lens can migrate either to the anterior chamber or become free-floating in the posterior vitreous or become subluxed and remain partially within the lens fossa. Vision is blurred if the lens is dislocated out of the line of vision; however, if the dislocation is partial the visual prognosis is favorable. Iritis and glaucoma (pupillary block) are common complications. Nonsurgical corrective lenses usually are the treatment needed to accommodate for the refractive error. Indications for surgery include:

> **NOTE** *A quivering iris may be a symptom of lens dislocation, due to the lack of lens attachment and support.*

- Anterior chamber dislocation
- Uveitis
- Glaucoma
- Lens opacification with poor visual function
- Refractive error not amenable to optical correction

Symptoms include:

- Monocular diplopia
- Injected painful eye in cases of trauma

ANATOMY

It behooves the reader to review the eye's basic anatomy and then learn its appearance on normal sonography. Only then can bedside ultrasonography be utilized to quickly and competently ensure rapid eye pathology diagnosis (**Figure** 30.3).

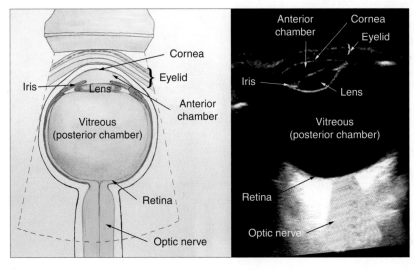

FIGURE 30.3 Normal eye anatomy sketch and ultrasound images side by side with similar labels.

- Cornea
  - Most anterior image below the skin
- Anterior chamber
  - Fluid-filled area between the cornea and the lens
  - Anechoic
- Iris
  - Rounded and beneath the cornea and anterior to the lens
- Lens
  - Posterior to the iris
  - Hyperechoic image
    - Posterior reflection waves seen

- Posterior chamber
  - Fluid-filled area posterior to the lens
  - Anechoic
- Vitreous body
  - Filled with vitreous gel
    - Encased on a vitreous membrane
  - Allows the eye to maintain its spherical structure
- Sclera
  - Outermost portion of the eye
- Choroid
  - Medial to the sclera and lateral to the retina
  - The choroid is the vascular layer and provides oxygen and nourishment to the outer layers of the retina
- Retina
  - Innermost portion
  - In the normal eye, the retina, choroid, and sclera are seen sonographically as one layer
  - Arising from a splaying of the posteriorly derived optic nerve and is composed of photoreceptors
    - Responsible for vision
    - Oxygen dependent on the adjacent lateral (medial to the sclera) choroid layer
- Macula
  - Lateral to the optic nerve
  - Indentation of the retina
  - Highest concentration of photoreceptors
  - Responsible for central vision
- Fovea
  - Most central part of the macula
  - Highest number of photoreceptors in the macula
- Optic nerve
  - Posterior to the retina
  - Hypoechoic
  - By use of ultrasound measurement one can obtain a high sensitivity for detecting elevated intracranial pressure (see Chapter 55, "Lumbar Puncture").

CONTRAINDICATIONS
- None

RELATIVE CONTRAINDICATIONS
- Globe rupture
  - It is imperative that the clinician does not place any pressure with the ultrasound probe on the globe itself, which may further increase the extrusion of intraocular contents.
  - Use adequate gel interface and do not exert probe pressure on the eye.

The literature argues that ultrasound may be especially useful when periorbital edema and pain interfere with the examination of the posttraumatic eye. Chandra et al. (2009) have shown that emergency residents were able to sonographically examine traumatically ruptured ocular globes with a relatively high sensitivity while inducing a minimal increase in intraocular pressure of 5%.

- Diagnosis should be avoided via this modality:
    - CT availability
    - Obvious clinical diagnosis

SPECIAL CONSIDERATION

Use the paper clip method to evaluate the globe when lids are swollen (**Figure** 30.4).

PROCEDURE PREPARATION

- Bedside ultrasound machine
- Linear array high-frequency ultrasound probe (vascular)
- Ultrasound gel
    - Use a thick layer of gel so that the probe minimally or does not touch the eye.
    - Lubricating jelly may be less irritating.

PROCEDURE

- Place the patient in the supine position.
- Place at least 1 to 2 cm of gel on the closed lid.
- Hold the probe like a pencil, resting your fingers and not holding the probe on the patient's cheek and brow.
- Have the patient keep the eye in a neutral position to start.
- The ultrasound marker should be in the lateral orientation with the image to the left.
- Scan horizontally, vectoring fully, superiorly, and inferiorly throughout the entire retina.
    - To visualize the entire retina, have the patient look up, then you scan superiorly and look down while you scan inferiorly.
- It is important to make use of a *kinetic examination.*
    - Have the patient move the eyes around at some point in order to help differentiate mimicking other posterior pathologies.

For added sensitivity, rotate the probe marker to the up position and scan in the vertical plane, scanning fully side to side (Figure 30.5) (**Video 30.1**).

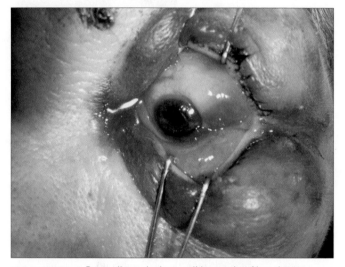

FIGURE 30.4 Paper-clip method on eyelid retraction. Note that no pressure is exerted on the globe itself and full examination is accomplished.

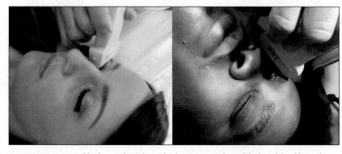

FIGURE 30.5 Horizontal and vertical eye scanning side by side. Note the thick layer of gel over the patients closed eyelid.

- To visualize the entire retina, have the patient look medially and angle the probe medially, then have the patient look laterally and angle the probe laterally.

Specific Pathologic Findings
Retinal Detachment (Figure 30.6)

- Clinician will see the retina separated/detached from the choroid, as the dissecting hypoechoic vitreous fluid will be evident.
- The free retina will move about in a serpentine/membrane-like manner upon kinetic examination.

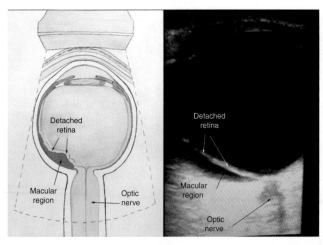

FIGURE 30.6 Ultrasound image of a retinal detachment next to a labeled sketch. Note the detachment is just lateral to the optic nerve and therefore is a "mac off" type. This means that the macula has been detached; therefore, urgent treatment is less critical.

- No matter how large the tear is, the retina will always be tethered at the optic nerve and the ora serrata.
- May see an accompanying vitreous hemorrhage.

Vitreous Detachment (Figure 30.7)

- Use the kinetic examination to delineate from retinal detachment
  - The congealed material "tumbles" around

Vitreous Hemorrhage (Figure 30.8) (Video 30.2)

- Hyperechoic "snow flakes" or "speckles" represent vitreous blood
- May have to increase the gain for full visualization

Globe Rupture (Figures 30.9 and 30.10)

- Loss of normal circular shape
- Decrease in the size of the globe
- Anterior chamber collapse
- Loss of the normal demarcation between the anterior and posterior chambers
  - Lens may be displaced or not identified

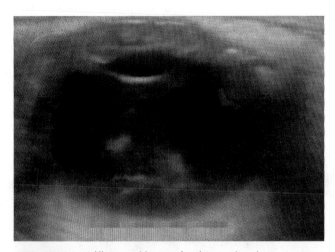

FIGURE 30.7 Ultrasound image of a vitreous detachment. Note congealed-like vitreous material in the vitreous body and the nonpresence of "speckles" or a retinal detachment.

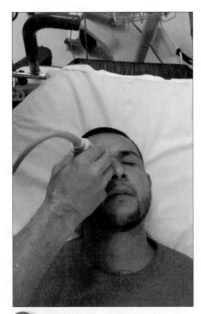

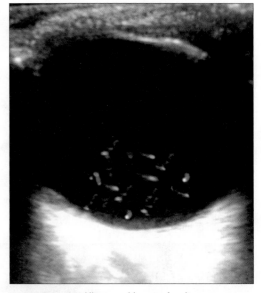

VIDEO 30.1 Horizontal and vertical eye scanning.
springerpub.com/campo

FIGURE 30.8 Ultrasound image of a vitreous hemorrhage.

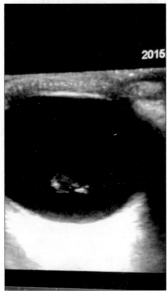

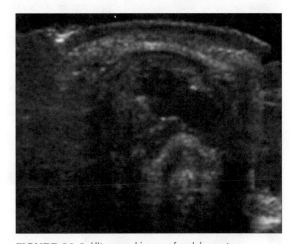

FIGURE 30.9 Ultrasound image of a globe rupture.

VIDEO 30.2 Vitreous hemorrhage.
springerpub.com/campo

- Echogenicity of the normal anechoic posterior chamber
- Buckling of the sclera
- CT has higher sensitivity (**Figure 30.10**).

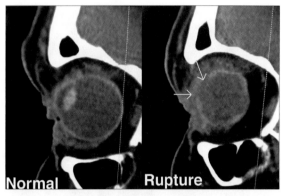

FIGURE 30.10 CT of globe rupture. Note the regular round appearance of the normal globe and the irregular appearance/indentation of the ruptured globe.

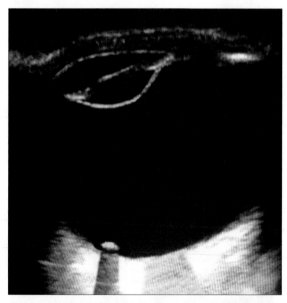

FIGURE 30.11 Ultrasound identification of intraocular foreign body.

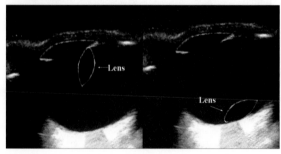

FIGURE 30.12 Lens subluxation and a posterior lens dislocation, side by side.

Intraocular Foreign Body (Figure 30.11)

- Bright echogenic acoustic profile of the foreign body
- Shadowing or reverberation artifacts may be seen
- CT has higher sensitivity

Lens Dislocation (Figure 30.12)

POST-PROCEDURE CONSIDERATIONS

- Ensure all the gel is removed from the patient.
- Clean the probe as previously described.
- A firm protective eye shield should immediately and properly be placed wtih diagnosis of a globe rupture.

EDUCATIONAL POINTS

- When sonographically evaluating anterior structures, have the depth set to limit posterior viewing.
- Practicing and learning the ultrasound appearance of normal eye structures is key to confidently and rapidly diagnosing intraocular pathology.
- Initial gain setting should be low, but expect to increase it during exam, especially when evaluating possible blood in the posterior or anterior chamber.
- The direct ophthalmoscope is insufficient for comprehensive examination because of the lower magnification and illumination, absence of stereopsis, and incomplete view of the retina.
- Though floaters are a nonspecific symptom, the sudden onset of large floaters in the center of the visual field may indicate posterior vitreous detachment.
- If a retinal detachment is just lateral to the optic nerve, it probably involves the macula and, in such cases, the visual acuity may be severely reduced.

- "Mac on" retinal detachments require urgent ophthalmological evaluation.
- A physical exam finding of a full-thickness laceration to the cornea or sclera, evidence of extruded intraocular contents, or an irregular/teardrop pupil signifies an open globe perforation and an immediate ophthalmology consultation is in order.

PEARLS

- Any separation of the retina is considered a retinal detachment.
- In retinal detachment, time lost means photoreceptors and hence vision lost/loss.
- Retinal tissue is stimulated by light and traction, so when the vitreous membrane separates from the retina or the retina tears one experiences photopsia (the sensation of light).
- Any debris, speckles, or material seen sonographically in the vitreous humor is considered pathologic.
- Upon kinetic ultrasound eye examination, posterior vitreous detachment appears as congealed material tumbling about, similar to clothes in a dryer.
- Globe rupture can present occultly because the most frequent sites are not easily visualized, and more superficial injuries may hinder examination of the posterior segment.
- Metal on metal contact injuries constitute a major risk for missile intraocular foreign bodies and one must maintain a high index of suspicion in such cases.

RESOURCES

Acerra, J. R. (2014). *Globe rupture*. Retrieved from http://emedicine.medscape.com/article/798223-overview#showall

Chandra, A., Mastrovich, T., Ladner, H., Ting, V., Radeos, M. S., & Samudre, S. (2009). The utility of bedside ultrasound in the detection of a ruptured globe in a porcine model. *Western Journal of Medicine, 10*(4), 263–266. Retrieved from http://www.ncbi.nlm.nih.gov/pmc/articles/PMC2791730/

Foos, R. Y. (1972). Posterior vitreous detachment. *Transactions of the American Academy of Ophthalmology and Otolaryngology, 76*, 480–497.

Pandya, H. P. (2014). *Retinal detachment*. Retrieved from http://emedicine.medscape.com/article/798501-overview#showall

Sonosite e-learning. (n.d.). *Sonosite e-learning*. Retrieved from https://www.sonosite.com/education/learning-center/58/9567 & https://www.sonosite.com/education/learning-center/58/9568

Thelen, U., Amler, S., Osada, N., & Gerding, H. (2012). Outcome of surgery after macula-off retinal detachment—Results from MUSTARD, one of the largest databases on buckling surgery in Europe. *Acta Ophthamologica Scandinavica, 90*(5), 481–486. doi:10.1111/j.1755-3768.2010.01939

UNIT **X**

**Procedures for Managing
Common Nasal Conditions**

CHAPTER 31

Procedures for Controlling Epistaxis

Larry Isaacs

BACKGROUND

Epistaxis, or nose bleeding, is a common condition, usually self-limited, with a peak incidence from ages 2 to 10 and 50 to 80. Bleeding usually occurs when the mucosa erodes into superficial blood vessels. More than 90% of bleeding comes from the anterior area (Kiesselbach's plexus); posterior bleeds are harder to control, with increased risk of airway compromise and aspiration. With the exception of trauma, anterior epistaxis is most often unilateral. Posterior bleeding tends to be present in older patients and may cause bilateral epistaxis. The patient often complains of blood going down the back of the throat.

PATIENT PRESENTATION

- Bleeding from the nose and/or mouth
- Dizziness
- Skin is pale and sweaty
- Anxiety

TREATMENT

The treatment for epistaxis can be direct pressure, vasoconstrictors (phenylephrine), cautery (silver nitrate), or packing. Before any of these techniques, to alleviate anxiety, reassure the patient; explain that identification of the source is imperative.

CONTRAINDICATIONS AND RELATIVE CONTRAINDICATIONS

- Significant facial fractures with suspected or confirmed basilar skull fracture

SPECIAL CONSIDERATIONS

Patients who are currently on antiplatelet agents (aspirin, nonsteroidal anti-inflammatory drugs [NSAIDs], clopidogrel) or blood thinners (i.e., warfarin, clopido-grel bisulfate, enoxaparin) and patients with uncontrolled hypertension are at greater risk for epistaxis. Treatment of underlying hypertension and coagulopathies will have an impact on the treatment.

PROCEDURE PREPARATION

- Personal protective equipment (gown, gloves, mask/eye shields)
- Absorbent pad
- Small or large basin
- Gauze
- Nose clip
- Cotton balls
- Vasoconstrictor
  - Oxymetazoline, phenylephrine, or 4% cocaine solution
- Lidocaine 4% or lidocaine 2% with epinephrine-soaked gauze
- Silver nitrate cautery
- Nasal packing/tampon
  - Ribbon gauze impregnated with petroleum jelly
  - Commercially prepared (Rhino Rocket, Gelfoam, Surgicel, and Floseal)
- Bayonet forceps

PROCEDURE

- Place absorbable pad on the upright patient's chest and place a basin on the lap.
  - The basin is useful if patient spits up any blood or to place any used gauze and so on.
- Have the patient blow the nose to remove any clots.
- Have the patient hold direct, firm pressure on the external naris for 5 to 20 minutes, tilting the head forward (to prevent swallowing of blood).
- Instill a vasoconstrictor.
  - Leave in for 10 to 15 minutes.
  - This often temporarily stops the bleeding, giving you a view of the culprit vessel for definitive hemostasis.
- Instill anesthesia.
  - Lidocaine 4% or lidocaine 2% with epinephrine-soaked gauze.
  - Leave in place for 5 to 10 minutes.
- If the culprit vessel is seen, you can try to inject the area with a 27-gauge syringe using lidocaine 2% with epinephrine to achieve hemostasis.

When hemostasis is achieved:

- The simplest way to achieve definitive treatment is by using silver nitrate cautery.
- Locate the vessel/area of the bleeding.
- Using one stick at a time, roll the tip on the mucosa until a dark gray eschar is formed.
- Be sure to tell the patient that he or she may need to sneeze, so have the patient turn his or her head away from you and to sneeze through the mouth.

If silver nitrate is unable to achieve hemostasis, the site of bleeding is too difficult to locate, or the bleeding is too diffuse, the next step is some type of nasal packing/tampon:

- Layer the ribbon gauze from bottom to top.
  - Layering the gauze (impregnated with petroleum jelly), from bottom to top, does work, but it is time consuming.

Commercial Product (Figure 31.1)

- With slow, gentle pressure, push the device into the naris on a horizontal plane, until the entire device is inside.
- If the device has a balloon, have the patient tell you when he or she begins to feel the pressure as you inflate; that is when you stop.
- Too much pressure can lead to pressure necrosis of the septum.

Coat the dry packing devices with antibiotic ointment, rather than placing them dry. This helps with comfort and helps prevent toxic shock syndrome (having a tampon/packing in place puts the patient at risk for toxic shock).

- After the device is placed, examine the posterior pharynx.
- Some blood behind the uvula is normal, and should stop; however, a constant flow of blood suggests a posterior bleed.
- Posterior bleeds are more dangerous (because of aspiration risk and difficulty controlling the source).
- There are some commercial devices that control posterior bleeds but understand that posterior bleeds should be admitted to the hospital.
- Thrombin kits are available, although they require mixing a thrombin powder with the saline diluent prior to use.
  - After it is drawn up in a 5-mL syringe, a special nasal drug delivery device is attached.
  - The contoured tip is inserted into the naris, and the solution is sprayed as a fine mist across the nasal mucosa.
  - Approximately half (2.5 mL) should be used initially and the remainder utilized after 3 to 5 minutes if bleeding persists.

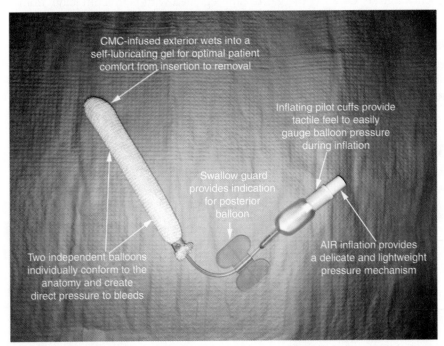

FIGURE 31.1 Commercially available inflatable balloons. This Rhino Rocket product is composed of an inflatable balloon coated with a carboxymethylcellulose hydrocolloid compound that acts as a platelet aggregator and also forms a lubricant on contact with water.

POST-PROCEDURE CONSIDERATIONS

- Antibiotic prophylaxis
  - Though used frequently, evidence is lacking in support of prophylactically preventing sinusitis and systemic infections.
- Antistaphylococcal coverage
  - Cephalexin or amoxicillin-clavulanate
  - Clindamycin or amoxicillin-clavulanate
- Refer to an otolaryngologist for packing removal in 2 to 3 days

EDUCATIONAL POINTS

- Do not remove the packing.
- Do not blow the nose.
- Sneeze with the mouth open.
- Keep head elevated, avoid bending below the waist for 2 to 3 days.

COMPLICATIONS

- Bleeding

PEARLS

- Using ribbon gauze with bayonet forceps was, in the past, the standard way to pack a nose. Layering the gauze (impregnated with petroleum jelly), from bottom to top, does work, but it is time consuming.
- One of the many commercial devices (i.e., Rapid Rhino, Rhino Rocket, Gelfoam, Surgicel, or Floseal) is certainly quicker and easier to use than ribbon gauze.
- Follow the directions that come with the device (for the tampons). For products like Gelfoam/Surgicel, place a small piece of the product on the bleeding septum.

RESOURCES

Gifford, T. O., & Orlandi, R. R. (2008). Epistaxis. *Otolarngologic Clinics of North America*, 41(3), 525–536. http://www.acep.org/Clinical—Practice-Management/Focus-On–Treatment-of-Epistaxis

Kucik, C. J., & Clenney, T. (2005). Management of epistaxis. *American Family Physician*, 71(2), 305–312.

CHAPTER **32**

Procedures for Removing Nasal Foreign Body

Larry Isaacs

BACKGROUND

This is usually a problem in young children, as adults are rarely leaving objects deep in their nose (except for psychiatric and mentally disabled adults). The history given by a parent or a caregiver, or the presence on evaluation of significant unilateral nasal discharge, should prompt a search for a foreign body.

Nasal foreign bodies can be organic or nonorganic—they are commonly toys, beads, paper, nuts, and food. Button batteries can cause tissue erosion and ulceration and, if left in place for prolonged periods of time, can lead to necrosis and septal perforation.

PATIENT PRESENTATION

- Pain
- Discharge
- Visible foreign body
- Anxiety

TREATMENT

Removal of the foreign body is necessary but not always achieved in the office, urgent, or emergency settings and referral to an otolaryngologist is required. Some food, such as candy, usually dissolves before removal is possible.

CONTRAINDICATIONS AND RELATIVE CONTRAINDICATIONS

None

SPECIAL CONSIDERATIONS

Procedural sedation and sometimes the operating room/short procedure unit are required to remove deep objects.

PROCEDURE PREPARATION

Prior to beginning the procedure you will need to discuss the procedure, potential complications, risks, and benefits with the patient. You will also need to discuss the importance of follow-up and the expected time to return to the treatment area or primary care provider for re-evaluation. Consent should be obtained based on your institution's policies and procedures.

You will need the following:

- Nasal speculum
- Good lighting
- Bayonet forceps or ear loop
- Vasoconstrictor
    - Oxymetazoline or phenylephrine
- Cyanoacrylate glue
- Cotton-tipped applicator (use the wooden end)
- 12-Fr Foley catheter

PROCEDURE

- Using a nasal speculum is useful here, as is good lighting (either with an assistant holding a flashlight, good overhead lighting, or a headlamp).
- The proper way to hold the nasal speculum is to insert it into the naris with the handles horizontal (parallel to the floor).
- If you are able to visualize the object, using bayonet forceps or an earwax removal tool (with the tip bent at 90 degrees) can often remove it.
- If there is too much nasal discharge or bleeding, using a vasoconstrictor will help dry the naris of blood and/or mucus.
- Topical anesthesia (lidocaine 4%) is helpful for patient comfort and cooperation.

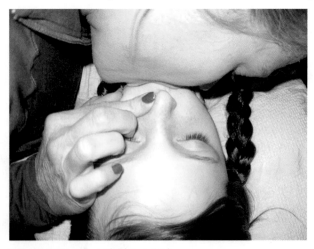

FIGURE 32.1 Parent's kiss method.

Parent-assisted technique is the "parent's kiss": A technique that often works well is one that requires the parent's help. It works better with larger objects (beans, large beads, etc.) (Figure 32.1).

- Inform the parent that it may get a little "messy" when the object gets expelled. Having a chuck on the patient's chest will help this somewhat.
- With the patient being held by the parent (supine), have the parent occlude the unaffected naris and blow with a strong puff into the patient's mouth.
- This will often result in the object being expelled from the naris.

Removal with 12-Fr Foley catheter

- Apply vasoconstrictor and topical anesthetic.
- Slide the tip of the catheter into the naris beyond the object.
- Slowly inflate the balloon with approximately 2 mL of air or water.
- Slowly withdraw the catheter with the balloon inflated and remove the object.

Cyanoacrylate glue (i.e., dermabond)

- Be sure the naris is as dry as possible (using the vasoconstrictors).
- Place a drop of adhesive on the wooden tip of a cotton-tipped applicator.
- Touch the foreign body with the wooden end and gently pull out of the naris.

POST-PROCEDURE CONSIDERATIONS
Try to be certain that all objects have been removed.

EDUCATIONAL POINTS
Unilateral foul-smelling nasal discharge in a young child/toddler indicates the presence of a nasal foreign body until proven otherwise.

COMPLICATIONS
There is sometimes some epistaxis afterward—control as usual.

PEARLS

- Having the patient supine, in a parent's lap if necessary, is important. You will need some help holding the patient's head still. Note that sometimes procedural sedation may be necessary.
- Commercial products can also be used for the removal of a nasal foreign body. The foreign-body remover consists of a syringe connected to a thin catheter with a balloon at the tip. Once the catheter is inserted past the object, the balloon can be inflated and the foreign body removed.

RESOURCES
Feied, C., Smith, M., Handler, J., & Gillam, M. (n.d.). Nasal foreign bodies. Retrieved from http://www.ncemi.org/cse/cse0309.htm

Fischer, J. (2015). Nasal foreign body. Retrieved from http://emedicine.medscape.com/article/763767-overview

Purohit, N., Ray, S., Wilson, T., & Chawla, O.P. (2008). The "parent's kiss": An effective way to remove paediatric nasal foreign bodies. Retrieved from http://www.ncbi.nlm.nih.gov/pmc/articles/PMC2645753

UNIT **XI**

Procedures for Managing Common Ear Injuries

CHAPTER 33

Procedures for Cerumen Removal

Theresa M. Campo

BACKGROUND

Cerumen, or earwax, moisturizes as well as repels water in the auditory canal and is bacteriocidal and fungicidal. It is composed of lipids, complex proteins, and sugars. Cotton-tipped applicators that are used to clean the ears push the cerumen into the canal and pack it down, leading to obstruction. Patients usually do not present for treatment until they experience a "clogged" sensation, decreased or loss of hearing, fullness, and/or dizziness. Cerumen may partially or completely block the tympanic membrane and should be removed for a thorough examination.

Indications for this procedure include difficulty visualizing tympanic membrane, cerumen impaction, and debris removal associated with otitis externa.

PATIENT PRESENTATION

- Fullness in ear
- Blocked or clogged sensation
- Dizziness
- Loss of hearing
- Tinnitus
- Painless; if pain present, suspect other origin (i.e., infection or perforation)

TREATMENT

There are three methods of cerumen removal: curette, gentle suction, and warm-water irrigation. Curette and irrigation are the most common and easily performed removals. Manual removal with curette is a simple procedure to perform to remove hard cerumen or large pieces. However, this can be painful to the patient. Warm water irrigation is painless, easy, and more often used.

Ceruminolytic agents can also be used to soften and aid in the removal of cerumen. There are three types of ceruminolytic agents: water-based, oil-based, and non-water/

non-oil-based. These agents can be used alone or as pretreatment for curette or water irrigation removal.

CONTRAINDICATIONS

- History or suspicion for perforated tympanic membrane, severe canal swelling
- Previous pain with irrigation
- Previous surgery to middle ear
- History of middle ear disease
- Sharp or organic foreign bodies
- Tinnitus
- Vertigo
- Radiation therapy to external or middle ear, skull base, or mastoid
- Patient with a history of mastoidectomy and hypersensitivity of the underlying structures

SPECIAL CONSIDERATIONS

- Patients who have previous surgery to the middle ear or mastoidectomy
- Diabetic patients should be carefully evaluated for the development of otitis externa after any manipulation of the ear and/or canal
- Irrigation should never be performed if a ruptured tympanic membrane is suspected or confirmed
- Jet irrigators can be used but care should be given not to rupture the tympanic membrane

PROCEDURE PREPARATION
Curette

- Flexible plastic or wire loop curette or plastic scoop
- Suction tip catheter or Frazier suction
- Gauze pads

Warm Water Irrigation

- Large-volume syringe (30–60 mL) or ear irrigator tip and syringe
- Large-gauge angiocatheter with needle removed (16 or 18 gauge)
- Warm water or normal saline
- Hydrogen peroxide
- Kidney basin
- Absorbent pad
- Towels

Light Source

- Otoscope or headlamp

PROCEDURE

Curette

- Gently straighten the canal by pulling the pinna back and upward (downward for children).
- Visualize the canal and wax with the otoscope.
- *Gently and slowly* insert the loop curette and remove the cerumen (Figure 33.1).

Warm-Water Irrigation

- Place an absorbent pad over the patient's shoulder.
- Have the patient sit up with the kidney basin below the ear and held snug against the neck to prevent water running down onto the neck and shoulders.
- Visualize the canal and wax with the otoscope.
- Fill the syringe with warm water.
  - Use warm water to prevent discomfort and dizziness.
  - Mix warm water and hydrogen peroxide (1:1 concentration).
- Gently straighten the canal by pulling the pinna back and upward (downward for children).
- Have the patient tilt his or her head so that the affected ear is facing the ground.
- Place the tip of the catheter at the opening of the canal. The tip should not be placed past the lateral one third of the ear canal.
- Instill the water gently and then allow it to run into the kidney basin (Figure 33.2).
- Repeat the irrigation until the cerumen is removed or the patient verbalizes complaints of pain, vertigo, and so on.
- Use the curette to help remove cerumen that is pushed to the canal entrance.
- Once completed, instill several drops of isopropanol in the canal to evaporate any residual moisture and prevent infection.

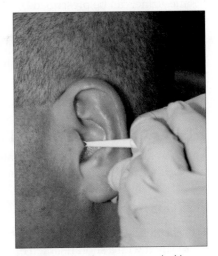

FIGURE 33.1 Cerumen removal with curette.

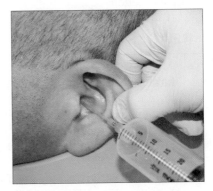

FIGURE 33.2 Cerumen removal with warm water irrigation.

POST-PROCEDURE CONSIDERATIONS

Pain

- The ear is very sensitive to pain.
- Topical ear drops, such as antipyrine and benzocaine, can be given for pain relief.

Tympanic Membrane

- Visualize the tympanic membrane to be sure it is intact and not perforated.

Vertigo

- Have the patient lie down until the dizziness resolves, which usually takes a few minutes.
- If the vertigo persists, a short dosing period of antivertigo medications, such as meclizine, can be prescribed.

Ear Canal Abrasion and/or Irritation

- Instillation and prescription of topical ear drops (i.e., fluoroquinolones) can be prescribed for the patient for a few days to help prevent infection and soothe the ear.

EDUCATIONAL POINTS

- Do not use cotton-tipped applicators inside the ear canal.
- Regular checkups with the primary care provider for evaluation and irrigation.

COMPLICATIONS

- Diabetes and immunosuppression
  - Treat with a short regimen of topical antibiotic ear drops (i.e., fluoroquinolones) for a few days.
- Complications arising from either curette or irrigation are usually benign and of brief duration.

PEARLS

- Always try to have the patient assist in the removal by holding the basin and turning the head. It helps the patient feel as though he or she is helping with the removal.
- Suction tip catheters can aid in the removal of the cerumen with either method. Use with caution in children.
- Pretreatment with ceruminolytics can help with an easy and quick removal of cerumen.
- A mixture of warm water and hydrogen peroxide (1:1) can be used prior to irrigation. Have the patient lie on the unaffected side with the ear facing the ceiling for 5 to 10 minutes prior to irrigation.

RESOURCES

McCarter, D. F., Courtney, U., & Pollart, S. M. (2007). Cerumen impaction. *American Family Physician, 75*(10), 1523–1528, 1530.

Morrissey, T., & Lissoway, J. B. (2013). Ear emergencies. In *Emergency medicine: Clinical essentials* (2nd ed.). Philadelphia, PA: Elsevier. Retrieved from https://www.clinicalkey.com/#!/content/book/3-s2.0-B9781437735482000276?scrollTo=%23hl0000528

O'Handley, J. G., Tobin, E., & Tagge, B. (2010). Otorhinolaryngology: Disorders of the external ear. In E. T. Bope, R. E. Rakel, & R. D. Kellerman (Eds.), *Conn's current therapy 2010* (1st ed.). Philadelphia, PA: Elesvier. Retrieved from http://www.mdconsult.com/das/book/body/188187220-3/965596089/1481/281.html#4-u1.0-B978-1-4160-2467-5..50027-0–cesec69_1222

Riviello, R. J. (2014). Otolaryngologic procedures. In J. R. Roberts & J. R. Hedges (Eds.), *Clinical procedures in emergency medicine* (6th ed., pp. 1189–1192). Philadelphia, PA: Saunders Elsevier. Retrieved from https://www.clinicalkey.com/#!/content/book/3-s2.0-B978145570606800063X

Riviello, R. J., & Brown, N. A. (2010). Otolaryngologic procedures. In J. R. Roberts & J. R. Hedges (Eds.), *Clinical procedures in emergency medicine* (5th ed., pp. 1189–1192). Philadelphia, PA: Saunders Elsevier.

VanWyk, F. C., Modayil, P. C., & Selvedurai, D. K. (2014). *Cerumen impaction removal*. Retrieved from http://emedicine.medscape.com/article/1413546-overview

CHAPTER **34**

Procedures for Foreign-Body Removal From the Ear Canal and Lobe

Theresa M. Campo

BACKGROUND

Foreign bodies in the external auditory canal are common complaints among children and adults. Foreign bodies can include insects, beads, rocks, sand, dirt, berries, vegetables, popcorn kernels, toys, cotton, erasers, and paper. The most common foreign body found in the ear is an insect. Because of sensory fibers, removal of these foreign bodies is easier in the lateral canal than in the medial canal.

Removal of foreign bodies can be distressing to the patient, especially a child. Limited attempts at removal should be made to help decrease anxiety and a painful, traumatic removal. Button batteries in the ear canal can cause significant tissue damage within hours, so immediate referral to an otolaryngologist should be done if prompt removal cannot be completed. Foreign bodies located in the medial canal should also be referred to a specialist.

Occasionally, earring backs become embedded in the ear lobe. Inflammation from irritation or infection causes swelling of the lobe, which occurs around the earring back, especially if worn tightly. Removal by the patient is usually difficult because of anxiety and pain. Foreign-body removal from the canal as well as the ear lobe will be discussed in this chapter.

PATIENT PRESENTATION

- Pain
  - Pain is severe if an insect is lodged in the canal
- Verbalization by a child to the parent or other person
- Fullness
- Vertigo
- Feel and hear something "moving" or "buzzing"

TREATMENT

There are numerous methods used to remove foreign bodies. The type of method used may depend upon the particular object you are attempting to remove. Irrigation, as discussed in Chapter 33, is most helpful for removal of dirt, sand, or small objects lying near the tympanic membrane. Irrigation should not be used for removal of organic material, such as vegetables, seeds, and so on, because the water causes the object to swell, making removal more difficult. Suction-tip catheters can be used for removal of difficult-to-grab objects such as beads and other smooth, round objects. These round objects become lodged in the canal because of the oval shape of the ear canal. Manual removal with various types of curettes can be used to remove small objects; the curette can be passed along the side of the object and gently pulled out of the canal. This method can be uncomfortable because of the sensitivity and nerve innervations of the canal. Alligator forceps can be used to remove objects that are easily grabbed, for example, insects, paper, cotton, and so on. Glue (cyanoacrylate) can also be used for removal of dry, smooth, and round objects in the lateral canal.

CONTRAINDICATIONS AND RELATIVE CONTRAINDICATIONS

- Irrigation should not be performed if suspicion or confirmation of tympanic membrane rupture or perforation is present.

SPECIAL CONSIDERATIONS

- Patients who are extremely anxious
  - To avoid traumatic removal, consider conscious sedation or referral to an otolaryngologist for these patients.

PROCEDURE PREPARATION
All Procedures

- Gloves
- Gauze pads
- Absorbent pads

Suction-Tip Catheter

- Suction-tip catheter (Frazier suction)

Manual Removal

- Flexible or rigid curette (loop or scoop)
- Alligator forceps

Insect Removal

- Mineral oil
- Lidocaine solution (2% or 4%)
- Alligator forceps and/or curette

Glue (Cyanoacrylate)

- Paper clip, cotton-tipped applicator, or very thin paint brush can be used
- Glue

PROCEDURE

Suction-Tip Catheter

- Inform the patient of the suction catheter noise so he or she is prepared and not startled.
  - Allowing the patient to hear the suction beforehand can alleviate fear.
- Place the suction between 100 and 140 mmHg.
- Gently straighten the canal by pulling the pinna back and upward for adults or downward for children.
- Gently place the suction tip onto the object and begin to suction and pull the object out of the canal (Figure 34.1).
  - Keep the tip away from the canal wall.

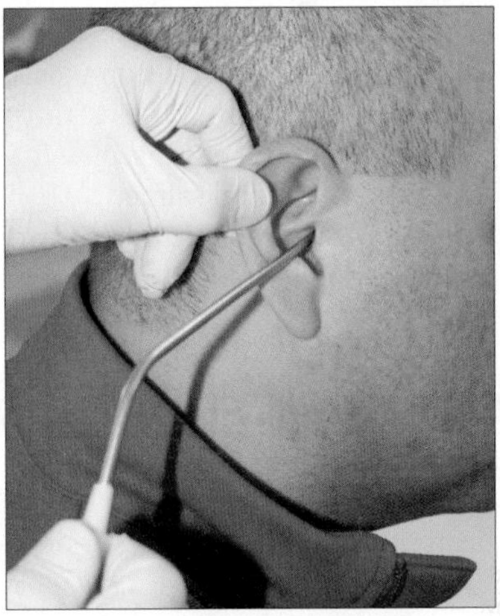

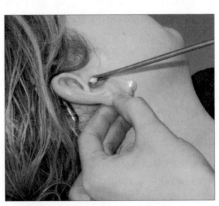

FIGURE 34.1 Foreign-body removal from the ear with a suction tip catheter.

Manual Removal

- Gently straighten the canal by pulling the pinna back and upward for adults or downward for children.
- Visualize the canal and foreign body with the otoscope.
- *Gently and slowly* insert the loop curette and remove the foreign body (Figure 34.2).

Insect Removal

- Instill either mineral oil and/or lidocaine (2% or 4%).
  - Mineral oil has been shown to be more effective.
- Once the insect is dead, removal with the mechanical technique can be performed.

FIGURE 34.2 Manual removal of a foreign body from the ear.

Glue (Cyanoacrylate)

- Place a small amount of glue on the tip of either a straightened paper clip, blunt/wooden end of a cotton-tipped applicator, or a very thin paintbrush.
- Once the glue is tacky, straighten the canal, as described earlier, and place the tip against the object and gently pull out of the canal.

This procedure is best used in cooperative adults. Glue can possibly spill or drip into the canal or the end of the applicator can adhere to the canal. Precision and patience are key with this procedure.

Earring Back in Earlobe

- Wipe the area clean with gauze and normal saline.
- Grasp the earlobe with both thumbs and index fingers.
- Gently, but firmly, push the anterior side toward the posterior side allowing the earring back to rise between your thumbs.
- Remove the back from the earring post.
- Remove the entire earring.
- Irrigate with normal saline.
- Apply topical antibiotic if necessary.
- Patients should not replace the earring until healed.

POST-PROCEDURE CONSIDERATIONS

- Minor abrasions usually heal without complications.
- Topical antibiotic drops can be prescribed to help prevent infection but have not been proven to be effective or necessary.

EDUCATIONAL POINTS

- Children
  - Do not put anything in the ears, nose, or other "holes" in their bodies.
  - Do not put anything smaller than your elbow in the ear.
- Adults
  - Do not use cotton-tipped applicators.
- Insects
  - Pest control should be advised for those patients with lodged insects that occur while sleeping or in the home.
  - Some insects just "fly in" especially during the warmer months.

COMPLICATIONS

- Tympanic rupture/perforation can occur either from the foreign body or from a traumatic removal.

PEARLS

- If a patient presents with a chronic dry cough that is not resolving, check the external canal for a foreign body. It may be pressing on the tenth cranial nerve, causing the cough.
- Always evaluate the other ear and nose for additional foreign bodies in children.
- Always perform and document your evaluation before and after removal, including removal failure.
- Cooperation and immobilization are key to a successful foreign-body removal.

RESOURCES

Heim, S. W., & Maughan, K. L., (2007). Foreign bodies in the ear, nose, and throat. *American Family Physician, 76*(8), 1185–1189.

Mantooth, R. (2009). *Foreign bodies, ear*. Retrieved from http://emedicine.com/article/763712-overview and http://emedicine.com/article/763712-treatment

Mantooth, R. (2013). *Ear foreign body removal in emergency medicine*. Retrieved from http://emedicine.medscape.com/article/763712-overview

Morrissey, T., & Lissoway, J. B. (2013). Ear emergencies. In *Emergency medicine: Clinical essentials* (2nd ed.). Philadelphia, PA: Elsevier. Retrieved from https://www.clinicalkey.com/#!/content/book/3-s2.0-B9781437735482000276?scrollTo=%23hl0000528

O'Handley, J. G., Tobin, E., & Tagge, B. (2010). Otorhinolaryngology: Disorders of the external ear. In E. T. Bope, R. E. Rakel, & R. D. Kellerman (Eds.), *Conn's current therapy 2010* (1st ed.). Philadelphia, PA: Elsevier. Retrieved from http://www.mdconsult.com/das/book/body/188187220-3/965596089/1481/281.html#4-u1.0-B978-1-4160-2467-5..50027-0–cesec69_1222

On-Kee Kwong, A., & Provataris, J. M. (2014). *Ear foreign body removal procedures*. Retrieved from http://emedicine.medscape.com/article/80507-overview

Riviello, R. J. (2014). Otolaryngologic procedures. In J. R. Roberts & J. R. Hedges (Eds.), *Clinical procedures in emergency medicine* (6th ed., 1189–1192). Philadelphia, PA: Saunders Elsevier. Retrieved from https://www.clinicalkey.com/#!/content/book/3-s2.0-B978145570606800063X

Riviello, R. J., & Brown, N. A. (2010). Otolaryngologic procedures. In J. R. Roberts & J. R. Hedges (Eds.), *Clinical procedures in emergency medicine* (5th ed., pp. 1194–1195). Philadelphia, PA: Saunders Elsevier.

CHAPTER **35**

Procedures for Managing an Auricular Hematoma

Theresa M. Campo

BACKGROUND

An auricular hematoma occurs from direct, blunt trauma to the ear causing a shearing force. It is commonly seen in wrestlers, rugby players, and after an assault or altercation. The shearing of the anterior auricle leads to separation of the perichondrium and the underlying vessels, leading to hematoma formation and compromise to the avascular cartilage. This injury needs immediate treatment to prevent the development of cauliflower ear and infection. Cauliflower ear is the development of new chaotic cartilage formation, which leads to a chronic and permanently deformed ear.

PATIENT PRESENTATION

- Anterior auricular tenderness, swelling, and/or deformity following trauma

TREATMENT

Treatment should be immediate to prevent complications. Needle aspiration and incision and drainage are the treatments of choice. Consideration should be given to needle aspiration as recurrence and difficulties producing full evacuation are considerable concerns. Treatment goals are to completely drain and evacuate the hematoma and prevent reaccumulation of the hematoma with a pressure dressing. Needle aspiration and incision and drainage techniques are discussed in this chapter.

Regardless of technique, patients should be placed on antistaphylococcal antibiotics and close follow-up should be discussed with the patient and family members.

CONTRAINDICATIONS AND RELATIVE CONTRAINDICATIONS

- Hematoma more than 7 to 10 days old
- Recurrent or chronic hematoma

SPECIAL CONSIDERATIONS

- Pediatric patient
  - Conscious sedation may be necessary for deep-seated or difficult-to-manage areas because of movement or severity.
  - Each case should be considered independently.
- Immunocompromised patients or those who have comorbidities
  - Patients with organ transplant, HIV/AIDS, diabetes, and/or cancer
- Pregnancy
- Antibiotics that are considered to be safe in pregnancy should be prescribed if necessary.

PROCEDURE PREPARATION
Needle Aspiration
- 18- to 20-gauge needle
- 10-mL syringe
- Topical antibiotic ointment

Incision and Drainage
- 3-mL syringe with 23- to 27-gauge needle—anesthesia
- Lidocaine 1% *without* epinephrine—anesthesia
- No. 11 or No. 15 blade scalpel
- 20-mL syringe with 18-gauge angiocatheter and normal saline for irrigation
- Topical antibiotic ointment

Compression Dressing
- 4 × 4 gauze
- Stretch bandage/roll gauze
- Dry cotton
- Vaseline gauze, 1/4 in., plain packing, or saline-soaked gauze

Sutured Dental Rolls
- Dental rolls
- 4-0 nylon suture material
- Suture kit

PROCEDURE
Small Hematoma
Needle Aspiration
- Prepare the site with skin cleanser and dry with a 4 × 4 gauze.
- Attach the 18- to 20-gauge needle to the 10-mL syringe.
- Insert the needle into the hematoma (Figure 35.1).
- "Milk" the hematoma between your thumb and forefinger until the contents are completely drained.

- Withdraw the needle from the ear.
- Apply a simple compression dressing to the ear to prevent reaccumulation (see the Compression Dressing section).

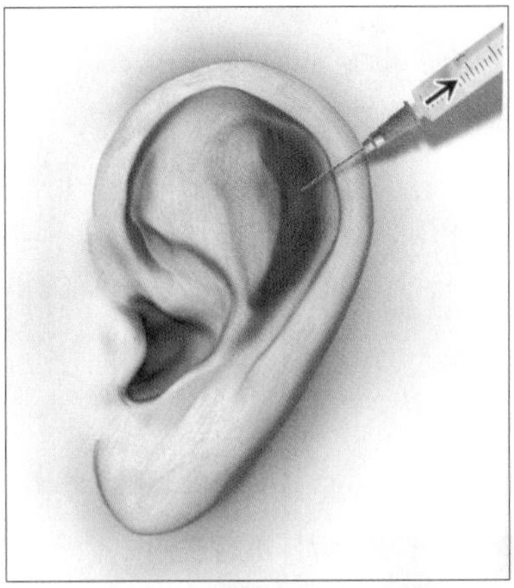

Incision and Drainage

- Place the patient in the lateral decubitus position with the affected ear facing upward.
- Prepare the area with skin cleanser.
- Dry the area with a 4 × 4 gauze.
- Perform local infiltration with the lidocaine 1% *without* epinephrine (an auricular block can also be performed; see Chapter 9).
- Using the scalpel, incise along the natural skin fold of the anterior auricle following the curve of the pinna (Figure 35.2).
- Gently peel the skin and perichondrium off the hematoma.
- Completely evacuate the hematoma (suction may be used if necessary).
- Draw the saline into the large syringe.
- Apply the splash shield to the end of the syringe.
- Irrigate the area.
- Dry thoroughly.
- Apply topical antibiotic ointment and approximate the wound edges.
- Apply a pressure dressing or suture dental rolls to the ear; both are described in the following sections.

Compression Dressing

- Insert dry cotton into the ear canal.
- Mold the conforming gauze into the convolutions of the ear (vaseline, saline, or packing).
- Cut a "V" shape into the 4 × 4 gauze to allow for a snug and comfortable fit behind the ear and place behind the entire ear.
- Place multiple layers of gauze over the ear.
- Wrap stretch bandage/roll gauze around the head to secure the dressing in place (Figure 35.3)

FIGURE 35.1 Needle aspiration of an auricular hematoma.

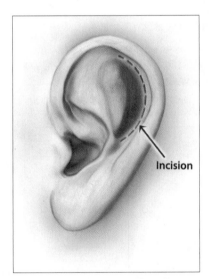

FIGURE 35.2 Incision and drainage of an auricular hematoma.

Sutured Dental Rolls

- With 4-0 nylon suture material, pass over the hematoma through the entire thickness of the ear.
- Place the dental roll on the posterior aspect of the ear and wrap the suture material over it.

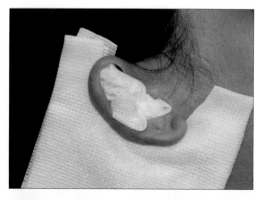

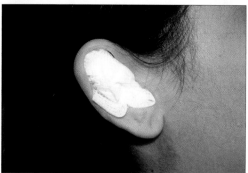

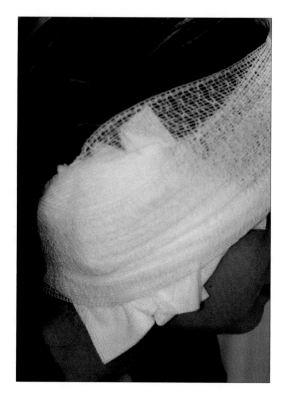

FIGURE 35.3 Applications of compression dressings.

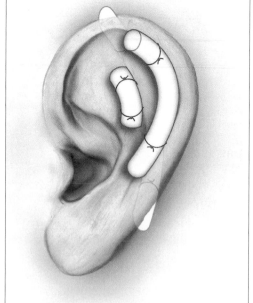

FIGURE 35.4 Suture dental rolls.

- Pass the suture needle back through the pinna such that it comes out anteriorly.
- Place another dental roll on the anterior aspect of the pinna over the incision.
- Wrap the suture material over the dental roll and tie into place (Figure 35.4).
- Remove the dressing in 7 days.

POST-PROCEDURE CONSIDERATIONS
Recurrence

Drainage may need to be repeated if fluid reaccumulation occurs.

- Referral to specialist is indicated.

EDUCATIONAL POINTS

- Close follow-up every 24 hours is necessary to assess for recurrence, infection, and vascular compromise.
- Aspirin, nonsteroidal anti-inflammatory medication, or anticoagulant medications should be avoided to prevent recurrence.

COMPLICATIONS

- Reaccumulation of the hematoma is the most common complication seen.
- Infection, chondritis, and scar formation
- Early drainage and close monitoring can help prevent the development of scar tissue (cauliflower ear). However, it may still develop.
- Recurrence and infection are indications for surgical treatment and intravenous antibiotics.

PEARLS

- Discuss the possibility of reoccurrence and development of cauliflower ear with the patient.
- Premedicate with oral analgesia medication.
- Reassurance should be given to patients of any age.
- Drainage should be performed on all hematomas unless older than 7 days.
- The use of lidocaine with epinephrine has generally been contraindicated for the outer ear. However, recent literature suggests that the use of epinephrine does not block the circulation to this area of the ear and, therefore, does not cause necrosis. The decision to use epinephrine for local infiltration of the outer ear is at the clinician's discretion and should be based on the most up-to-date evidence practice. Epinephrine is also acceptable for regional block of the ear.

RESOURCES

Leybell, I. (2009). *Drainage, auricular hematoma*. Retrieved from http://emedicine.com/article/82793-overview and http://emedicine.com/article/82793-treatment

Leybell, I. (2014). *Auricular hematoma drainage*. Retrieved from http://emedicine.medscape.com/article/82793-overview

O'Handley, J. G., Tobin, E., & Tagge, B. (2010). Otorhinolaryngology: Disorders of the external ear. In E. T. Bope, R. E. Rakel, & R. D. Kellerman (Eds.), *Conn's current therapy 2010* (1st ed.). Philadelphia, PA: Elsevier. Retrieved from http://www.mdconsult.com/das/book/body/188187220-3/965596089/1481/281.html#4-u1.0-B978-1-4160-2467-5..50027-0–cesec69_1222

Riviello, R. J. (2014). Otolaryngologic procedures. In J. R. Roberts & J. R. Hedges (Eds.), *Clinical procedures in emergency medicine* (6th ed., 1189–1192). Philadelphia, PA: Saunders Elsevier. Retrieved from https://www.clinicalkey.com/#!/content/book/3-s2.0-B978145570606800063X

Riviello, R. J., & Brown, N. A. (2010). Otolaryngologic procedures. In J. R. Roberts & J. R. Hedges (Eds.), *Clinical procedures in emergency medicine* (5th ed., pp. 1195–1197). Philadelphia, PA: Saunders Elsevier.

UNIT **XII**

Procedures for Examination and Management of Common Oral Injuries

CHAPTER 36

Dental Anatomy, Examination, and Anesthetics

Theresa M. Campo

DENTAL ANATOMY

The tooth is composed of the crown and root. The crown is the visible part and is covered with enamel. It projects above the gingiva and consists of three layers. The outer layer is the enamel, which is the hardest structure of the tooth with increased mineralization. The center layer is the dentin, a bone-like material, and the pulp is the inner hollow layer.

The root system is also composed of three layers: the cementum (outer layer), dentin (middle layer), and the pulp canal (the center). Blood vessels and nerves enter the pulp through the apical foramen and pulp canal. The pulp supplies the dentin with nutrients. Periodontal ligaments act as a sling or hammock holding the tooth in the socket and cushioning the tooth during mastication. These ligaments secure the tooth to the alveolar bone (Figure 36.1).

FIGURE 36.1 Tooth anatomy

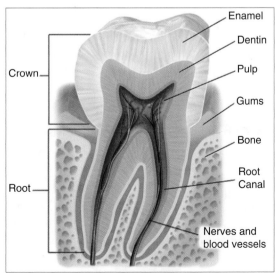

There are primary and secondary teeth. Primary teeth, also known as milk or baby teeth, consist of 20 teeth that begin to erupt at around 6 months of age and are complete at about 2 years of age. These teeth begin to shed between age 6 and 12 years and are complete around the 18th birthday. Secondary teeth, or permanent teeth, consist of 32 teeth: 8 incisors, 4 canine, 8 premolars, and 12 molars.

The teeth can be divided into two areas: the upper and lower arches (maxillary and mandibular teeth). These areas can be further divided into the four areas of upper and lower, right and left. They are referenced to the patient (i.e., patient's right upper or left lower). There are four groups of teeth: the incisors, canines, premolars, and molars.

The incisors are the four most anterior maxillary and mandibular teeth and are responsible for cutting and biting food. They have one root. There are four canine teeth (maxillary and mandibular), which are just distal to the incisors. They are responsible for ripping and tearing food and are the longest and most stable of the teeth. They have one root.

The next teeth are the premolars with four each in the maxilla and mandible. They have sharp points and a broad base for ripping, chewing, and grinding food. The premolars have one root but the first maxillary may have two roots. The molars are the farthest back, with six each in the maxilla and mandible. They consist of a broad surface for crushing, chewing, and grinding food. They may have one to four roots. The third molars in both maxillary and mandibular are called wisdom teeth.

DENTAL EXAMINATION

A thorough examination of the oral cavity should be done with any complaints of facial swelling, sore throat, sinus pressure, neck or oral pain, swelling, or drainage. Before starting an examination, the patient should be asked to remove any dentures or removable appliances for full visualization.

Inspection
- External features of the face and neck
- Jaw movement for symmetry
- Lips

Intra-Oral
- Mucosa and tissue including frenula
  - Torn frenulum can be a sign of abuse

Gingiva
- Inflammation could be a sign of systemic disease (i.e., diabetes) or pregnancy.

Teeth
- There are 32 permanent teeth. Numbering begins with the right upper molar (No. 1) counting across to the left upper molar (No. 16) followed by the left lower molar (No. 17) and finishing at the right lower molar (No. 32) (Figure 36.2).
- Discoloration can occur because of medications or poor hygiene.

Tongue

- Inspect for lesions, cuts, or bleeding

Hard and Soft Palate

- Lesions
- Have patient say "ahhh" and note symmetrical rise of uvula/palate

Palpation

- Periauricular, submandibular, submental, and cervical lymph nodes
- Temporalmandibular joint
    - Symmetry of movement
    - Clicking or crepitus
- Intra-oral tissue including the frenula
- Gingiva
- Teeth
    - Chipping, breakage, roughness, and mobility
- Express Wharton's duct
    - Located under tongue
    - Fluid should be clear
- Hard and soft palate
    - Masses

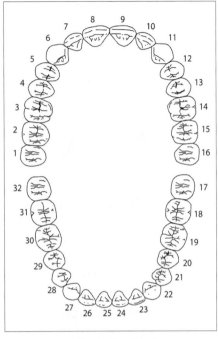

FIGURE 36.2 Numbering of teeth.

ANESTHETICS

Background

Dental anesthesia is used for many dental, oral, and maxillofacial procedures, including odontalgia (toothache) and lacerations. Dental blocks do not distort soft tissue needing repair and are a safe way to control pain without the use of narcotics.

Profound anesthesia can be achieved through infiltration or depositing anesthetic apically to a particular tooth. This can be accomplished for all teeth in the mouth with the exception of the lower molars. The lower molars usually require a mandibular block (inferior alveolar infiltration/lingual nerve). Infiltration typically provides profound anesthesia to the pulp in approximately 4 minutes and can last about 7 minutes with soft tissue numbness lasting 2 to 3 hours. The mandibular block can take up to 15 minutes to achieve profound anesthesia and can last 4 to 5 hours or longer depending on the anesthetic used.

Treatment

Dental anesthesia can be helpful with the following:

- Odontalgia and pulpitis
- Dental impaction

- Periodontal abscess
- Laceration repair of the tongue, lip, and oral mucosa
- Dental, mandibular, and/or maxillary fractures and trauma

Contraindications and Relative Contraindications

- Hypersensitivity or allergies to anesthetic agents
- Uncooperative patients
- Infected tissue
- Bleeding disorders
- Valvular heart disease

Special Considerations

- Be cognizant of organ dysfunction (i.e., liver), which can increase the l = half-life of Lidocaine twofold, as well as stress ailing pathology. Always consult product information. (In general, local anesthetics are quite safe.)
- Proper documentation of a patient with a history of neurovascular damage

PROCEDURE PREPARATION

- Lidocaine 5% or benzocaine 20% solution for topical application
- Nonsterile gloves
- Absorbent pads
- Gauze
- Cotton-tipped applicator(s) or cotton balls
- Lidocaine 1% or 2% or bupivacaine 0.25% with or without epinephrine
- Dental aspirating syringe, if available
- 3-mL syringe with 1.5-in. needle
- Small-gauge needle (25–27-gauge)
- Suction setup with Yankauer suction tip

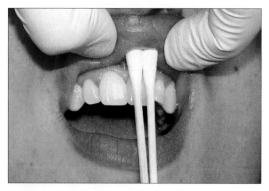

FIGURE 36.3 Topical anesthesia

PROCEDURE
Topical

Topical anesthesia can be beneficial to reduce the pain experienced with injectable anesthesia.

- Dry mucosa with gauze.
- Place lidocaine 5% or benzocaine 20% solution on the tip of applicators or cotton balls.
- Place on mucosa where needle is to be inserted for 3 to 5 minutes (Figure 36.3).

Injectable

Injectable anesthesia can be used for laceration repair, mandibular fractures, toothache, and abscess. Lidocaine 1% or 2% with or without epinephrine can be used for lacerations (short term) or bupivacaine 0.25% with or without epinephrine can be used for mandibular fractures or toothaches (long term) for their respective durations.

Supraperiosteal Infiltration (Local)
Individual Tooth Pain or Toothache

- Apply topical anesthetic described previously.
- Have the patient relax their facial muscles as much as possible by asking to close his or her mouth.
- Fully extend the mucous membrane for visualization by either pulling gently out and down (mandibular) or out and up (maxilla).
- Dry the area with gauze and visualize the mucobuccal fold.
- Insert the needle into the mucous fold, in front of the affected tooth, with the bevel of the needle facing the bone (Figure 36.4).
- Aspirate
- Inject 1 to 2 mL of anesthetic at the apex of the tooth.
- Withdraw the needle.
- Give patient gauze to hold pressure.
- If the procedure fails to anesthetize the area, inject the palatal side of the tooth.

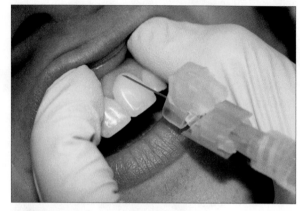

FIGURE 36.4 Supraperiosteal infiltration.

> **NOTE** *Maxillary first bicuspids and maxillary molars may require small palatal infiltration at approximate area of root tip.*

Anterior Superior Alveolar Block

Canine and incisors (lateral and medial):

- Apply topical anesthetic.
- Have the patient relax the upper lip by closing the jaw slightly.
- Retract the lip anteriorly.
- Insert the needle at the apex of the canine tooth at a 45-degree angle (Figure 36.5)
- Aspirate.
- Inject 2 mL of anesthetic.
- Withdraw the needle.
- Give patient gauze to hold pressure.

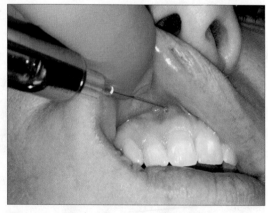

FIGURE 36.5 Anterior superior alveolar block.

Middle Superior Alveolar Block

Mediobuccal root of maxillary first molar and maxillary bicuspids:

- Apply topical anesthetic.
- Have the patient open his or her mouth about halfway.
- Retract the cheek laterally.

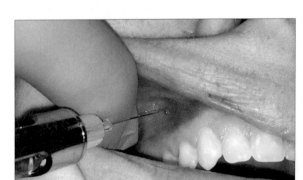

FIGURE 36.6 Middle superior alveolar block.

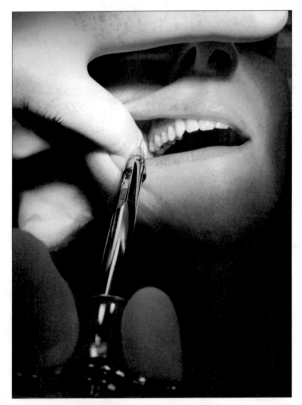

FIGURE 36.7 Posterior superior alveolar block.

- Position and insert the needle at the junction between the second premolar and first molar at a 45-degree angle (Figure 36.6).
- Aspirate
- Inject 2 to 3 mL of anesthetic.
- Withdraw the needle.
- Give patient gauze to hold pressure.

Posterior or Superior Alveolar Block

Maxillary molars:

- Apply topical anesthetic.
- Have the patient open the mouth about halfway.
- Retract the cheek laterally.
- Position the needle to the posterior aspect of the second molar and insert toward the maxillary tuberosity (upward, backward, and inward) along the curvature of the tuberosity approximately 2 to 2.5 cm (Figure 36.7).
- Aspirate
- Inject 2 to 3 mL of anesthetic.
- Withdraw the needle.
- Give patient gauze to hold pressure.
- Occasionally, the first molar will not be anesthetized with this technique alone and will need an additional technique (middle superior alveolar [MSA]).
- Puncture of the pterygoid plexus and hematoma formation can occur if aspiration is not performed.
- Cranial nerve V can be blocked if the needle is inserted too far posteriorly.

Upper molars and upper first premolars may require a palatal injection because these teeth possess a palatal root. Determine approximately where the root tip would be in the palate and press with a blunt object with gentle pressure (such as the blunt end of the dental mirror). At the same time, insert the needle into the tissue near the mirror handle. Slowly express a small amount of anesthetic into the site. Only use a small amount (few drops), and tissue blanching is a good indication of enough anesthetic. Too much anesthetic with the pressure applied can result in necrosis. This procedure is well tolerated because of the Gate theory of pain, which states that the larger pressure nerve fibers will override the smaller pain nerve fibers. This is why rubbing your head after you hit it is soothing (Figure 36.7).

Inferior Alveolar Infiltration (With Lingual Nerve Block)

This is the most common type of dental nerve block used to anesthetize the mandibular teeth to midline, the floor of the mouth, lower lip, chin, and anterior two thirds of the tongue. Although this technique may be considered more complex than previous methods, once mastered, it is a highly effective block. It should be performed only after reading and reviewing procedural resources and with supervision until one is proficient in this technique.

- Have the patient lie down with the back of the head firmly against the stretcher or in a reclining position in a dental chair, if available.
- Stand on the side opposite the area to be injected.
- Palpate the coronoid notch and then place the thumb over the notch (retromolar fossa—anterior ramus of the mandible).
- Place the index finger just anterior to the ear (external ramus).
- Retract the tissue toward the cheek and visualize the pterygomandicular triangle (see Figure 36.8).
- Apply topical anesthetic.
- Hold the syringe parallel to the mandibular teeth at an angle to the medial ramus with the distal end of the syringe lying between the first and second premolars on the opposite side of the mouth.

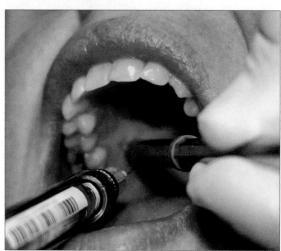

FIGURE 36.8 Inferior block.

- In children, the syringe will need to be held at a slightly higher angle, not parallel, because of the difference in anatomy (mandibular foramen is lower).
- Insert the needle into the triangle approximately 1 cm above the level of the teeth until the end of the needle hits the bone (usually no more than 2.5 cm).
- Withdraw the needle slightly, aspirate, and then instill the anesthetic.
- 5 mL

The lingual nerve can also be anesthetized as it branches off of the inferior alveolar nerve at this point.

Patients may experience jaw soreness after the injection for a few days. Be sure to include this information in your instructions.

Mental Nerve Infiltration

This block is most commonly used for lower lip lacerations. The mental nerve is an extension of the inferior alveolar nerve through the mental foramen. This nerve block can be performed either intra-orally or extra-orally. However, the intra-oral technique will only be covered in this book as it is considered to be less painful to the patient.

- Palpate the mental foramen by placing a gloved finger over the labial fold over the mandible approximately 1 cm inferior and anterior to the second premolar (usually not palpable).

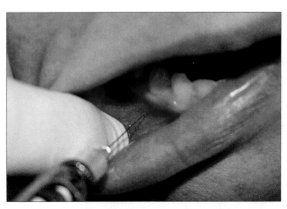

FIGURE 36.9 Mental block.

- Between the first and second premolar in adults
- Between the first and second primary molars in children
- Apply topical anesthetic.
- Insert the needle at a 45-degree angle using the supraperiosteal technique.
  - Do not inject directly into the foramen as this can cause nerve damage.
- Aspirate and then instill 2 to 3 mL of anesthetic while "fanning out" (see Figure 36.9).

EDUCATIONAL POINTS

- Rinse with warm salt water.
- Use caution chewing and swallowing food because of the anesthesia.
- Use caution swallowing fluids because of the anesthesia.

COMPLICATIONS

- Pain
- Infection
- Allergic reaction
- Anxiety

PEARLS

- Distraction through imagery can help to decrease the patient's anxiety.
- Have the parent at the bedside for comfort.
- Massaging the injection site can help increase the speed of absorption.
- Make sure the periosteum is encountered when performing inferior alveolar nerve anesthesia.
- Recent literature shows a link between periodontal and myocardial infarctions as the increased inflammatory activity in atherosclerotic lesions may represent a link between periodontal infection and cardiovascular disease.
- An apprehensive patient or a patient with pulp infection may require additional anesthetic.

RESOURCES

Amsterdam, J. T., & Kilgore, K. P. (2014). Regional anesthesia of the head and neck. In J. R. Roberts & J. R. Hedges (Eds.), *Clinical procedures in emergency medicine* (6th ed.). Philadelphia, PA: Saunders Elsevier. Retrieved from https://www.clinicalkey.com/#!/content/book/3-s2.0-B9781455706068000306

Bahekar, A. A., Singh, S., Saha, S., Molnar, J., & Arora, R. (2007). The prevalence and incidence of coronary heart disease is significantly increased in periodontitis: A meta-analysis. *American Heart Journal, 154*(5), 830–837. doi: 10.1016/j.ahj.2007.06.037

Benko, R. (2010). Regional anesthesia of the head and neck. In J. R. Roberts & J. R. Hedges (Eds.), *Clinical procedures in emergency medicine* (5th ed., pp. 503–506, 1217–1219). Philadelphia, PA: Saunders Elsevier.

Hermann, H. J., & Laskin, D. M. (2007). In P. S. Auerbach (Ed.), *Wilderness medicine* (5th ed.). Philadelphia, PA: Mosby Elsevier. Retrieved from http://www.mdconsult.com/das/book/body/188210824–3/0/1483/238.html?tocnode=54235634&fromURL=238.html#4-u1.0-B978–0-323–03228-5..50031–8_1433

Knight, J. (2009). Dental basics for primary care NPs. *American Journal for Nurse Practitioners, 13*(3), 36–41.

Scheinfeld, N. S. (2009, May 17). *Nerve block, inferior alveolar*. Retrieved from http://emedicine.medscape.com/article/82622.-overview and http://emedicine.medscape.com/article/82622.-treatment

Scheinfeld, N. S. (2014). *Inferior alveolar nerve block*. Retrieved from http://emedicine.medscape.com/article/82622-overview

Van Meter, M. W., & Dave, A. K. (2009, April 5). *Nerve block, oral*. Retrieved from http://emedicine.medscape.com/article/82850-overview and http://emedicine.medscape.com/article/82850-treatment

Van Meter, M. W., & Dave, A. K. (2014). *Oral nerve block*. Retrieved from http://emedicine.medscape.com/article/82850-overview

CHAPTER **37**

Procedures for Managing Dental Injuries

Theresa M. Campo

Dental pain and injuries are commonly seen in the emergency and urgent care settings and less frequently in the office setting. They can be anxiety producing for the patient and family members. Dentoalveolar abscesses, odontalgia (toothache), dental fractures, and luxations are the most common problems requiring quick interventions. Other problems encountered by providers are pulpitis, gingivtis, pericoronitis, cellulitis, and periodontitis, and are not covered in this chapter.

In the United States in 2008, dental services accounted for $101.2 billion of the $2.3 trillion spent on health care. Direct costs accompanied by the indirect costs of days lost at school and work are not only a burden financially on the individual and family, but also on society. Providers can address these problems early and efficiently through procedures, medical treatment, and referral to dentists and oral surgeons.

DENTOALVEOLAR ABSCESS
Background
Dentoalveolar abscesses are a collection of pus in the structures surrounding the teeth. In children, the abscess is usually periapical from dental caries invading the protective layer and the pulp. The infection causes pulpitis (inflammation of the pulp) and may lead to necrosis. The abscess is formed when the infection reaches the alveolar bone. A periodontal abscess is more common in adults and involves the periodontal ligaments and bone (support structures). This type of abscess can occur secondary to foreign body in children. Infections are polymicrobial with anaerobic gram-negative rods and gram-positive cocci, facultative and microaerophilic *streptococci*, and *viridans streptococci* (Figure 37.1)

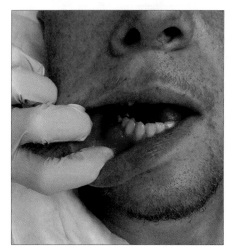

FIGURE 37.1 Dental abscess.

Deep-space infections present with fever, trismus, toxic appearance, chills, pain, and difficulty with speech and/or swallowing. The infection can spread into the deep spaces of the face and neck. These spaces include buccal, maxillary sinus, parapharyngeal, retropharyngeal, sublingual, submandibular, submasseteric, and temporal. The sublingual space can cause elevation of the base of the tongue and floor of the mouth, causing dysphagia and airway compromise.

Patient Presentation

- Pain (buccal and/or facial; local or along facial planes)
- Swelling (intraoral and/or extraoral)
- Common locations and associated causes of facial swelling are given in Table 37.1.
- Fever
- Gingival bleeding
- Pus drainage
- Regional lymphadenopathy (submental, submandibular, cervical)
- Fluctuant mass (buccal or palatal)
- Mobile tooth/teeth
- Severe infection—trismus, dysphagia, airway compromise, and necrotizing fasciitis

TABLE 37.1 Facial Swelling

Region	Location/Cause	Presentation
*Sublingual	Mandibular Canine Lateral and medial incisors Premolar First molar	Pain Dysphagia Unilateral elevation floor of mouth and/or base of tongue Airway compromise
*Submandibular	Mandibular Second molar Third molar	Pain Swelling—triangle of neck around angle of jaw (below mandible) Trismus Tender to palpation
*Submental	Mandibular Incisors	Pain Firm Midline swelling beneath chin

(continued)

TABLE 37.1 Facial Swelling (*continued*)

Region	Location/Cause	Presentation
Retropharyngeal (more common in children of 4 years and younger)	Maxillary or mandibular First molar Second molar Third molar	Stiff neck Sore throat Dysphagia Voice change Stridor (sever case involving mediastinum)
Buccal	Maxillary or mandibular Premolar Molar	Pain Swollen cheeks Trismus
Masticator	Mandibular Third molar	Pain Trismus Large abscess may require intubation while awake (can lead to parapharyngeal space)

* Infection in these areas can lead to Ludwig's angina (sensation of choking and suffocation). The majority of cases originate from tooth infection with approximately 75% originating from second or third molar.

Treatment

The treatment of dentoalveolar abscesses is dependent on the extent of the infection as well as the involvement of deep spaces. If the infection is localized and easily accessible, then it can be treated with either needle aspiration or incision and drainage. If the infection is more complex and widespread, involving the deep spaces, or the patient has respiratory compromise, then rapid referral to an oral surgeon and anticipation of a surgical intervention in the operating room should be done.

Special Considerations

- Pediatric patients.
  - Conscious sedation may be necessary for deep-seated or difficult-to-manage areas because of movement or severity.
- Each case should be considered independently.
- Patients who are immunocompromised or have comorbidities such as organ transplant, HIV/AIDS, diabetes, and/or cancer should be treated more aggressively and with a lower index of suspicion for abscess and infection.
- Patients with artificial heart valves and prosthetic joints should be prophylaxed based on the current American Heart Association/American College of Cardiology guidelines.

Procedure Preparation

Topical anesthesia and injectable anesthesia (see Chapter 36)
- Gauze
- Nonsterile gloves
- Kidney basin for patient to spit into
- Culture swab for culture and sensitivity

Needle Aspiration

- 3- or 5-mL syringe
- 21-gauge needle
- Hydrogen peroxide and water (50:50 solution)

Incision and Drainage

- Hemostat
- Scalpel (No. 11 or No. 15 blade)
- Normal saline for irrigation
- Packing material (1/4-in. gauze)
- Fenestrated Penrose drain

Procedure

- Dry oral mucosa.
- Apply topical anesthesia (see Chapter 31).
- Perform either a local or nerve block (see Chapter 36).

Needle Aspiration

- Insert needle into fluctuant area.
- Aspirate
- Withdraw contents.
- Obtain culture.
- Have patient rinse the mouth with hydrogen peroxide and water.

Incision and Drainage (See Chapter 21 for Illustrations of the Procedure)

- Make a small incision over the fluctuant area.
  - Direct the point of the scalpel blade toward the alveolar surface.
- Insert the tip of the hemostat into the incision.
- Gently perform blunt dissection of the area to break up loculations.
- Place the culture swab into the incision.
- Irrigate with normal saline.
  - Have the patient lean forward or to the side to prevent aspiration and choking.
- Insert packing if the wound is large enough.
  - You can suture the end of the packing to the mucosa with an absorbable suture to prevent aspiration.

Some abscesses can extend from intraoral to extraoral and may need to be incised through the facial skin. Incision and drainage should be performed intraorally when at all possible to minimize scarring. If the abscess needs an extraoral approach, please follow the procedure for subcutaneous abscesses in Chapter 25.

Post-Procedure Considerations
Pain

- Pain medication should be prescribed based on the patient's pain level and tolerance.
- Relieving the abscess can significantly reduce the pain.

Infection
- Oral antibiotics should be prescribed (amoxicillin–clavulanate, clindamycin).

Educational Points
- Perform frequent warm salt water rinses for wounds without packing.
- Proper intraoral hygiene and regular visits to the dentist are important for the prevention of further caries and infection.
- Follow up within 1 to 2 days with either a dentist or oral surgeon.

Complications
- Cavernous sinus thrombosis
- Fistula formation—chronic infection
- Ludwig's angina
- Maxillary sinusitis
- Osteomyelitis

PEARLS

- Frequent reassurance can help with anxious patients.
- Instruct the patient to spit out any drainage and to try not to swallow.
  - Give the patient a kidney basin and gauze.

DENTAL FRACTURE
Background
Dental trauma is commonly seen in office, urgent, and emergency care settings. The majority of injuries occur from contact sports but many occur from altercations, falls, or motor vehicle or motorcycle crashes. Fractures of the posterior teeth can occur from whiplash-type injury or striking of the chin, closing jaw forcibly.

Many dental injuries can be accompanied by intraoral lacerations. Careful probing of the laceration is required to make sure chips and fragments are not in the laceration(s). If a tooth fragment cannot be located, radiographs need to be performed to rule out aspiration or ingestion of the tooth or large fragment.

Crown fractures can be classified as uncomplicated or complicated. The root fractures are difficult to diagnose and often require radiographs for definitive diagnosis and should always be referred to a dentist, orthodontist, or oral surgeon for prompt treatment and follow-up. Crown fractures can be placed in a three-category classification system known as the Ellis classification (Figure 37.2). Please see Table 37.2 for classification, presentation, and treatment of fractures.

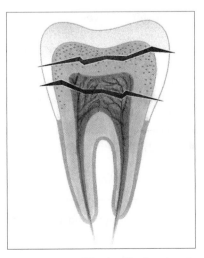

FIGURE 37.2 Ellis classification of tooth fracture.

TABLE 37.2 Ellis Classification of Crown Fractures

Ellis Class	Complicated or Uncomplicated	Fracture Location	Presentation	Treatment
Ellis I	Uncomplicated	Enamel	Sharp edges of tooth Little to no sensitivity	Smooth rough edges with emery board
Ellis II	Uncomplicated	Enamel Dentin	Sensitivity to temperature and air Yellow or pink tint to dentin	Supraperiosteal block Cap tooth with composite
Ellis III	Complicated	Enamel Dentin Pulp	Pain Dentin pink Frank bleeding	Supraperiosteal block Cap tooth with composite Immediate referral to dental specialist

Special Considerations

- Children are at increased risk of infection with Ellis II and III fractures because of the increased pulp-to-dentin ratio. Dental referral should be within 24 hours of the injury.
- Patients who are immunocompromised are at increased risk for infection because of the decreased immune response. Antibiotic therapy and close follow-up are required with these patients.

Procedure Preparation

- Topical anesthesia and injectable anesthesia (see Chapter 36)
- Gauze
- Nonsterile gloves
- Kidney basin for patient to spit in
- Calcium hydroxide, zinc oxide, or glass ionomer composites
- Dental spatula
- Tongue depressor (if dental spatula is not available for mixing the composite)
- Cotton-tipped applicators (if dental spatula is not available for application onto tooth)
- Aluminum foil (Aluminum foil can be placed on top of a cap, although this is not necessary if referral to the dental specialist is within 24 hours.)
- Emery board

Procedure
Ellis I

- Smooth rough surface with emery board.

Ellis II and Ellis III

- Dry oral mucosa.
- Apply topical anesthesia.
- Perform either a local or nerve block.
- Mix the catalyst and base of the composite material as directed on the label with the dental spatula (1:1 ratio).
  - A tongue depressor can be used in place of a spatula.
- Dry the tooth using gauze (have the patient bite down on the gauze).
- Apply the mixture to the tooth with the dental spatula.
- Allow the mixture to dry per the composite material instructions (usually a few minutes).

Post-Procedure Considerations
Aspiration/Ingestion

- Tooth and tooth fragments have the potential to be swallowed or aspirated. Care should be given to avoid this.

Educational Points

- Eat soft foods.
- Avoid chewing on affected side/tooth.
- Risk of pulp necrosis, color change, and/or root reabsorption with any fracture is a possibility.

Complications

- Pulp death
- Decreased dental arch
- Ankylosis
- Color change
- Abscess
- Disruption of permanent tooth with fracture to primary tooth

---

PEARL

- Reassure the patient to alleviate anxiety.

SUBLUXATION AND LUXATION
Background

Dental trauma can result in a subluxation (i.e., mobile tooth or teeth), or luxation (i.e., partial or complete displacement of the tooth or teeth). Mobile or displaced teeth can be divided into four categories or types (Table 37.3).

TABLE 37.3 Luxation Categories: Type, Mechanism, and Treatment

Type	Mechanism	Treatment
Extrusive	Tooth lifted up partially out of socket	Splint Dental referral
Intrusive	Tooth pushed down into the socket The apex of the tooth may be crushed or fractured	Radiographs Dental referral within 24 hours
Lateral	Tooth displaced laterally may be facial, lingual, or medial May be associated with alveolar wall injury	Splint Dental referral within 24 hours
Complete	Tooth forced completely out of socket Also known as avulsion	Supraperiosteal block Replace tooth in socket Splint or temporary suture Immediate dental referral Soft or liquid diet depending on severity and treatment Antibiotic prophylaxis

Patient Presentation

- Pain
- Mobile tooth/teeth
- Missing tooth/teeth
- Bleeding

Treatment

The treatment of subluxation and luxation depends on the degree of mobility and extent of the injury. The goal of treatment is to secure the tooth in place as soon as possible and refer to the dentist within 24 hours of the injury. Pulp necrosis, color change, and necrosis of the alveolar ligaments can result from the trauma.

Subluxation of a primary tooth should not require any intervention unless the tooth is interfering with occlusion. The periodontal paste (Coe-Pak) can be used to secure a grossly mobile tooth/teeth until seen by a dental specialist within 24 hours. However, primary teeth that have a complete luxation (avulsion) should not be replaced in the socket.

A complete luxation of permanent tooth/teeth requires prompt attention and replacement of the tooth/teeth into the respective socket. The alveolar ligament cells can begin to die as early as 60 minutes after injury. The use of milk or commercial "save a tooth" preparations can increase this time significantly. If the preparations are not available to the patient, then the patient should be encouraged to place the tooth in mouth with his or her saliva.

The use of periodontal paste to splint the tooth/teeth into place as well as a temporary suture technique are discussed in this section.

Contraindications and Relative Contraindications

- Fractured tooth
- Severe maxillofacial trauma/injury
- Extended period of time after complete luxation
- Contamination
- Special considerations
- Immunocompromised patients, diabetics

Procedure Preparation
Replacing the Tooth/Teeth Into the Socket

- Gauze
- Absorbent pads

Topical and supraperiosteal block materials (see Chapter 36)

- Frazier suction tip
- Suction apparatus
- Normal saline

Splinting

- Nonsterile gloves
- Gauze
- Lubricant
- Periodontal paste (Coe-Pak)

Temporary Suture

- Suture kit
- Gauze
- Sterile gloves
- Absorbable suture material

Procedure
Replacing the Tooth/Teeth Into the Socket

- Topical and supraperiosteal block (Chapter 36)
- Check the oral cavity for trauma (i.e., fracture).
- Gently suction the socket for blood clots, being careful not to suction the wall of the socket.
- Irrigate the area with normal saline.
- Gently rinse off the tooth holding it by the crown only.
    - Never scrub or rub the tooth, especially the root.
- Gently, but firmly, replace the tooth in the socket.
    - The position does not have to be perfect but should be anatomically correct.
- Splint or suture if the tooth is too mobile after insertion.

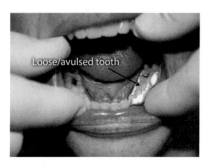

FIGURE 37.3 Securing loose-avulsed tooth with compound.

Splinting (Figure 37.3)

- Grossly mobile or replaced tooth/teeth.
- Replace the tooth/teeth into the socket as described previously.
- Mix the periodontal paste per the instructions.
- Mix base with catalyst to make a moderately sticky paste.
- Completely dry the enamel and gingiva with gauze.
- Place lubricant on gloved fingers.
- Place the paste over the affected tooth/teeth and the adjacent teeth.
  - Be sure you apply the paste to the grooves between the teeth.

Temporary Suture (Figure 37.4)

- Replace tooth/teeth into the socket as described previously.
- Insert the suture needle into the gingiva at the border of the replaced tooth.
- Bring the suture straight down behind the tooth, coming out in front of the tooth.
- Cross the tooth with the suture.
- Insert the suture needle into the gingival on the opposite tooth border.
- Bring the suture straight down behind the tooth, coming out in front of the tooth.
- Cross the tooth with the suture.
- Tie a square knot.

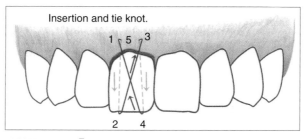

FIGURE 37.4 Temporary suture

Post-Procedure Considerations

If the tooth/teeth do not remain in place or are too mobile with splinting, then the temporary suture technique should be used. The patient should be medicated for pain and prophylaxed with antibiotics (penicillin or clindamycin).

Educational Points

- Minimally mobile tooth/teeth
  - Soft diet
- Dental specialist follow-up
- Grossly mobile or complete luxations

  - Liquid to soft diet
  - Dental specialist follow-up within 24 hours

Complications

- Loss of tooth/teeth
- Decreased dental arch
- Ankylosis
- Color change
- Abscess
- Disruption of permanent tooth with fracture to primary tooth

PEARL
■ Always be honest with the patient and/or parent about the potential outcome.

RESOURCES

Amsterdam, J. T., & Kilgore, K. P. (2014). Regional anesthesia of the head and neck. In J. R. Roberts & J. R. Hedges (Eds.), *Clinical procedures in emergency medicine* (6th ed.). Philadelphia, PA: Saunders Elsevier. Retrieved from https://www.clinicalkey.com/#!/content/book/3-s2.0-B9781455706068000306

Benko, R. (2010). Regional anesthesia of the head and neck. In J. R. Roberts & J. R. Hedges (Eds.), *Clinical procedures in emergency medicine* (5th ed., pp. 1220–1225 & 1229–1233). Philadelphia, PA: Saunders Elsevier.

Chow, A. W. (2010). Orofacial odontogenic infections. In G. L. Mandell, J. E. Bennett, & R. Dolin (Eds.), *Principles and practice of infectious diseases*. New York, NY: Churchill and Livingstone. Retrieved from http://www.mdconsult.com/book/player/book.do?method= display&type=bookPage& decorator=header&eid=4-u1.0-B978-0-443-06839-3..00060-6-s0040&displayedEid=4-u1.0-B978-0-443-06839-3..00060-6-s0045&uniq=188210824&isbn=978-0-443-06839-3&sid=965655401#lpState=open&lpTab=contentsTab&content=4-u1.0-B978-0-443-06839-3..00060-6%3Bfrom%3Dtoc%3Btype%3DbookPage%3Bisbn%3D978-0-443-06839-3

Douglass, A. B., & Douglass, J. M. (2003). Common dental emergencies. *American Family Physician, 67*(3), 511–516.

Drezner, J. A., Harmon, K. G., & O'Kane, J. W. (2007). Sports trauma to the teeth, face and eye. In R. E. Rakel (Ed.), *Textbook of family medicine* (7th ed.). Philadelphia, PA: Saunders Elsevier. Retrieved from http://www.mdconsult.com/das/book/body/188210824-5/0/1481/482.html?tocnode= 53394272&fromURL=482.html#4-u1.0-B978-1-4160-2467-5..50043-9–cesec26_2486

Gampel, N. E., Narang, V., & Shah, D. (2014). *Management of dental trauma*. Retrieved from http://emedicine.medscape.com/article/1799897-overview

Hermann, H. J., & Laskin, D. M. (2007). Wilderness dentistry and management of facial injuries. In P. S. Auerbach (Ed.), *Wilderness medicine* (5th ed.). Philadelphia, PA: Mosby Elsevier. Retrieved from http://www.mdconsult.com/das/book/body/188210824-3/0/1483/238.html?tocnode=54235634&fromURL=238.html#4-u1.0-B978-0-323-03228-5..50031-8_1433

Kliegman, R. M., Behrman, R. E., Jenson, H. B., & Stanton, B. F. (Eds.). (2007). Dental trauma. In *Nelson textbook of pediatrics* (18th ed.). Philadelphia, PA: Saunders Elsevier. Retrieved from http://www.mdconsult.com/das/book/body/188210824-8/965665260/1608/772.html#4-u1.0-B978-4160-2450-7..50313-3_6366

Matijevic, S., Lazic, Z., Kuljic-Kapulica, N., & Nonkovic, Z. (2009). Empirical antimicrobial therapy of acute dentoalveolar abscess. *Vojnosanitetski Pregled: Military Medical & Pharmaceutical Journal of Serbia, 66*(7), 544–550.

Nguyen, D. H., & Martin, J. T. (2008). Common dental infections in the primary care setting. *American Family Physician, 77*(6), 797–802, 806.

Peng, L. F., Cheng, C., Kazzi, A. A., & Peng, W. (2013). *Fractured tooth*. Retrieved from http://emedicine.medscape.com/article/763458-overview

Peng, L. F., Kazzi, A. A., & Peng, W. (2013). *Displaced tooth*. Retrieved from http://emedicine.medscape.com/article/763378-overview

Peng, L. F., Kazzi, A. A., Peng, W., & Cheng, C. (2008). *Dental, displaced tooth*. Retrieved from http://emedicine.medscape.com/article/763378-overview and http://emedicine.medscape.com/article/763378-treatment

Peng, L. F., Kazzi, A. A., Peng, W., & Cheng, C. (2009a). *Dental, avulsed tooth*. Retrieved from http://emedicine.medscape.com/article/763291-overview and http://emedicine.medscape.com/article/763291-treatment

Peng, L. F., Kazzi, A. A., Peng, W., & Cheng, C. (2009b). *Dental, fractured tooth*. Retrieved from http://emedicine.medscape.com/article/763458-overview and http://emedicine.medscape.com/article/763458-treatment

Peng, L. F., Kazzi, A. A., Peng, W., & Cheng, R. (2014). *Avulsed tooth*. Retrieved from http://emedicine.medscape.com/article/763291-overview

Scheinfeld, N. S. (2014). *Inferior alveolar nerve block*. Retrieved from http://emedicine.medscape.com/article/82622-overview

Van Meter, M. W., & Dave, A. K. (2014). *Oral nerve block*. Retrieved from http://emedicine.medscape.com/article/82850-overview

CHAPTER 38

Peritonsillar Abscess (Quinsy)

Theresa M. Campo

ANATOMY

One cannot have a discussion regarding peritonsillar abscess (PTA) without an understanding and review of the anatomy of this region. The palatine tonsils arise from the second pharyngeal pouch as buds of endodermal cells during embryonic development and continue to grow until between the ages of 6 and 7 years. There are two palatine tonsils, each located on the lateral walls of the oropharynx. These lie within a depression between the anterior and posterior tonsillar pillars. The tonsillar pillars are comprised of glossopalatine and pharyngopalatine muscles. Around the tonsils is a surrounding covering and in the medial portion this provides a pathway for blood vessels and nerves. The space between the tonsil and capsule is where the majority of PTA forms. Weber glands, which are mucous salivary glands located superior to the tonsils in the soft palate and posterior to the tongue, assist in clearing debris from the tonsils. If these glands become inflamed it is possible to develop infection, cellulitis, and ultimately abscess formation. It is important to note the proximity of the carotid sheath, which encompasses the carotid artery and jugular vein (see Figure 38.1).

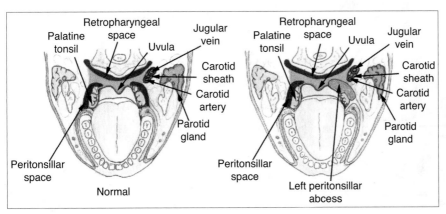

FIGURE 38.1 Tonsillar anatomy

BACKGROUND

PTA, also known as Quinsy, is one of the most common deep-space infections of the neck and head regions, accounting for approximately 30% of soft tissue abscesses in these regions. This particular infection is a continuum of a tonsillar/peritonsillar infection that then develops in the peritonsillar space. It most commonly occurs in adolescent and young adults with an incidence of 1:10,000. The infection spreads past the tonsillar capsule and invades the space between the lateral aspect of the tonsil capsule and the superior constrictor muscle of the pharynx. If the infection is left untreated or is undertreated, then it can progress to a cellulitis and ultimately an abscess may develop. Predisposing factors include dental infections, chronic/recurring tonsillitis, smoking, and infectious mononucleosis. PTA can occur in persons who have had a complete tonsillectomy as it most commonly occurs in the peritonsillar space.

If a PTA is left untreated, sepsis, thrombophlebitis, airway obstruction, deep neck infections, mediastinitis, and possibly invasion of the carotid artery may occur. PTA most often occurs in the superior pole but can also be found in the mid- and lower/inferior poles (see Figure 38.2).

The differential diagnosis should include infectious mononucleosis, cervical adenitis, peritonsillar cellulitis, parapharyngeal abscess, tracheitis, Ludwig angina, leukemia, lymphoma, epiglottitis, reropharyngeal abscess, internal carotid artery aneurysm, psudoaneurysm, neoplasm, and tubercular granuloma. Infectious origins manifest more rapidly than chronic etiologies. Any chronic mass or pulsatile mass should be investigated with further evaluation and imaging in a rapid manner.

The most common organisms found to cause PTA are:

Aerobic

- Group A *Streptococcus/Streptococcus pyogenes*
- *Staphylococcus aereus*
- Neisseria
- Corynebacterium
- Respiratory anaerobes

Anaerobic

- Fusobacterium
- Prevotella

PATIENT PRESENTATION

- Progressive tonsillitis
- Increased pain, usually unilateral
- Dysphagia
- Odynophagia
- Otalgia (affected side)
- Change of voice
- Fever
- Malaise
- Headache
- Neck pain
- Drooling

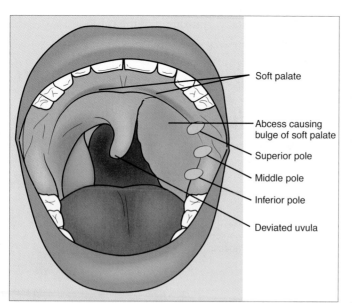

Soft palate

Abcess causing bulge of soft palate

Superior pole

Middle pole

Inferior pole

Deviated uvula

FIGURE 38.2 Peritonsillar abscess.

CLINICAL FINDINGS

- Trismus, which may be severe
- Voice changes—"hot potato voice"
- Anterior cervical lymphadenopathy
- Erythematous mucosa
- Purulent exudate
- Unilateral swelling and displacement of inferior tonsil and soft palate toward midline with deviation of uvula to the contralateral side
- Hardness or fluctuance over the peritonsillar region with a gloved finger
- Consider ordering a complete blood count (CBC) with differential, mononucleosis screening, and electrolytes

DIAGNOSTIC IMAGING

- Foremost a clinical diagnosis
- Radiologic imaging usually for unclear cases
- Ultrasound is diagnostic and therapeutic coupled with abscess evacuation.

CT Scan

- Scan with intravenous contrast
- Not used as standard of care in uncomplicated cases.
- Can be beneficial in complicated cases:
  - If suspicion for infection and need to differentiate cellulitis from abscess
  - May be beneficial in identification of infection beyond the peritonsillar space especially for the patient with disproportionate presentation with clinical findings
- Sensitivity 100%
- Specificity 75%

MRI

- Improved soft tissue detail as well as assessment of carotid sheath are major advantages. However, this modality is costly, time consuming, and not widely available.

Ultrasonography

- Used for diagnosis and guided treatment of PTA
- Intraoral sonography is very beneficial and is an effective method to assess difference between cellulitis and abscess.
- Limitations—user dependent, patient dependent (cooperative, presence of trismus, etc.)

TREATMENT
Hydration

Patients may present with moderate to severe dehydration because of dys/odynophagia resulting from throat pain. Hydration via intravenous fluid replacement should be promptly initiated. Crystalloid solutions, such as lactated Ringers or normal saline (0.9%), should be given at a rapid rate for hydration and electrolyte stability.

Pain and Fever Management

Intravenous NSAIDs and/or narcotic analgesics should be liberally administered as well as antipyretics for fever control.

Antibiotics

Antibiotics should be used prior to any surgical intervention. Penicillin is the first line treatment for PTA and has been shown to be clinically effective when used alone or in combination with other antibiotics. However, some studies show that more than 50% of cultures grow beta-lactamase producing anaerobes and broad-spectrum coverage should be considered. Clindamycin (Cleocin) is also used as a first-line treatment especially in patients with a penicillin allergy. The combination therapy of penicillin and metronidazole are shown to be effective in 98% of patients treated. This combination covers anaerobic as well as increasing penicillin anaerobic coverage. Erythromycin can also be used in patients with a penicillin allergy. Common medication preparations used are:

- Penicillin G benzathine (Bicillin L-A)
- Metronidazole (Flagyl) combined with penicillin
- Clindamycin (Cleocin)
- Nafcillin (Unipen)
- Erythromycin (E.E.S)
- Zosyn

It is important to check your local and regional resistance data for updated antibiotic recommendations.

Glucocorticoid Steroids

Steroids are commonly used as an adjunct to other therapies for relief of symptoms, especially swelling and pain. Current evidence is inconsistent regarding the benefits of this particular treatment. However, there is no documented significant risk or complication and it is felt to be a reasonable therapy in the empirical treatment of adults. Some studies demonstrate steroid use as effect in decreasing recovery time, decreasing hospital time/admission, and improving symptom relief overall. Further studies are necessary for the use of steroids in children, as well as the cost effectiveness in all populations.

Surgical Intervention

There are three methods of surgical intervention. They are needle aspiration, incision and drainage, and immediate tonsillectomy. Needle aspiration and incision and drainage with and without ultrasound guidance are further discussed in this chapter.

CONTRAINDICATIONS AND RELATIVE CONTRAINDICATIONS

- Severe trismus
- Absence of a PTA
- Coagulopathy
- Uncooperative patient

SPECIAL CONSIDERATIONS

- Immunocompromised and diabetic patients
- Very young and elderly

PROCEDURE PREPARATION

- Patient should be upright with head properly supported.

Needle Aspiration

- Light—head lamp is optimal
- Tongue blade(s)
- Gauze
- Kidney or large basin
- Patient drape or Chux pad
- Wall suction with Frazier or Yankauer tip
- 25- to 27-gauge long needle (1″ or longer)
- 16- to 18-gauge long needle (spinal needle if available)
- 3-mL syringe
- 12-mL syringe
- Topical anesthetic (Cetacaine spray)
- Viscous lidocaine
- Injectable anesthetic (lidocaine 1% with epinephrine)
- Saline or dilute hydrogen peroxide in a cup

Incision and Drainage

- Same as needle aspiration
- #11 or #15 blade
- Tape
- Kelly clamp or hemostat

Intraoral Ultrasonography

- Ultrasound machine with a high frequency (4–9 MHz) intracavitary transducer (vaginal or intraoral transducer)
- Transducer (probe) cover
- Small amount of gel

PROCEDURE
Needle Aspiration

- *Parenteral narcotic pain relief and/or minor sedation may be necessary for this procedure.
- *Place a patient drape or Chux pad over the patient's chest to just under the chin.
- *Don head lamp or adjust overhead lighting to assist with proper visualization and lighting.

There are several methods to assist with visualization of the peritonsillar area. You can either use tongue blades, a curved laryngoscope blade, or a dismantled vaginal speculum with light to hold the tongue out of the way and give light intra-orally. One may also tape two tongue blades together, side by side, for an enhanced view and to further keep the tongue from protruding superiorly and obstructing the pharyngeal view.

There is a new device called the reciprocating procedure device (RPD). An RPD allows for one-handed aspiration (see Figure 38.3). This device is a two-syringe pulley system that allows for injection and aspiration. When the thumb depresses one plunger, the syringe injects; when the accessory plunger is pressed down, then the other syringe aspirates. This allows for better needle control; safer, more accurate aspiration; and decreased complications.

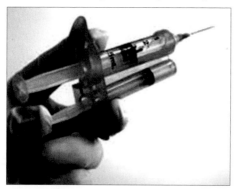

FIGURE 38.3 Reciprocating procedure device (RPD). Used with permission from Avanca Medical Devices.

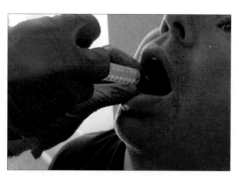

FIGURE 38.4 Proper positioning for needle aspiration of peritonsillar abscess.

- *Position yourself so you can easily visualize the area and manage the needle and syringe safely (Figure 38.4).
- *Manually palpate the peritonsillar area to ascertain the fluctuant area.
- *Have the patient gargle repeatedly with viscous lidocaine at least 15 minutes prior to the procedure in a repetitive manner and ensure all is spit out.
- *Apply topical anesthetic (Cetacaine) to fluctuant area.
- *If injectable anesthetic is required, use the 25- to 27-gauge long needle to inject intramucosally. You can move the tongue if needed with your finger. Be careful not to increase the size of the abscess while injecting anesthetic. It is normal for the area to blanch during the injection.
- *Attach the long 16- to 20-gauge needle to the 12-mL syringe.
- Take the needle cover and cut the distal 0.5 to 1 cm of the needle cover and then replace over the needle attached to the syringe. Be sure that no more than 1 cm of needle is exposed beyond the needle cover. This will help avoid penetration too far, especially if the patient inadvertently moves forward, and risk carotid sheath penetration and injury (Figure 38.5). Remember, this is a safe buffer, as studies have shown that the carotid artery's depth is an average of 25 mm deep to the pharyngeal wall, though aberrancy does exist.

- Insert the needle into the area of fluctuance along the sagittal plane. Do not angle laterally toward the carotid artery and do not insert the needle into the tonsil itself. The needle should be in the peritonsillar space only. Do not go further than 1 cm even if no pus is returned.
- Have an assistant stand on the other side of the bed holding a Yankauer suction device (this can also aid in keeping the mouth optimally open).
- Continue to aspirate pus and remove as much pus as possible.
- It is normal to remove 2 to 6 mL of pus from a PTA and it can be common to remove > 8 mL of pus. However, when large amounts of pus are removed there is a higher incidence of recurrence and often repeat aspiration, incision, and drainage or tonsillectomy may be warranted based on the individual case.
- If no pus is returned, remove the needle and attempt again in the middle pole of the space. If still no pus, then remove the needle and make a final attempt in the inferior pole of the space. Make no more than these three attempts.
- Keep the needle position in the same sagital plane when redirecting in lower poles.
- A negative aspirate does not rule out a PTA. Further diagnostic imaging may be warranted.
- Stopping the procedure on a negative aspiration in the superior pole will miss up to 30% of the cases.

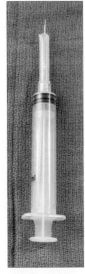

FIGURE 38.5 Needle and syringe with cut cover tip.

Incision and Drainage

- Follow the same steps used for needle aspiration marked with an asterisk in the preceding procedures.
- Tape all but the distal end of the scalpel tip to prevent deep penetration (Figure 38.6).
- Advise the patient that he or she will notice the flow of pus/blood in the mouth and to expectorate it and not swallow.
    - Have an assistant hold the suction tip in their mouth to help with the drainage.
- Incise 0.5 cm of mucosa in a posterior to anterior direction, being careful not to exceed the taped area of the scalpel.
    - A stab incision with the #11 scalpel blade is acceptable as well.
- Take the Kelly clamp or hemostat and insert into the opening while the clamp is closed. Once inside the incision, gently open the clamp, breaking up any loculations.
- Have the patient rinse, gargle, and spit the saline or peroxide mixture.
- Packing is not used in this procedure.

Intraoral Ultrasonography

- Follow the same steps used for needle aspiration marked with an asterisk in the preceding procedures.

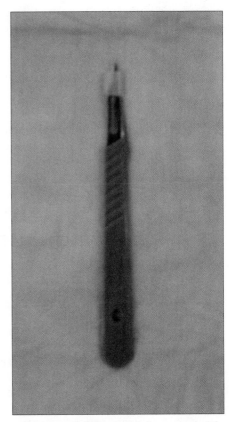

FIGURE 38.6 Incision and drainage—scalpel tip.

- Place a protective sheath or condom over the tranducer.
- Place a small amount of gel on the inside and outside of the sheath/condom. However, the moisture from the oral mucosa can allow for sufficient transmission without the gel.
- Topical anesthetic should be sprayed on the posterior pharynx
- Injectable anesthetic should not be necessary for diagnosing an abscess but may be necessary if needle aspiration and/or incision and drainage are indicated.
- Place the transducer over the tonsillar tissue.
- Begin scanning in a systematic manner along two orthogonal planes. This will allow visualization of the tonsil and allow you to determine the size of the tonsil. You will also be able to determine whether a fluid collection is present or not.
- Next evaluate the soft palate in both a sagittal and transverse plane to determine the superior and inferior ends of the abscess, the depth and proximity to the carotid sheath and artery.
- Color Doppler should now be used to identify and characterize adjacent structures such as the carotid artery.
- Color Doppler can also show hypervascularity in areas of inflammation.
- Be sure to scan the inferior pharynx for pus collection, which may occur in the mid- and lower pole of the tonsil.
- Comparison to the contralateral tonsil should now be done.
- If an abscess is identified, then needle aspiration or incision and drainage should be done using the guidance of ultrasound (follow those steps, respectively).

If moderate to severe trismus is present and intraoral ultrasound cannot be completed, consider using a transcutaneous approach using a high-frequency linear transducer to scan the pharynx. Please note this method may not be as accurate in diagnosing and treating a PTA. Although the literature is limited in this modality to case reports, at the time of this writing, CT imaging should be considered.

POST-PROCEDURE CONSIDERATIONS

Patients should be observed for at least 1 hour post-procedure for bleeding and reaccumulation of pus. Patients may require admission to the hospital for hemorrhage, further surgical intervention, intravenous antibiotics (toxic patients), hydration, and pain management, although a successful evacuation usually is synonymous with a discharge home with close ear, nose, and throat specialist follow-up. Consultation with an otolaryngologist is also required for close follow-up.

EDUCATIONAL POINTS

Frequently rinse, gargle, and spit with saline or dilute hydrogen peroxide post-procedure.

- Encourage completion of the full course of antibiotics and discuss the risks of stopping prematurely.
- Report any bleeding or reaccumulation of pus to the provider or return to the emergency department.
- The pus collection does not accumulate in the palatine tonsil itself; it accumulates in between the tonsillar capsule and the pharyngeal wall (superior constrictor muscle and the palatopharyngeus muscle).
- Standard ultrasound vaginal probes, familiar to most clinicians, can be used as an intra-oral device when evaluating a proper needle position in cases of PTA.

- Intra-oral sonography helps avoid up to 24% of the false negative rates with blind needle aspiration; ensure the diagnosis and identify the carotid artery.

COMPLICATIONS

- Aspiration of blood or pus
- Hemorrhage
  - Coagulopathy
  - Carotid aneurysm or pseudoaneurysm aspirated
- Poor healing
  - Too small or too large of an incision
- Inadequate treatment of abscess
  - May cause airway obstruction, tissue necrosis, carotid sheath hemorrhage, extension of infection into deep neck tissue or posterior mediastinum (chest wall)
- Cervical abscess, cerebral abscess
- Sepsis
- Jugular vein thrombosis
- Carotid artery injury
  - Data shows that this is a rare occurrence (< 10%) but extreme care must be given during any of these procedures.
- PTA is not an indication for a tonsillectomy.

PEARLS

- You can place the patient in the Trendelenburg position and sit at the head of the bed to enhance visualization.
- Gargling with viscous lidocaine for 10 minutes may avoid infiltrative anesthesia.
- Infiltrative anesthesia may distort ultrasound image, so if needed, administer after sonography.
- Taping together two tongue blades side by side may improve pharyngeal view.
- A dry tap does not rule out PTA.
- The abscess does not usually occur within the tonsil itself but within the space between the tonsil and the wall, so do not direct the needle in the medial positioned tonsil.
- The carotid artery lies posterior and lateral to the PTA while the pus collection is medially positioned relative to the carotid artery.
- Imaging is usually unnecessary.
- Antibiotics alone will not treat a PTA; evacuation of pus does.
- Avoidance of this needed procedure in cases of PTA, for fear of inadvertently puncturing the caratid artery, is unfounded in the literature.

RESOURCES

Adams, J. G., Barton, E. D., Collings, J., DeBlieux, P. M. C., Gisondi, M. A., & Nadel, E. S. (2013). *Emergency medicine clinical essentials* (2nd ed., chap. 29). Philadelphia, PA: Elsevier Saunders.

Adhikari, S. R. Ultrasound guide for emergency physicians. Retrieved from http://www.sonoguide.com/smparts_ent.html

Cosby, K. S., & Kendall, J. L. (2014). *Practical guide to emergency ultrasound* (2nd ed). Philadelphia, PA: Wolters Kluwer/LWW.

Deutsch, M. D., Kriss, V. M., & Willging, J. P. (1995). Distance between the tonsillar fossa and internal carotid artery in children. *Archives of Otolaryngology Head and Neck Surgery, 121*(12), 1410-1412. Retrieved from http://www.ncbi.nlm.nih.gov/pubmed/7488372

Flores, J., Tan, A. J., & Mehta, N. (2014). *Peritonsillar abscess in emergency medicine.* Retrieved from http://emedicine.medscape.com/article/764188-overview#showall

Hidaka, H., Ishida, E., Suzuki, T., Matsutani, S., Kobayashi, T., & Takahashi, S. (2014). Unusual parapharyngeal extension of peritonsillar abscess to the masticator space: Successfully drained by extraoral and intraoral endoscopic approaches. *Annals of Otology, Rhinology & Laryngology, 123*(5), 333–337.

Ishii, K., Aramaki, H., Aray, Y., Uchimura, K., Nishida, M., & Yoda, K. (2002). Evaluation of safe surgical treatment of peritonsillar abscess using computed tomography. *Nihon Jibiinkoka Gakkai Kaiho, 105*(3), 249–256.

Powell, J., & Wilson, J. A. (2012). An evidence-based review of peritonsillar abscess. *Clinical Otolaryngology, 37*, 136–145.

Rehrer, M., Mantuani, D., & Nagdev, A. (2013). Identification of peritonsillar abscess by trancutaneous cervvical ultrasound. *American Journal of Emergency Medicine, 31*(1), 267. Retrieved from http://www.ncbi.nlm.nih.gov/pubmed/22795424

Roberts, J. R., Custalow, C. B., Thomsen, T. W., & Hedges, J. R. (2014). *Roberts and Hedges' clinical procedures in emergency medicine* (6th ed). Philadelphia, PA: Elsevier Saunders.

Scott, P. M., Loftus, W. K., Kew, J., Ahuja, A., Yue, V., & van Hasselt, C.A. (1999). Diagnosis of peritonsillar infections: A prospective study of ultrasound, computerized tomography and clinical diagnosis. *Journal of Laryngol Otol, 113*, 229–232.

Seckin, O. U., Koral, K., Margraf, L., & Deskin, R. (2013). Management of intratonsillar abscess in children. *Pediatrics International, 55*, 455–460.

U.S. National Cancer Institute. (n.d.). *Tonsils.* Retrieved from https://commons.wikimedia.org/wiki/File%3ATonsils_diagram.jpg

CHAPTER 39

Reducing Mandibular Dislocations

Theresa M. Campo

BACKGROUND

Mandibular dislocation can occur from numerous mechanisms but the most common is from opening the jaw widely during activities, such as yawning, dystonic reactions, laughing, taking large bites, oral sex, seizures, trauma, vomiting, and intraoral and dental procedures. Less likely, it can also occur from facial trauma. Mandibular dislocations occur when the condylar head completely displaces out of the mandibular fossa and cannot be reduced by the patient. A thorough history and physical examination are imperative to assess for accompanying injury and to properly diagnose the injury. Diagnostic imaging will also aid in the diagnosis and determination of treatment necessary. Plain radiographs, such as a panorex and/or complete mandible, can be performed but CT scan is more widely used, especially with traumatic injuries, to visualize overlying structures that may not be easily visualized on the plain radiograph. Keep in mind, however, this is a bedside diagnosis as few entities have similar clinical presentations.

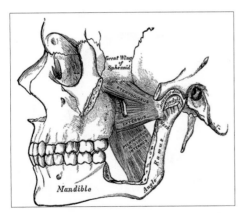 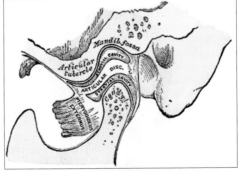

FIGURE 39.1 Normal anatomy of the mandible.

Before we further discuss mandibular dislocations, it is important to review the anatomy and the mechanism for dislocation. The temporomandibular joint (TMJ) is the articular surface between mandibular condyles and temporal bone and is a combination hinge and sliding movement and, as such, is classified as a ginglymoarthrodial joint. The mandibular condyles slide or glide along the mandibular fossa in combination with a hinge action. The temporomandibular, sphenomandibular, and capsular ligaments provide joint support. Nerve and blood supply are from the branches of the auriculo-temporal and masseteric divisions of the mandibular nerve and superficial temporal branch of the external carotid artery, respectively. Jaw opening occurs from lateral traction of the mandibular neck by the lateral pterygoid muscles. Jaw closure occurs from the action of the strong masseter muscle along with the medial pterygoid, and temporis muscles. The actions of these muscles are coordinated to first retract the mandible and condyles posteriorly to the temporal articular eminence, followed by elevation and placement of the condylar head into the mandibular fossa. Jaw protrusion and lateral movement are performed by the medial and lateral pterygoid muscles. Figure 39.1 demonstrates the normal anatomy of the mandible in an open and closed position.

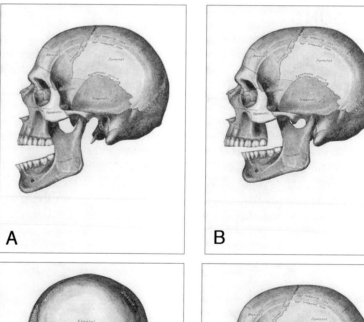

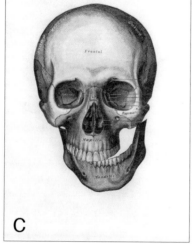

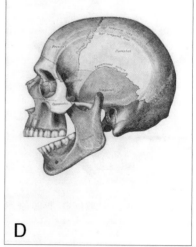

FIGURE 39.2 Mandible dislocation. A. anterior; B. posterior; C. superior; D. lateral

Mandibular dislocations can be anterior, posterior, lateral, or superior and are classified based on the location of condyle in comparison to the temporal articular eminence (Figure 39.2). Anterior mandible dislocations are the most commonly occurring. The focus of this chapter covers anterior dislocations, although all types are briefly discussed.

Anterior

The mandible elevates before retraction, which displaces the condyle head out of the mandibular fossa anterior to the temporal articular eminence. Chronic dislocation secondary to repetitive weakening of the joint capsule can occur from repeated dislocations, congenital malformation, and hypermobility syndrome.

Posterior

The mandibular condyle is displaced caudal out of the mandibular fossa toward the mastoid process. This usually occurs from a blow to the chin or mandible and may cause auditory canal injury. May also be associated with a condylar neck, base-of-skull fracture or basilar skull fracture.

Lateral

The mandibular condylar head moves laterally and superiorly into the temporal space. Clinically, and unlike anterior or posterior dislocations, the patient's chin is deviated to the side. This injury is associated with mandibular fracture(s).

Superior

This rare type of superior dislocation is also known as "central dislocations." The mandibular condyle is displaced superiorly into the middle cranial fossa and because of such may be associated with a mandibular fossa fracture and/or dislocation of the mandible into the middle skull base. It can occur from a direct blow with the mouth partially open. Depending on the mechanism of injury, this injury may have accompanying injury to the facial nerve, cranial nerve VIII injury (which may cause deafness), intracranial hematoma, cerebral contusion, and cerebrospinal fluid leakage.

PATIENT PRESENTATION
- Acute jaw pain
- Difficulty speaking and swallowing
- Trismus (difficulty opening or the inability to open the mouth)
- Malocclusion
- Mouth open with prominent jaw

CLINICAL FINDINGS
- Tongue blade test—a tongue blade is placed between the molars. Ask the patient to bite down. If the patient can stabilize the tongue blade while it is simultaneously being twisted by the provider, then mandibular fracture is unlikely.
- Unilateral—deviation of the jaw/chin away from the dislocation

- Bilateral—open mouth with prominent jaw giving the appearance of an underbite with pain over the TMJ
- Anterior—visible and palpable preauricular depression from condyle displaced out of mandibular fossa
- Lateral—condylar head may be felt

Physical examination should include the following:

- Basal skull fracture (battle sign, raccoon eyes, etc.)
- Cerebrospinal fluid leakage
- Cranial nerve deficit, specifically CN V and VIII
- Hearing
- External auditory canal for abnormalities
- Oral cavity for lacerations indicating an accompanying fracture

CONTRAINDICATIONS AND RELATIVE CONTRAINDICATIONS

- Accompanying injury as discussed
- Noncooperative patient may require sedation

PROCEDURE PREPARATION

Conscious sedation is usually necessary during the reduction to alleviate pain, muscle spasm, and anxiety that causes the inability of the patient to relax the muscles enough to allow reduction to occur. Again, the strong masseter muscles will be in spasm and, until they are in a more relaxed state, it will be difficult to counter-oppose their force and redirect the condylar head inferior and posterior to the articular eminence. Policies and guidelines of your institution should be followed.

Local Anesthetics

- 25- to 30-gauge needle
- 3- or 6-mL syringe with needle
- Lidocaine 1%
- Skin cleanser

Reduction

- Head rest/support
- Tongue depressor
- Gauze
- Gloves
- Bite block

PROCEDURE

The key to any successful mandible reduction is masticator muscle relaxation. The patient may be able to relax enough to facilitate the reduction. If the patient is not able to provide muscle relaxation, conscious sedation may be indicated. It is important to take measures to protect your thumb and fingers during the reduction utilizing any of the discussed methods. Without such protection, they may be injured during normal jaw closing because of involuntary muscle spasm at the time of reduction. To prevent injury, put on protective gloves and ask an assistant wrap gauze around each thumb to act as a cushion and to protect your thumbs. You can also use a bite block in the patient's mouth (manufactured or by wrapping gauze around the end of a tongue blade). Make sure you remove any dentures prior to starting any of the reduction methods.

Local Anesthesia
Temporomandibular Space

- Prepare skin with cleanser anterior to the ear.
- At the palpable preauricular depression insert the needle (into the TMJ space).
- Direct the needle anterior and superior onto the inferior surface of the glenoid fossa.
- Inject approximately 2 mL of lidocaine directly into the lateral ptyerygoid muscle.
- Palpate the maxillary tuberosity.
- Insert the needle and inject 2- to 3-mL of lidocaine into the lateral pterygoid muscle, which is posterior to the maxillary tuberosity.

Supine Reduction

- Place patient in a sitting position with the head supported.
- Stand in front of the patient, facing the patient.
- Put on gloves.
- Ask an assistant to wrap gauze around each thumb.
- Place thumbs on the inferior molars as far back as possible.
- Cup your fingers around the mandible.
- Apply constant and steady downward and posterior pressure on the mandible using the thumbs to slightly open the mouth (Figure 39.3).

Recumbent

- Place the patient in a supine position.
- Stand behind the patient, facing the patient.
- Put on gloves.
- Ask an assistant to wrap gauze around each thumb.
- Place thumbs on the inferior molars as far back as possible.
- Apply downward and backward pressure on the mandible until reduced (Figure 39.4).

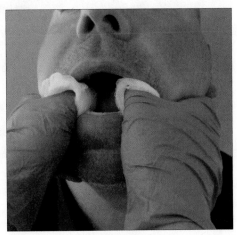

FIGURE 39.3 Supine/sitting reduction

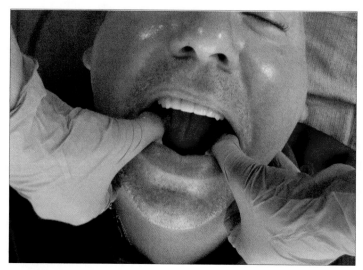

FIGURE 39.4 Recumbent. Note that gauze should be wrapped around the fingers during the procedure, although it is not worn in some of these photos. The photos are for demonstration only.

Wrist Pivot

- Place patient in a sitting position with the head supported.
- Stand in front of the patient, facing the patient.
- Grasp the mandible at the apex of the mentum with both hands.
- Place fingers on the inferior molars.
- Apply cephalad force with thumbs and caudal pressure with fingers.
- Pivot the wrists to reduce the mandibular condyle (Figure 39.5).

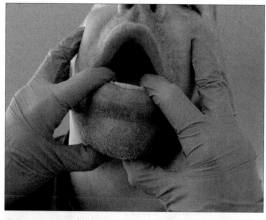

FIGURE 39.5 Wrist pivot.

Ipsilateral (Three Maneuvers: External, Intra-oral, and Combined External)

External/Ipsilateral (Figure 39.6)

- Place patient in a sitting position.
- Stand behind patient supporting the head with the nondominant hand.
- Use the dominant hand to apply downward pressure on displaced condyle, which is inferior to the zygomatic arch.

If this fails:
Intraoral

- Stand in front of the patient facing the patient.
- Apply downward pressure on ipsilateral lower molars.

If this fails:

Combined external

- Apply downward pressure on molars with gauze-wrapped fingers while your other hand applies pressure on the displaced condyle.

Gag Reflex

This method uses jaw relaxation with transient decent of the mandible inferiorly:

- With the patient awake and relaxed, apply tactile stimulation to the soft palate with a tongue blade.

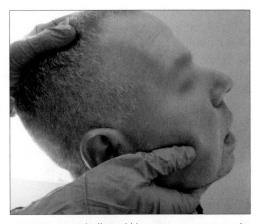

FIGURE 39.6 Ipsilateral (three maneuvers: external, intra-oral, and combined external).

- The stimulation will induce the gag reflex, causing muscle relaxation, and allow the mandible to descend caudally, moving the condyle inferiorly, and reducing it back into place.

Unified Hand Technique

This is a new method for reduction of a unilateral dislocation (Figure 39.7).

- Place patient in a sitting position with the head supported.
- Stand in front of the patient, facing the patient.
- Place both thumbs wrapped in gauze on the affected molar occlusal surface.
- Apply inferior and posterior pressure.

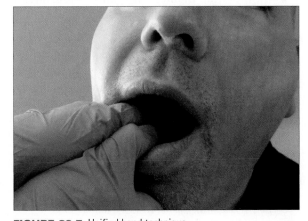

FIGURE 39.7 Unified hand technique.

COMPLICATIONS

Complications may occur from the trauma of the dislocation or from the reduction procedure and may include any of the following:

- Fracture
- Recurrence
- Injury to internal carotid artery and/or facial nerve
- Posterior dislocation—injury to the external auditory canal that can result in deafness

- Superior dislocation—surrounding structure injury
- Provider thumb injury
- Joint injury
- Ligamentous or muscular injury
- Intraoral injuries (i.e., fracture or luxed tooth/teeth, lacerations, abrasions)

POST-PROCEDURE EDUCATION

- Do not open mouth wide for at least 1 week.
- Eat soft foods.
- Nonsteroidal anti-inflammatory drugs
- Muscle relaxants
- Warm compresses
- Soft collar may be considered to support the TMJ post-reduction

---

PEARLS

- This is an "across the room" diagnosis.
- In traumatic and/or recurrent cases, imaging may be avoided.
- Successful reduction usually warrants conscious sedation, as the masseter muscle force is difficult to overcome when it is in a state of spasm.
- Acute dystonia may have a similar presentation.
- Always wrap thumbs with gauze before attempting reduction.
- Masseter muscle spasm is associated with much pain and apprehension.

RESOURCES

Akinbami, B.O. (2011). Evaluation of the mechanism and principles of management of temporomandibular joint dislocation. Systemic review of literature and a proposed new classification of temporomandibular joint dislocation. *Head and Face Medicine, 7,* 10. doi: 10.1186/1746-160x-7-10. Retrieved from http://www.ncbi.nlm.nih.gov/pmc/articles/PMC3127760

Bontempo, L. J. (2013). Maxillofacial disorders. In J. G. Adams (Ed.), *Emergency medicine: Clinical essentials* (2nd ed.). Philadelphia, PA: Saunders Elsevier.

Chan, T. C., Harrigan, R. A., Ufberg, J., & Vilke, G. M. (2008). Mandibular reduction. *Journal of Emergency Medicine, 34*(4), 435–440.

Chaudhry, M. (2014). *Mandible dislocation.* Retrieved from http://emedicine.medscape.com/article/823775-overview#showall

Cheng, D. (2010). Unified hands technique for mandibular dislocations. *Journal of Emergency Medicine, 38*(3), 366–367.

Cohen, L., & Kim, D. J. (2014). New facial asymmetry: A case of unilateral temporomandibular joint dislocation. *Journal of Emergency Medicine, 47*(1), e11–e13.

Procedures for Managing Common Musculoskeletal Conditions and Injuries

CHAPTER 40

Procedures for Arthrocentesis

Keith A. Lafferty

BACKGROUND

Joints allow free movement between two bone surfaces; the movement of the bones causes friction and generates heat. The cartilaginous articular surfaces (composed of collagen and proteoglycan substances) at the end of bones are highly compressible and well lubricated by synovial fluid, which is secreted by cells of the synovial membrane lining the joint space. The synovial fluid helps dissipate heat and allows smooth motion of the joint. These cells also participate in the inflammatory cascade and contain lysosomes in their cytoplasm. The high concentration of hyaluronic acid in the synovium gives it its high viscosity. Finally, a capsule encircles the entire joint, which is further supported by its surrounding ligaments, tendons, and muscle. The synovial membrane, periosteum, and joint capsule are rich in sensory nerve fibers. Of note, polymorphonuclear cells release hyaluronidase from their lysosomes, which enzymatically destroy hyaluronic acid, thereby decreasing the synovial fluid viscosity in inflammatory joint conditions. This thinning of the synovial fluid can be tested grossly by placing the drawn synovial fluid between the gloved thumb and index finger and, upon separating the fingers, measuring the fluid length, otherwise known as the string sign (Figure 40.1).

The inflamed joint can be a diagnostic challenge to even the most experienced provider. Furthermore, the clinical signs and symptoms that distinguish septic arthritis from other arthritides can have much overlap.

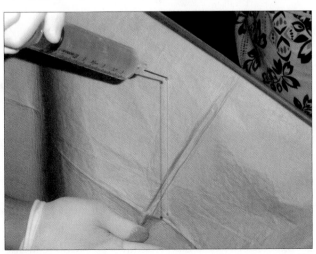

FIGURE 40.1 String sign.

Diagnostic reasons aside, arthrocentesis can be a therapeutic benefit, providing relief from traumatic hemarthrosis and chronic arthritides.

DIFFERENTIAL DIAGNOSIS
- Cellulitis
- Bursitis
- Tendonitis
- Baker's cyst
- Deep vein thrombosis

PATIENT PRESENTATION
- Pain
- Swelling
- Possible erythema

TREATMENT

Clothing should be removed and the affected joint exposed. Aspirate as much fluid as possible for diagnostic and therapeutic reasons. It is paramount to rule out septic arthritis. The approach for arthrocentesis is usually on the extensor surfaces. This is secondary to the fact that extensor surfaces are generally more superficial, expose more of the joint, and the neurovascular structures are usually embedded in the flexor surface.

Fluid analysis should consist of a Gram stain and culture, cell count, and crystals. Note that a negative Gram stain does not rule out septic arthritis. In general, cell counts more than 50,000 white blood cells (WBCs)/mm^3 warrant treatment for septic arthritis. Gout and pseudogout have crystal formation and usually induce less than 50,000 WBCs/mm^3. However, up to 20% of these arthrotides can induce a WBC count greater than 50,000 WBCs/mm^3. Rheumatoid arthritis and the seronegative arthritides also usually induce less than 50,000 WBCs/mm^3. Osteoarthritis has less than 4,000 WBCs/mm^3.

CONTRAINDICATIONS
- Overlying cellulitis

RELATIVE CONTRAINDICATIONS
- Bleeding
- Diatheses
- Bacteremia
- Prosthetic joint

PROCEDURE PREPARATION
- Protective gown and sterile gloves
- Sterile drapes
- Skin cleanser with chlorhexidine or providone iodine
- Local anesthetic agent
- 10- to 60-mL syringe, depending on joint size

- 18- to 22-gauge needle depending on joint size
- Red, purple, and green test tubes for lab analysis
- Sterile technique is mandatory and aseptic technique is paramount.

PROCEDURE
Knee

- Position towels under the knee to give 15 degrees of slight flexion.
- For the medial approach, identify the medial midpatellar area; the site of entry should be just below this.
- Direct an 18-gauge needle slightly cephalic toward the intercondylar femoral notch (Figure 40.2 and **Video 40.1**).
- Keep it just under the posterior surface of the patella.
- Make sure that the needle stays parallel to the floor.
- A lateral approach may be used as well.

Radiohumeral Joint (Elbow)

- Patient should be sitting upright in bed.
- Elbow flexed at 90 degrees on the table with the forearm in pronation.
- Identify the lateral epicondyle and the head of the radius.
- Using a 22-gauge needle, enter the joint in a medial matter, perpendicular to the joint (Figure 40.3).

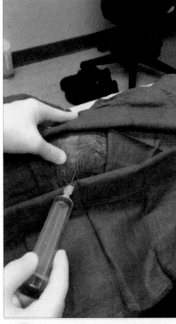

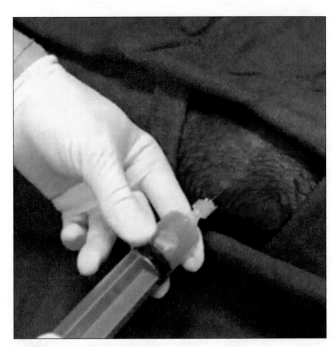

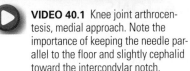
VIDEO 40.1 Knee joint arthrocentesis, medial approach. Note the importance of keeping the needle parallel to the floor and slightly cephalid toward the intercondylar notch.
springerpub.com/campo

FIGURE 40.2 Knee arthrocentesis.

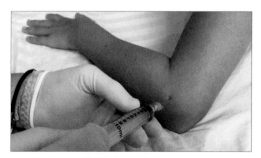

FIGURE 40.3 Radiohumeral arthrocentesis.

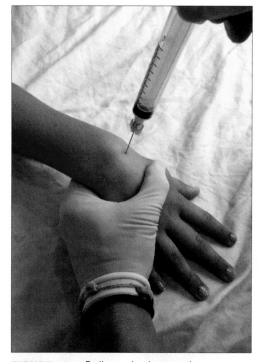

FIGURE 40.4 Radiocarpal arthrocentesis.

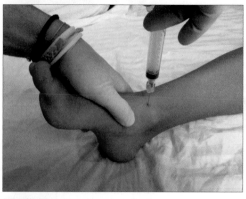

FIGURE 40.5 Tibiotalar arthrocentesis.

Radiocarpal Joint (Wrist)

- Patient should be sitting upright in bed.
- Forearm/wrist prone on the table with the wrist flexed at 30 degrees with slight traction.
- Identify the dorsal radial tubercle (it is a prominence of the distal dorsal radius).
- The extensor pollicis longus tendon runs radial to this tubercle and makes the dorsal tendon border the snuff box.
- Enter the joint space with a 22-gauge needle distal to the radial tubercle and on the ulna side of the extensor pollicis longus tendon, where a sulcus can be palpated perpendicular to the skin (Figure 40.4).

Tibiotalar Joint (Ankle)

- Patient should be supine on the bed.
- Foot in plantar flexion.
- Identify the medial malleolar sulcus (lateral to the medial malleolus).
- The lateral margin of the sulcus is bordered by the anterior tibial tendon (best seen by active dorsiflexion).
- Insert a 20- or 22-gauge needle dorsally (perpendicular to the fibular shaft) into the medial malleolar sulcus (Figure 40.5).

Glenohumeral Joint (Shoulder)

- Patient should be sitting on stretcher with hands on the lap.
- Identify the coracoid process medially and the humeral head laterally.
- Insert a 20- or 22-gauge needle in the sulcus bordered by the coracoid and the humeral head.
- Needle is inserted inferiorly and laterally to the coracoid and directed posteriorly (Figure 40.6).

COMPLICATIONS

- Infection
- Hemarthrosis
- Corticosteroid-related complications

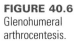

FIGURE 40.6
Glenohumeral
arthrocentesis.

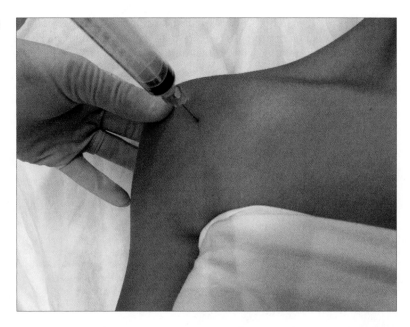

PEARLS

- Active and passive range of motion will always elicit pain in articular disease, while rarely being elicited in periarticular disease.
- Relaxation of muscles is of paramount importance because their contraction narrows the joint surface.
- Fat globules in the synovial fluid are diagnostic of a fracture.
- Arthrocentesis of the acute traumatic hemarthrosis not only provides symptomatic relief of pain, but also allows proper assessment of ligamentous stability.
- A dry tap is rare and, if it occurs, one should question the proper position of the needle.
- If minimal fluid returns, synovial culture trumps other lab tests.
- Ultrasound guidance may be of benefit in localizing difficult joint spaces.
- Because of the action of hyaluronidase on hyaluronic acid, viscosity can be tested by dripping a small amount of fluid from the syringe needle and measuring the length of the string created. In inflammatory conditions, especially in infectious etiologies, the "string sign" will be much less than 10 cm.
- Note that extracapsular disease can mimic articular diseases such as bursitis, tendonitis, and cellulitis.

RESOURCES

Lowery, D. W. (2006). Arthritis. In J. Marx, R. Hockberger, & R. Walls (Eds.), *Rosen's emergency medicine concepts and clinical practice* (pp. 1780–1781). Philadelphia, PA: Mosby Elsevier.

Ma, L., Cranney, A., & Holroyd-Leduc, J. M. (2009). Acute monoarthritis: What is the cause of my patient's painful swollen joint? *Canadian Medical Association Journal, 180*(1), 59–65.

Parrillo, S. J., & Fisher, J. (2004). Arthrocentesis. In J. Roberts & J. Hedges (Eds.), *Clinical procedures in emergency medicine* (pp. 1042–1056). Philadelphia, PA: Saunders Elsevier.

Siva, C. (2003). Diagnosing acute monoarthritis in adults: A practical approach for the family physician. *American Family Physician, 68*(1), 83–90.

Wise, C. (2008). Arthrocentesis and injection of joints and soft tissue. In G. S. Firestein, E. D. Harris, R. C. Budd, I. B. McInnes, & S. Buddy (Eds.), *Firestein: Kelley's textbook of rheumatology.* Philadelphia, PA: W. B. Saunders.

CHAPTER 41

Procedures for Therapeutic Joint Injection

Keith A. Lafferty

BACKGROUND

This modality has been used since the 1950s and its use has been increasing in recent years. Injured joint tissue leads to a proliferation of the inflammatory cascade, in part from the synovial cells themselves and also from circulating polymorphonuclear leukocytes. This proliferation of cytokines increases blood flow, induces pain and swelling, and decreases range of motion. Corticosteroids suppress this inflammatory cascade by decreasing capillary permeability and by attenuating many of the cytokine effects.

The ideal steroid for injection should have a long duration of activity, have little or no postinjection pain, and should possess minimal side effects. Different agents have not been studied in a comparable manner. The duration of the effect is related to the solubility of the agent, with lower solubility corticosteroids having an increased joint duration. Because long-acting agents are in a crystalline solution, they can cause a postinjection flare that does not occur when using a short-acting solution. Combining two such agents together offsets each other's shortcomings. Also, mixing the solution with a long-acting anesthetic agent provides even earlier relief of symptoms and dilutes the solution. Also, in general, larger joints require more corticosteroids than smaller joints (up to 10 mL should be instilled into the knee joint) (Figure 41.1).

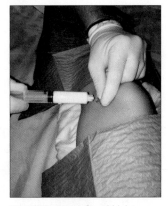

FIGURE 41.1 Steroid joint injection using an angio-catheter.

PATIENT PRESENTATION
- Pain
- Tenderness
- Swelling
- Erythema
- Decreased range of motion

TREATMENT (TABLE 41.1)
Only after aspiration of synovial fluid and positively ruling out septic arthritis, therapeutic joint injection may be implemented. Basically any arthritic condition, except septic arthritis, is a candidate for this treatment modality such as, but not limited to, osteo, rheumatoid, gout, pseudogout, and autoimmune arthrotides.

TABLE 41.1 Summary of Treatment for Therapeutic Joint Infection

Medication	Large Joint (mg)	Small Joint (mg)	Potency	Solubility	Duration
Hydrocortosone acetate (Hydrocortone)	NA	NA	1	High	Low
Triamcinolone acetonide (Kenalog)	20	2–6	5	Intermediate	Intermediate
Triamcinolone hexacetonide (Aristospan)	20	2–6	5	Intermediate	Intermediate
Methylprednisolone acetate (Depo-Medrol)	40	3.5–0.5	5	Intermediate	Intermediate
Betamethasone acetate/sodium phosphate (Celestone Soluspan)	6	1.5–3	25	Low	High
Dexamethasone acetate (Decadron-LA)	5	0.5–1.5	25	Low	High

CONTRAINDICATIONS
- An infection of either articular or overlying periarticular tissue
- Acute fractures
- Prosthetic joints

RELATIVE CONTRAINDICATIONS
- Bleeding diathesis
- Bacteremia
- Chronic debilitating diseases such as tuberculosis

- Achilles/patella tendonopathies
- Two previous injections with failure

PROCEDURE PREPARATION

- See arthrocentesis on particular joints in Chapter 40
- Sterile gloves
- Sterile drapes
- Skin cleanser with chlorhexidine or providone iodine
- Local anesthetic agent
- 5- to 10-mL syringe, depending on joint size
- 18- to 22-gauge needle, depending on joint size
- Sterile technique is mandatory and aseptic technique is paramount.

PROCEDURE

Occasionally, a therapeutic joint injection immediately follows an arthrocentesis. In this situation, an angiocath may be used with the catheter left in place after the arthrocentesis. The corticosteroid-filled syringe can now be attached to the catheter and injection procedures may be followed (Figure 41.1). To view figures corresponding with anatomical landmarks, see Chapter 40.

Knee

- Position towels under the knee to give 15 degrees of slight flexion.
- For the medial approach, identify the medial midpatellar area; the site of entry should be just below this.
- Direct a 20-gauge needle slightly cephalic toward the intercondylar femoral notch.
- Keep the needle just under the posterior surface of the patella.
- Make sure the needle stays parallel to the floor.
- A lateral approach may be used as well.

Radiohumeral Joint (Elbow)

- Patient should be sitting upright in bed.
- Elbow flexed at 90 degrees on the table with the forearm in pronation.
- Identify the lateral epicondyle and the head of the radius.
- Using a 22-gauge needle, enter the joint in a medial manner, perpendicular to the joint.

Radiocarpal Joint (Wrist)

- Patient should be sitting upright in bed.
- Forearm/wrist prone on the table with the wrist flexed at 30 degrees with slight traction.
- Identify the dorsal radial tubercle (it is a prominence of the distal dorsal radius).
- The extensor pollicis longus tendon runs radial to this tubercle and also makes the dorsal tendon border the snuff box.
- Enter the joint space with a 22-gauge needle distal to the radial tubercle and on the ulna side of the extensor pollicis longus tendon where a sulcus can be palpated perpendicular to the skin.

Tibiotalar Joint (Ankle)
- Patient should be supine on the bed.
- Foot in plantar flexion.
- Identify the medial malleolar sulcus (lateral to the medial malleolus).
- The lateral margin of the sulcus is bordered by the anterior tibial tendon (best seen by active dorsiflexion).
- Insert a 20- or 22-gauge needle dorsally (perpendicular to the fibular shaft) into the medial malleolar sulcus.

Glenohumeral Joint (Shoulder)
- Patient should be sitting on a stretcher with hands on his or her lap.
- Identify the coracoid process medially and the humeral head laterally.
- Insert a 20- or 22-gauge needle in the sulcus bordered by the coracoid and the humeral head.
- Insert the needle inferiorly and laterally to the coracoid and directed posteriorly.

COMPLICATIONS
- Infection
- Subcutaneous atrophy and calcification
- Tendon rupture (repeated injections)
- Juxta-articular bone necrosis (repeated injections)
- Intra-articular bleeding
- Transient steroid flare

PEARLS
- If there is any suspicion of septic arthritis, abandon this treatment.
- Ultrasound guidance has been shown to improve intra-articular needle position, and hence improve the outcome.
- Limit injections to a span of 3 months apart.

RESOURCES
Carek, P. J., & Hunter, M. H. (2005). Joint and soft tissue injections in primary care. *Clinics in Family Practice, 7*(2), 359–378.

Lavelle, W., Lavelle, E. D., & Lavelle, L. (2007). Intra-articular injections. *Medical Clinics of North America, 91*(2), 241–250.

Stephens, M., & Beutler, A. (2008). Musculoskeletal injections: A review of the evidence. *American Family Physician, 78*(8), 971–976.

Wise, C. (2008). Arthrocentesis and injection of joints and soft tissue. In G. Firestein (Ed.), *Firestein: Kelley's textbook of rheumatology.* Philadelphia, PA: W. B. Saunders. Retrieved from http://www.mdconsult.com/das/book/body/217633773-3/1049214966/1807/344.html#4-u1.0-B978-1-4160-3285-4..10049-X_1409

CHAPTER 42

Procedures for Shoulder Dislocation

Keith A. Lafferty

BACKGROUND

Because the glenohumeral joint has the greatest range of motion of any joint in the body, it also is the most commonly dislocated joint. Contributing to this is an innately loose capsule, shallow glenoid fossa, lack of anterior muscular support, and a relatively thin anterior–inferior glenohumeral ligament (joint capsule), which is prone to tears. Shoulder dislocations are broadly divided into anterior and posterior types based on the position of the humeral head in relation to the glenoid fossa. Note that posterior dislocations occur 2% of the time and will only be briefly discussed. Anterior subluxations are subdivided into subcoracoid (most common), subglenoid (together these two represent 99% of all anterior dislocations), subclavicular, and intrathoracic (Figures 42.1 and 42.2). Rarely, and clinically obvious in its unique presentation, an inferior lie of the humeral head may present with the ipsilateral arm in a cephalad position (luxatio erecta).

Anterior

- The mechanism of injury in anterior types is usually an indirect force of abduction, extension, and external rotation.
  - Rarely, is it the result of a direct blow to the shoulder.
- In general, sporting activity in the young and falling in the elderly are the culprits.
- Patients younger than 30 years of age have more than an 80% recurrence rate, whereas those older than 40 years of age have a much lower recurrence rate (10%).
- Studies have shown an increase in the incidence of anterior–inferior glenohumeral ligament avulsions from the glenoid rim, now thought to be the primary factor for recurrent dislocations; it is amenable to arthroscopic surgical repair.
  - In fact, the current evidence suggests that younger athletic patients who are unwilling to modify their activities may benefit from stabilization after their initial dislocation to avoid recurrent instability.
  - Rotator cuff injuries are much more common and are reported in up to 15% in those who are older than 40 years of age (opposed to those patients younger than 30 years of age), as these tendons weaken as one ages.

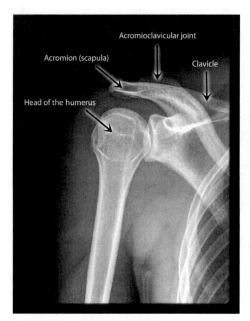

FIGURE 42.1 Normal shoulder joint.

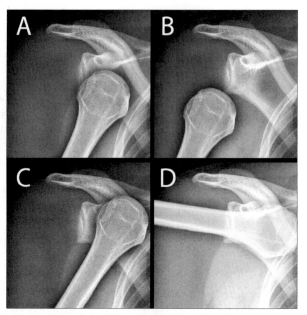

FIGURE 42.2 Types of anterior shoulder dislocation.

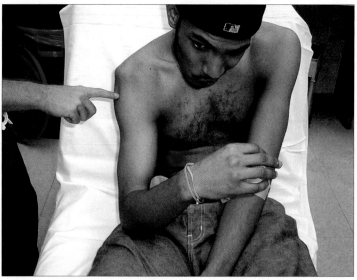

FIGURE 42.3 Testing of the axillary nerve.

- Axillary nerve injury secondary to traction neuropraxia is the most common neuronal injury and must be tested for in the pre- and post-reduction period (Figure 42.3).
  - Nerve function almost always returns to normal within time.
- Although there is a proximity with the axillary artery, disruption is rare but usually is clinically obvious in terms of coolness, severe persistent pain, and axillae hematoma/chest-wall hematoma formation.
  - This rare event usually occurs in older persons and warrants immediate arteriography.

- Associated fractures are common and are reported in up to 30% of cases, giving importance to pre-procedural x-rays.
  - Compression fracture of the humeral head caused by its impingement on the inferior glenoid rim causes the most common fracture, known as the Hill–Sachs deformity (Figure 42.4).
  - A corresponding fracture of this deformity of the inferior glenoid rim, known as the Bankart lesion, also occurs via the same mechanism.
  - The greater tuberosity is also susceptible to an avulsion-type fracture.
    - None of these fractures change treatment.

Posterior

- The mechanism is that of an internal rotation and adduction from an indirect force such as a seizure or electrical/lightning shock/strike.
- Note these forces are opposite to those inducing an anterior dislocation; rarely is direct blunt trauma to the anterior shoulder the culprit.
- These posterior types are often clinically missed because the anterior–posterior radiograph may not display any overlap of the humeral head and the glenoid fossa.
- Only the "Y" view can clearly demonstrate the dislocation type (Figure 42.5).
- There is a higher incidence of posterior glenoid rim and lesser tuberosity fractures.

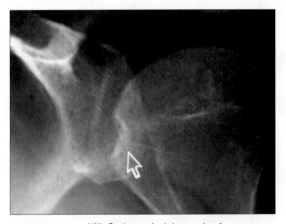

FIGURE 42.4 Hill–Sacks cortical depression fracture secondary to impaction of the humeral head against the anterior inferior glenoid rim.

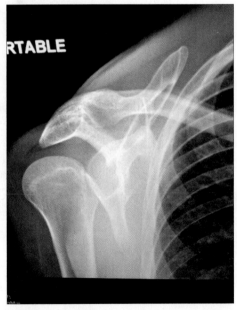

FIGURE 42.5 "Y" view showing the humeral head posterior to the glenoid fossa.

NOTE *that the AP x-ray misses this diagnosis 50% of the time though one can look for the following on a standard AP view: an internally rotated humeral head that appears round, known as the light-bulb sign, widening of the glenohumeral joint greater than 6mm, and loss of the normal half-moon overlap sign.*

Inferior

- The mechanism is extreme hyperabduction driving the humeral head through the inferior joint capsule.
- Higher incidence of rotator cuff tears.

PATIENT PRESENTATION

Anterior

- Severe pain
- Injured extremity held by the contralateral arm with slight external rotation and abduction.
- The normal rounded contour of the shoulder is flattened with a shelflike appearance, secondary to a now-prominent acromian process (Figure 42.6).
- Anterior shoulder appears full.
- Patient is unable to use the ipsilateral hand to palpate the contralateral shoulder, otherwise known as the scarf sign.

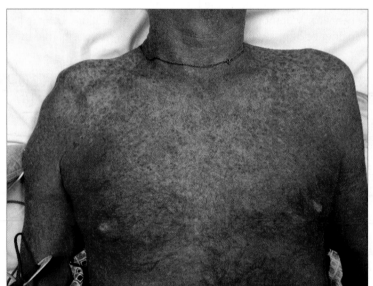

FIGURE 42.6
Anterior shoulder dislocation. Note obvious deformity and prominence of the acromion process, depression below this, and fullness in the anterior shoulder representing the displaced humeral head.

Posterior

- Severe pain
- Injured extremity held by the contralateral arm with slight internal rotation and adduction.
- The posterior shoulder appears full, while the anterior shoulder appears flat (Figure 42.7).

Inferior

- Severe pain
- Fully abducted humerus that appears in a locked position
- Elbow flexed
- Ipsilateral hand near or behind the patients head
- Humeral head may be palpated along the thoracic wall

FIGURE 42.7
Note depression in the anterior shoulder and prominence in the posterior shoulder representing the displaced humeral head. This type is clinically less obvious compared to anterior dislocations.

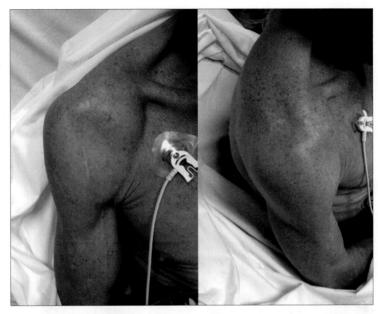

Reduction Techniques

Regardless of the technique used, the astute clinician should be familiar with multiple techniques as no technique carries a 100% success rate. Also, the literature is lacking in comparative studies in comparison techniques. In general, conscious sedation is recommended with the exception of the recurrent dislocation presenting immediately. Basically, all techniques involve a form of traction, leverage, or scapular manipulation. Essentially one is either moving the humeral head with the glenoid fossa remaining fixed or vice versa.

CONTRAINDICATIONS

- In patients with a contraindication to sedation, such as intoxicated patients, intra-articular anesthetic injection may be beneficial (see Chapter 34)
- Open dislocations

PROCEDURE PREPARATION/REDUCTION TECHNIQUE

- Prepare for conscious sedation (cardiac monitor, pulse oximeter, etc.)
- Assistant
- Two sheets

PROCEDURE

Anterior

Modified Traction–Countertraction

- Patient is supine with the arm abducted and elbow flexed at 90 degrees.
- Tie and wrap a sheet around the waist of the provider with the other end placed in the anticubital fossa of the patient at the flexed elbow.

- An assistant has another sheet wrapped across the chest of the patient at the level of the axillae, applying countertraction (Figure 42.8).
- The provider leans back (traction) and rotates the arm externally and possibly internally at the same time.
- Pressure applied to the head of the humerus may facilitate this technique.

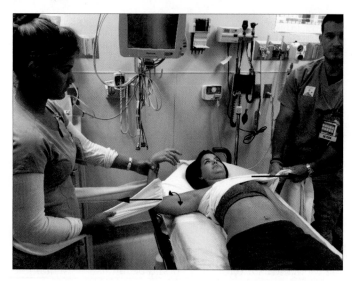

FIGURE 42.8 Modified traction counter traction method.

External Rotation

- Patient is supine with the arm adducted to the side.
- Gradually the elbow is flexed to 90 degrees while slow forearm external rotation is applied until the arm lies in the coronal plane (Figure 42.9).
- This should take place slowly, usually requiring more than 10 minutes.
- A "clunk" sound may not be appreciated by the provider or the patient.
- This technique may be attempted without sedation in the appropriate patient.
- Also of benefit, this technique requires only one provider.
- Pressure applied to the head of the humerus may facilitate this technique.

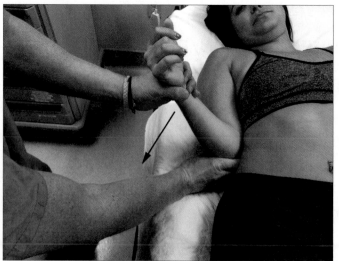

FIGURE 42.9 External rotation. Note the importance of keeping the humerus fully adducted and the elbow adhered to the patient's torso. Slow constant movement increases success.

Scapula Manipulation

Reduction is accomplished by repositioning the glenoid fossa rather than the humeral head. McNamara showed the success to be 86% and in two thirds of the patients studied, no pre-treatment medications were required.

- The patient is placed in the prone position.
- Traction is applied on the ipsilateral arm, which is hanging off the bed, with traction via an assistant or weights.
- May also be done with the patient sitting upright with the clinician behind the patient and an assistant in front applying traction on the outstretched arm while he or she is applying simultaneous countertraction on the ipsilateral clavicle (Figure 42.10).
- The provider pushes the inferior tip of the scapula with two thumbs medially and superiorly while stabilizing the superior scapula with the top hand, which causes the glenoid to move anteriorly and caudally to meet the humeral head.
- This technique may be attempted without sedation in the appropriate patient.
- This can be difficult in heavier patients as landmarks are diminished.

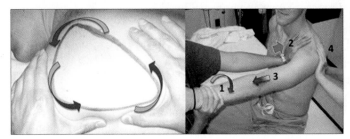

FIGURE 42.10 Scapular manipulation method. Prone and sitting techniques shown.

Milch

In the fully abducted and overhead position, the shoulder muscles are in an effusively relaxed locus.

- Patient is supine while the provider stands behind the stretcher and fully abducts and externally rotates the arm to the complete overhead position as if they were reaching for an apple from a tree by means of grasping the near fully extended elbow and wrist (Figure 42.11).
- Traction is applied in the longitudinal direction of the humerus.
- May apply upward pressure to the humeral head with the contralateral hand.

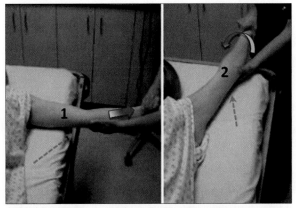

FIGURE 42.11 Milch technique for reduction in anterior shoulder dislocation. Note provider stands behind stretcher and the humerus is fully abducted and the elbow extended.

Posterior

- Patient is supine with the arm adducted.
- As in the modified traction–countertraction technique described in anterior dislocations, tie and wrap a sheet around the waist of the provider with the other end placed over the anticubital fossa of the patient at the flexed elbow.
- An assistant has another sheet wrapped across the chest of the patient at the level of the axillae, applying countertraction.
- The provider leans back and applies traction in the long axis of the humerus.
- An assistant applies anterior pressure to the posteriorly displaced humeral head.
- Lateral traction to the proximal humerus facilitates this technique.

Inferior

- Traction in an upward direction in line with the humerus similar to the Milch technique.
- An assistant has another sheet wrapped across the chest of the patient at the level of the axillae, applying countertraction.
- May employ cephalad pressure over the humeral head.

POST-PROCEDURE CONSIDERATIONS

- Typically, after reduction, all patients should be placed in a sling and swathe and should follow up with orthopedics.
- Note that current evidence suggests that the immobilization for 3 weeks of a first-time traumatic shoulder dislocation in external rotation reduces the risk of recurrent dislocation as compared to standard internal rotation immobilization.
- Proper analgesics should be given.
- Although most providers perform x-rays after reduction, if the patient displays stability of the joint with a normal neurological exam, and is able to take the ipsilateral hand and touch the contralateral shoulder, x-rays may be forgone.

The Quebec Decision Rule for Radiography in Shoulder Dislocation study has shown that by using certain clinical criteria, pre-reduction imaging can be reduced by 28% and post-reduction studies by 82%. The sensitivity and negative predictive value for ruling out a clinically significant fracture was shown to be 100% and 99.2%, respectively. The prospectively derived four risk factors warranting imaging include:

1. Age 40 years or older
2. Mechanism (motor vehicle collision, assault, sporting injury, fall from a distance greater than patient's height)
3. Presence of humeral ecchymosis
4. First episode of dislocation

PEARLS

- Younger patients usually redislocate, older patients usually do not.
- Older patients may injure their rotator cuff tendons, younger patients usually do not.
- Posterior dislocations are often missed radiographically. A "Y" view will show the anterior/posterior relation of the humeral head and the glenoid fossa.

- Gradual, gentle traction and rotation, along with maximal muscular rotation, are the cornerstones to successful reduction techniques.
- Avoid jerking forces because this increases complications and decreases success rates.
- If a patient can take the ipsilateral hand and touch the contralateral shoulder (scarf sign), there is no dislocation (Figure 42.12).
- Ultrasound is being used more often to complement clinical confirmation of dislocation and adequate reduction.
- Luxatio erecta (inferior) dislocations are always associated with an inferior joint capsule tear.

FIGURE 42.12
Scarf sign.

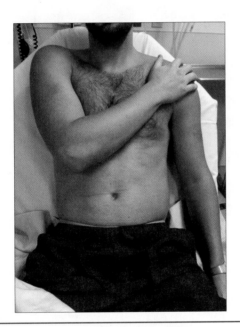

RESOURCES

Dodson, C. C., & Cordasco, F. A. (2008). Anterior glenohumeral joint dislocations. *Orthopedic Clinics of North America, 39*(4), 507–518.

Halberg, M. J. (2009). Bedside ultrasound for verification of shoulder reduction. *American Journal of Emergency Medicine, 27*(1), 503–504.

Hendey, G. W. (2000). Necessity of radiographs in the emergency department management of shoulder dislocations. *Annals of Emergency Medicine, 36*(2), 108–113.

http://www.ncbi.nlm.nih.gov/pubmed/19166638

http://www.ncbi.nlm.nih.gov/pubmed/8517564

McNeil, N. J. (2009). Postreduction management of first-time traumatic anterior shoulder dislocations. *Annals of Emergency Medicine, 53*(6), 811–813.

Newton, E. J. (2007). Emergency department management of selected orthopedic injuries. *Emergency Medicine Clinics of North America, 25*(3), 763–793.

Tintinalli, J., Meckler, G., Stapczynski, J., Ma, O. J., Cline, D., & Cydulka, R. (2010). *Tintinalli's emergency medicine: A comprehensive study guide* (7th ed.). New York, NY: McGraw-Hill

Ufberg, J., & McNamara, R. (2004). Management of common dislocations. In J. Roberts & J. Hedges (Eds.), *Clinical procedures in emergency medicine* (pp. 948–960). Philadelphia, PA: Saunders Elsevier.

CHAPTER **43**

Elbow Dislocation

Christopher Lee Plaisted and Keith A. Lafferty

BACKROUND

Anatomically, the elbow is considered a large hinge joint (similar to the knee) that is formed between the humerus and the ulna to allow for flexion and extension. However, this more complex joint has a second articulation, the radiohumeral joint, which allows for supination and pronation. The elbow is subjected to very strong forces and therefore contains distinctive bone structures and several strong accessory ligaments that strengthen its configuration.

In particular, the major lateral stabilizers are the radial collateral ligament (RCL) and the radial humeral joint. The primary medial stabilizer is the ulnar collateral ligament (UCL). The elbow relies more on its bony configuration rather than its ligamentous support in maintaining its integrity, specifically the articulation of the distal humerus' intercondylar groove and its housing in the olecranon fossa. The UCL and the RCL comprise the majority of the joint capsule and therefore are the main source of stability for the elbow. They can be disrupted partially or fully when there is a dislocation. The future stability/instability is dependent on the degree of initial injury to these stabilizing structures and subsequent healing after reduction. Because of this reinforcement, considerable force is necessary to dislocate the elbow. Furthermore, associated fractures of the radial head and coronoid process of the ulna are common and add to instability. Posterior elbow dislocations are the most common type, comprising 90%. Because the common mechanism is falling on the outstretched hand (FOOSH), sport activities account for up to 50% of elbow dislocations (Figure 43.1). As a result, this type of injury is more commonly seen in adolescents and young adults.

The most common sports associated with this injury are competitive cheer-leading, gymnastics, cycling, rollerblading, and skateboarding. This

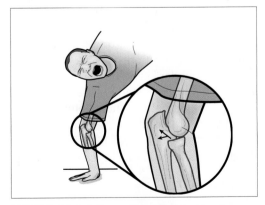

FIGURE 43.1 Falling on the outstretched hand.

joint is one of the most common joints dislocated, with an incidence of 6 to 13 per 100,000 and is second to the shoulder as the most common upper extremity dislocation. Note that children have a more immature/weaker distal humeral metaphysis in comparison to the ligamentous support and, although elbow dislocations are the most common type in children, the same mechanism of FOOSH may result in a supracondylar fracture in the pediatric age group.

ANATOMY

The elbow is a hinge-like joint formed by the humerus and ulna and the radius and ulna.

- Flexion up to 180 degrees and extension to 0 degree
  - Humeroulnar articulation
- Supination and pronation
  - Radiohumeral articulation

The elbow is an extremely stable joint and is typically resistant to disruption mainly because of its bony structure but also in part because of its ligamentous stabilizers (Figure 43.2).

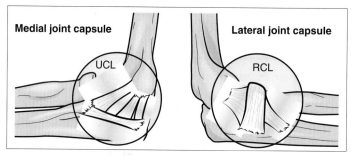

FIGURE 43.2
Elbow joint.

- UCL also known as MCL or medial collateral ligament
  - Consists of three main bands
    - Anterior oblique
      - Provides the most resistance to valgus stress, aiding in prevention of dislocation
    - Posterior oblique
    - Transverse
- RCL also known as lateral collateral ligament (LCL)
  - Consists of two main bands
    - Prevents varus stress
      - Provides the most resistance varus stress, aiding in the prevention of dislocation.
    - Annular ligament
      - Acts to stabilize the radial head to the ulna throughout the range of pronation and supination and, in doing so, preventing radial head dislocation.

Elbow dislocations are characterized and named according to the relationship of the distal dislocated bone in relation to the proximal joint (Figure 43.3).

Posterior

- FOOSH

FIGURE 43.3
Types of elbow
dislocations.

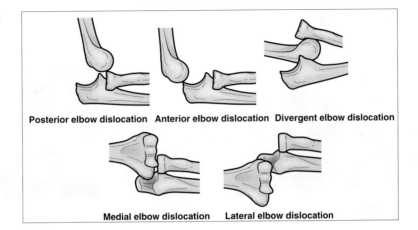

Posterior elbow dislocation   Anterior elbow dislocation   Divergent elbow dislocation

Medial elbow dislocation   Lateral elbow dislocation

Anterior

- Caused by a strong blow to the posterior aspect of a flexed elbow
- This force propels the olecranon anterior in relative to the humerus
- Anterior dislocations and any open fracture are commonly associated with disruption of the brachial artery and/or injury to the median nerve

Divergent

- Combination of axial compressive with rotational forces on an outstretched, pronated arm
- Very rare injury that is associated with significant high-energy trauma to the elbow

Medial/Lateral

- Associated with posterior dislocations

There are two main fascia inscribed compartments:

- Anterior
  - This is a concern, considering the proximity of the brachial artery along with the ulnar and medial nerves.
- Posterior

PATIENT PRESENTATION

In general, elbow dislocations are classified as follows:

- Simple—74%
  - No fracture
  - Closed
- Complex—26%
  - Fracture
    - Terrible triad requires surgery. May be grossly unstable and difficult to maintain reduction.
      - Dislocation
      - Radial head fracture
      - Coronoid fracture
  - May require CT scan if x-ray is inconclusive

Posterior

- Most common types of dislocation (Figure 43.4)

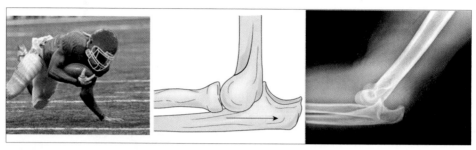

FIGURE 43.4 Posterior elbow dislocation next to gross sketch and x-ray.

- Deformity with a prominent olecranon creating a divot over the distal tricep
  - The olecranon is displaced from the plane of the epicondyles disparate to a supracondylar fracture, in which the epicondyles are palpable in the same plane as the olecranon
- Held in slight flexion
- Essentially no ROM
- Pain
- Swelling

Anterior

- Mechanism of injury is a direct posterior blow to a flexed elbow
  - Arm is extended
  - Upper arm appears shortened

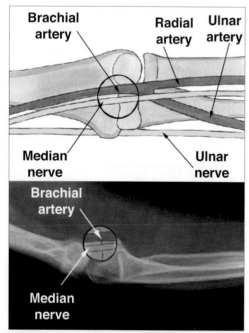

FIGURE 43.5 Anterior elbow dislocation.

- Forearm is elongated and supinated
- Essentially no ROM
- Tricep tendon may be disrupted
- Pain
- Swelling
  - Highest incidence of brachial artery disruption, especially with an associated fracture (Figure 43.5).

Medial/Lateral/Divergent

- These types of dislocation are rare with the mechanism of injury related to significant high-energy trauma to the elbow (Figure 43.6). The proximal radio ulnar joint is disrupted as the distal part of the humerus is driven between the radius and ulna, and the forearm dislocates posteriorly.
- Assessment for brachial artery disruption and/or entrapment of the ulnar (especially with associated medial epicondyle fractures) and median nerves needs rapid evaluation (Figure 43.5).

FIGURE 43.6 Divergent elbow dislocation x-ray with brachial/radial/ulnar artery and median/ulnar nerves.

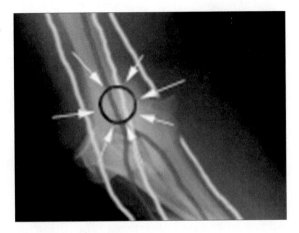

TREATMENT

Initial evaluation should focus on:

- Brachial artery integrity
  - Test the brachial artery itself as well as its two main tributaries: the radial and ulnar arteries
- Neuropraxia of the ulnar and medial nerves
  - Ulnar nerve injuries are reported in 14% of cases
    - Usually transient
  - Median nerve injuries are associated with brachial artery injuries considering their proximity
- PA and lateral radiographs should be performed prior to reductions in order to document possible fractures and confirm clinical diagnosis
  - Usually occur at
    - Radial head
    - Coronoid process
    - Olecranon
    - Humeral condyles
    - Capitellum
- If x-rays are inconclusive, consider CT scan for increased sensitivity (Figure 43.7)

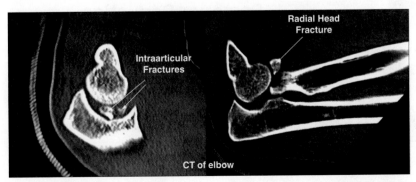

FIGURE 43.7 Complex elbow dislocation with intra-articular fracture fragment hindering successful reduction and not visualized on x-ray.

CONTRAINDICATIONS

■ Open dislocations
  ■ Orthopedic consultation to perform copious irrigation and take patient to the operating room

RELATIVE CONTRAINDICATIONS

■ Fracture
■ Incongruent reduction
  ■ Can be secondary to soft tissue interposition and/or loose body
  ■ May require surgical intervention to resolve

PROCEDURE PREPARATION

Administer intravenous/intramuscular analgesics early in the course prior to radiographs

■ Prepare for conscious sedation
  ■ Cardiac monitor
  ■ Pulse oximeter
  ■ NCO_2
  ■ Assistant
  ■ Potent and short-acting sedative
    • Propofol
    • Ketamine
    • Etomidate

PROCEDURE

Fundamental to the successful realignment of all reductions (displaced fractures as well) is the notion that the clinician cannot simply apply traction to the bones that are displaced. This may not only lead to multiple unsuccessful reduction attempts and frustration, but may also lead to iatrogenic fracture(s). The clinician must understand and conceptualize the need to apply the following three forces to all such cases:

■ Exaggeration
  ■ Actually amplify and make the dislocation worse
    • Causes the bone to clear any potential soft tissue or bony tuberosity
■ Distraction
■ Traction

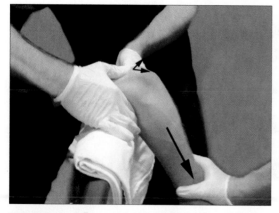

FIGURE 43.8 Prone method for posterior elbow reduction.

Posterior Reduction
Prone Method

■ Position patient in the prone position on the stretcher, assuring his or her head is turned and airway is not compromised.
■ Patient's arm is hung over the edge of the stretcher or padded side rail in the flexed position (Figure 43.8).
■ Distal pressure is applied via the clinician's two thumbs to the posterior aspect of the palpable and free olecranon (**Video 43.1**).

The assistant uses both hands and grasps the forearm and applies downward pressure.

- Slight flexion of the elbow may help relax/disengage the tricep muscle.
- Successful reduction is either heard or felt with an obvious "clunk."

Flex the patient's elbow 90 degrees to assure successful reduction.

Traditional Traction Method

- Place the patient in the supine position with assistant stabilizing the humerus.
- Grasp the affected wrist with the forearm in supination.
- Apply an exaggeration of the injury, distraction, and slow and steady in-line traction.
- Slight flexion of the elbow may help relax/disengage the tricep muscle.
- Successful reduction is either heard or felt with an obvious "clunk."
- Flex the patient's elbow 90 degrees to assure successful reduction.

Anterior Reduction

- Patient lies in the supine position.
- An assistant provides countertraction by grasping the humerus with both hands.
- The clinician holds the forearm with both hands and applies an exaggeration of the injury, distraction, and slow and steady in-line traction.
- Flex the patient's elbow 90 degrees to assure successful reduction.

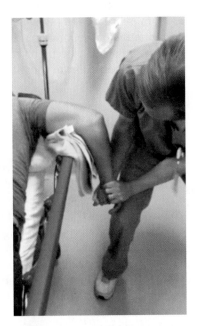

 VIDEO 43.1 Prone method for posterior elbow reduction. Note there should be an assistant applying distal pressure on the olecranon.
springerpub.com/campo

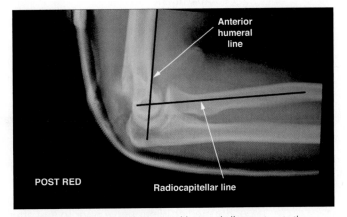

FIGURE 43.9 Postreduction x-ray with normal alignment; note the humeral olecranon fossa and radiocapitellar lines intact.

POST-PROCEDURE CONSIDERATIONS

- After reduction, reassess for any neurovascular abnormalities.
  - Immediate surgical consultation should be obtained for emergency arteriography if a pulse is diminished or absent.
- Order bedside postreduction x-ray (Figure 43.9).
- Put the elbow through gentle range of motion (ROM).
  - Greater than 20-degree extension of shoulder should be avoided as it may allow for the elbow to re-dislocate.

- Immobilize the elbow with a long arm splint with 90-degree flexion with slight pronation of the forearm.
  - After splint placement, reassess for any neurovascular abnormalities.
- Patients benefit from short-term immobilization and early ROM therapy.

COMPLICATIONS
Valgus Instability

- Patients will show a variable amount of UCL laxity, which correlates with a worse clinical and radiographic result.
- To minimize the stress on the UCL, the forearm should be placed in full pronation, which reduces the chances of recurrent posterolateral subluxation.
- Detrimental effects of prolonged immobilization:
  - Flexion contractures
  - Enhanced perception of pain
  - Increased duration of disability
- On long-term follow-up in simple closed reductions, Josefsson et al. have shown that one third of patients had what was described as "moderate loss of extension" at the elbow.
- Throughout the immobilization phase, wrist and shoulder function should be maintained through ROM and strengthening exercises.
- In anterior and divergent dislocations especially, compartment syndrome may occur after the acute phase of treatment and warrants observation.
  - Multiple evaluations of the neurovascular status to the anterior forearm compartment
    - Swelling
    - Pain
    - Passive finger flexion

EDUCATIONAL POINTS

- Open and anterior dislocations are associated with disruption of the brachial artery and/or injury to the median nerve and warrant a detailed neurovascular exam and orthopedic consultation.
- Significant soft tissue swelling and or hematoma formation or those who have vascular/neurologic compromise should have immediate orthopedic/vascular surgery consultation.
- Evaluation and documentation of the brachial artery and neurologic examination of the median/ulnar nerve prior to and after closed reduction are paramount.
- All dislocations are attended by at least some disruption of the joint capsule (UCL and/or RCL), and depending on the degree of this disturbance, coupled with any associated fracture(s), future stability/instability can be predicted.
- Complex elbow dislocation is dislocation when a fracture is present. CT scans are increasingly used to diagnose the degree and location of the fracture (Figure 43.7).
- FOOSH type of injury accounts for the majority of elbow dislocations.

PEARLS

- Exaggeration, distraction, and traction are the rule for successful elbow joint reduction coupled with proper sedation/analgesia.
- Open and anterior dislocations are associated with brachial artery injury.
- Although dislocations with a neurovascular compromise merit expedient orthopedic consultation, reduction should be done immediately as successful realignment often restores any such compromise.
- Anterior dislocations are rare and typically require orthopedic consultation, as they are associated with brachial artery injuries.
- Complex elbow dislocations require orthopedic consultation.
- Early analgesics are a must and should be given prior to radiographs.
- Conscious sedation is the rule.
- Neurovascular examination of ulnar/median nerves and the brachial artery should occur at the prereduction, postreduction, and the post-splint phases.
- Consider CT scan in instances where a reduction cannot occur or be maintained in order to detect subtle intra-articular fracture(s).
- Chronic pain and stiffness are a common long-term sequelae.
- Neurovascular compromise is not a reason not to do a reduction, but rather a reason to do a reduction.

RESOURCES

Chorley, J., Hergenroeder, A. C., Bachur, R. G., & Wiley, J. F. (2014). *Elbow dislocation in the child or adolescent athlete*. Retrieved from http://www.uptodate.com/contents/elbow-injuries-in-the-child-or-adolescent-athlete?source=search_result&search=elbow+dislocation&selectedTitle=1%7E11

Halstead, M., & Bernhardt, D. T. (2014). *Elbow dislocation*. Retrieved from http://emedicine.medscape.com/article/96758

Harnarayan, P., Cawich, S., Harnanan, D., & Budhooram, S. (2015). Brachial artery injury accompanying closed elbow dislocations. *International Journal of Surgery Case Reports, 8,* 100–102.

Horn, A., & Ufberg, J. (2014). Management of common dislocations. In J. Roberts & J. Hedges (Eds.), *Clinical procedures in emergency medicine* (6th ed., pp. 954–998). Philadelphia, PA: Saunders, Elsevier.

Josefsson, P. O., Johnell, O., & Gentz, C. F. (n.d.). Long term sequelae of simple dislocation of the elbow. *Journal Bone Joint Surgery, 66,* 927–930. Retrieved from http://emedicine.medscape.com/article/823277-clinical#showall

Keany, J. E., & McKeever, D. (2013). *Elbow dislocation in emergency medicine clinical presentation*. Retrieved from http://emedicine.medscape.com/article/823277

Kumar, A., & Ahmed, M. (1999). Closed reduction of posterior dislocation of the elbow: A simple technique. *Journal Orthopedic Trauma, 21*(3), 58–59.

CHAPTER 44

Procedures for Digit Dislocation

Keith A. Lafferty

BACKGROUND

Because of the high exposure of the hand, injuries are common, especially among athletes. A basic review of the articular anatomy is key to understanding and treating these common injuries.

The anatomic structure of the proximal interphalangeal (PIP), distal interphalangeal (DIP), and metacarpophalangeal (MCP) joints are fundamentally the same. Note that, however, the MCP joint is condyloid in shape, allowing some abduction and adduction, whereas the PIP/DIP joints are more hinge or tongue-and-groove joints, which do not allow lateral movement. The ligamentous supports of the MCP joints are thicker and are also reinforced by the deep transverse metacarpal ligament and hence are much less prone to injury.

The MCP/interphalangeal (IP) joints are stabilized laterally by the strong collateral ligaments and the flexor surface is supported by the vulnerable volar plate ligament (Figure 44.1). The extensor hood complex helps prevent volar dislocation. Because of this lateral–volar support, dorsal dislocations are more common and also, by definition, imply a disruption of the volar plate. Lateral dislocations have a disruption of one of the collateral ligaments and at least a partial tear of the volar plate. Dislocations are more common at the PIP joint than at the DIP joint secondary to the additional stability of the flexor and extensor tendon insertions at the distal phalanx.

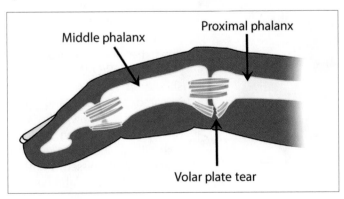

FIGURE 44.1 Volar and collateral ligament anatomy.

Middle phalanx

Proximal phalanx

Volar plate tear

Mechanistically, the usual force of dislocation is that of an axial load injury with hyperextension, with subsequent tearing of the volar plate and plus-or-minus collateral ligament injury. IP dislocations occur in the toe with the same axial load and hyperextension mechanistic forces that apply to the fingers.

Classification of dislocated MCP/IP joints is either simple or complex. Simple dislocation implies that no soft tissue (volar plate, tendon) is interposed or entrapped in the joint, allowing an easy closed reduction. Complex dislocation implies there is soft tissue entrapment in the joint, making a closed reduction nearly impossible with the probable need for operative repair. Many MCP dislocations are of the complex variety.

The first MCP joint is much more susceptible than the other MCP joints for injury, most important, this involves the ulna collateral ligament. This is known as a "game keeper's thumb." The integrity of this ligament is crucial for proper thumb opposition and normal grasping features of the hand. The patient may present with only localized tenderness along the ulna collateral ligament at the first MCP joint. Associated volar plate injuries are common. Early recognition of this injury through ulna collateral stress testing is key in identifying such an injury. Proper immobilization and immediate orthopedic follow-up decreases morbidity. Skiers are susceptible to such injury when they fall on an upright ski pole.

PATIENT PRESENTATION

Symptoms present as follows:

- Acute pain
- Swelling
- Deformity (Figure 44.2)
- Decreased range of motion

TREATMENT

Anesthesia can be performed using either a digital or metacarpal block for DIP/PIP dislocations or a wrist block (radial or ulna) for MCP dislocations. Closed reduction can be accomplished in most cases. Radiographs, before and after reduction, are used to identify fractures and confirm adequate reduction (Figure 44.3). The proper use of a methodical technique is paramount for successful reduction and, furthermore, to avoid causing a simple dislocation to become a complex one.

Open PIP/DIP dislocations should be reduced, copiously irrigated, sutured, and have immediate follow-up with orthopedics. Open MCP dislocations should be reduced, irrigated, and dressed, and then admitted for formal operative repair.

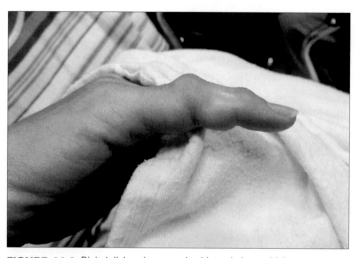

FIGURE 44.2 Digital dislocation—proximal interphalangeal joint.

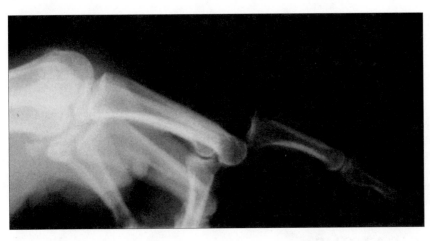

FIGURE 44.3 X-ray of dorsal proximal interphalangeal joint dislocation.

PROCEDURE PREPARATION

- Patient should be comfortable with the dislocated joint well exposed
- Local anesthetic agent
- Rubber gloves
- Finger splint, thumb spica, or buddy tape

PROCEDURE

PIP/DIP Closed Reduction

Exaggerate the deformity followed by hyperextension, longitudinal traction, and finally dorsal pressure (Figure 44.4).

MCP Closed Reduction

This is a more difficult procedure compared to IP reduction and has a higher chance of complex dislocation. If an improper method is used, the chance of converting a simple dislocation to a complex dislocation is increased.

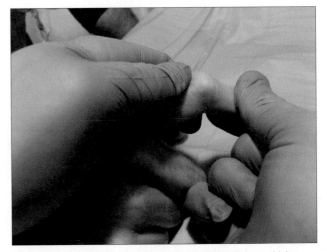

FIGURE 44.4 Closed reduction of proximal interphalangeal joint dislocation.

- Flex wrist in order to relax the stabilizing effects of the flexor tendons.
- Extend and apply longitudinal traction.
- Apply dorsal pressure.
- Unlike IP reductions, excessive hyperextension and excessive longitudinal traction should be avoided.

POST-PROCEDURE CONSIDERATIONS

- Postreduction radiographs are not necessary for uncomplicated reductions.
- DIP splints are applied with the DIP and PIP joint in 20 degrees of flexion.
- PIP reductions should be splinted or buddy taped with treatment for 2 to 3 weeks.
- Finger reductions should be splinted or buddy taped with treatment for 10 to 14 days.
- First MCP dislocations are treated with a thumb spika and 20 degrees of flexion for 4 weeks and immediate orthopedic follow-up.
- Other MCP joint reductions are treated in flexion using a volar splint for 3 to 4 weeks.
- Treatment of toe reductions is with buddy tape and a walking shoe for 2 to 3 weeks for the first toe and 10 to 14 days for the lesser toes.

COMPLICATIONS

- Fractures
- Conversion of a simple dislocation into a complex one

PEARLS

- Always remove rings from patients.
- Volar dislocations are rare and often require operative repair.
- Avoid long-term immobilization to eliminate the possible sequelae of joint stiffness and loss of flexion.
- A firm grip can be ensured if the provider wears a tight rubber glove.
- On reduction, always exaggerate the deformity first in order to lessen further injury and maximize successful reduction.
- Because extrinsic flexors of both IP joints are four times stronger than their extensor counterparts, proper range of motion is mandatory in postreduction care to prevent flexion contractures.

RESOURCES

Geiderman, J. M. (2006). General principles of orthopedic injuries. In J. Marx, R. Hockberger, & R. Walls (Eds.), *Rosen's emergency medicine concepts and clinical practice* (Vol. X, pp. 564–565, 784–786). Philadelphia, PA: Mosby, Elsevier.

Leggit, J. C. (2006). Acute finger injuries: Part II. Fractures, dislocations, and thumb injuries. *American Family Physician, 73*(5), 827–834.

Polansky, R., & Kwon, N. S. (2009). *Joint reduction, finger dislocation.* Retrieved from http://emedicine.medscape.com/article/109206-overview

Ufberg, J., & McNamara, R. (2004). Management of common dislocations. In J. Roberts & J. Hedges (Eds.), *Clinical procedures in emergency medicine* (pp. 948–960). Philadelphia, PA: Saunders Elsevier.

Young, G. M. (2008). *Dislocation, interphalangeal: Differential diagnosis & workup.* Retrieved from http://emedicine.medscape.com/article/823676-diagnosis

CHAPTER **45**

Procedures for Hip Dislocation

Christopher Lee Plaisted and Keith A. Lafferty

BACKGROUND

The femoroacetabular joint is one of the two ball-and-socket joints in the body, the other being the glenohumeral joint, with the hip being the largest and representing 5% of all joint dislocations. Because of this ball-and-socket structure, the femur can rotate freely through a 360-degree circle and can also swivel around its axis about 90 degrees. Secondary to this compact joint, with the ball situated deep within its socket, a strong, dense, and enclosing labrum, generous ligamentous support, and much surrounding muscular support, high energy is required to induce traumatic dislocations (Figure 45.1).

Because of this, these dislocations are often associated with other fractures and potential coincident life-threatening injuries that may take precedence in resuscitation. Not surprisingly, the physical findings of a hip dislocation may be overlooked on initial resuscitation of a patient with trauma, especially an unconscious one. Indeed, up to 95% of these patients have other associated traumatic injuries, including 88% having accompanying fractures. Leading mechanisms of hip luxation include frontal motor vehicle collisions (MVCs) (70%), auto versus pedestrian accidents, major falls from heights, and extreme contact sports. Because of the amount of dynamism required for native hip luxations and potential coexisting injuries, all such patients require hospitalization. This is not the case for prosthetic hip dislocations, as is discussed.

All acute hip dislocations require rapid diagnosis and reduction to prevent significant morbidity and associated

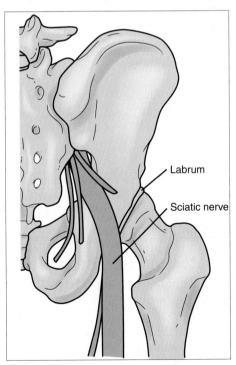

FIGURE 45.1 Hip anatomy with sciatic nerve.

long-term complications. Among the most serious is that of avascular necrosis (AVN), reported in as much as 15% of cases. Secondary to the blood circulation to the femoral head being somewhat precarious normally (highest incidence of AVN in the body), any disruption can result in rapid ischemia resulting in the death of marrow and osteocytes in as few as 6 hours. The arterial supply to the femoral head is principally provided by the deep branch of the medial femoral circumflex artery emanating many encroaching tributaries at the base of the femoral neck ascending to the femoral head (Figure 45.2). This arterial supply is well affixed to the femoral neck and is easily damaged with any femoral neck fracture displacement. Because of this, a reduction must occur promptly, as the incidence of subsequent AVN of the femoral head is a time-dependent phenomenon and most likely to occur if relocation is delayed beyond 6 hours (excluding prosthetic hips).

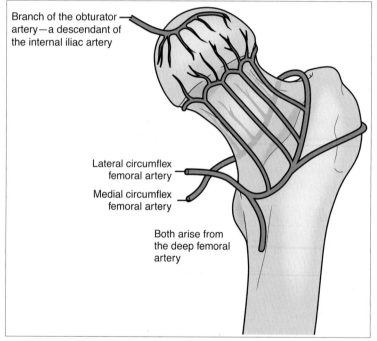

Branch of the obturator artery—a descendant of the internal iliac artery

Lateral circumflex femoral artery

Medial circumflex femoral artery

Both arise from the deep femoral artery

FIGURE 45.2 Arterial supply to the femoral head.

Other long-term sequelae include sciatic/peroneal nerve neuropraxia (as follows), osteoarthritis, and heterotropic bone deposition, which is the process by which bone tissue forms outside of the skeleton after traumatic long-bone injury and may become symptomatic.

Posterior Hip Dislocations

Posterior hip dislocations (PHDs) account for 90% of all cases. Unrestrained front-seat passengers are especially vulnerable to PHDs secondary to the anatomic positioning of knee flexion, hip flexion/adduction, coupled with a posteriorly displaced force. The more the hip is flexed on impact, the less chance there is for an associated acetabular fracture. On collision, the flexed knee strikes the dashboard and transmits a high forceful axial load along the femoral shaft up the flexed adducted femur through the femoral head, propelling it posteriorly through the acetabulum (Figure 45.3). Associated fractures of the posterior rim of the acetabulum can occur. Because of the proximity of the sciatic nerve, these have the highest incidence of inducing neuro-praxia (Figure 45.4). The incidence is approximately 10% in adults and 5% in children. The peroneal branch is most often injured via laceration, stretching, or compression, or later encased in heterotopic ossification. A focused neurological exam at the time of injury is extremely important because once a nerve injury is detected, prompt closed reduction must ensue. Often this relieves distortion of the nerve from a dislocated femoral head or displaced acetabular fracture and diminishes long-term sequelae. Full/partial recovery of nerve function occurs in 60% to 70% of patients.

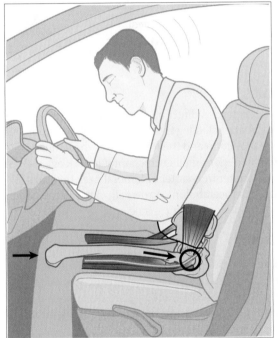

FIGURE 45.3 Posterior hip dislocation via motor vehicle accident.

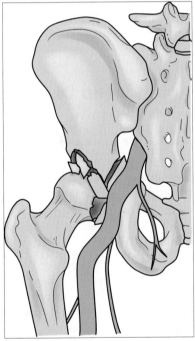

FIGURE 45.4 Sciatic nerve injury secondary to posterior hip dislocation.

Prosthetic Hip Dislocations

Another increasing cohort are patients' status post–total hip arthroplasty (THA). A recent study has shown that from the years 2000 to 2010, the number of such procedures has more than doubled to 310,800. The number grew by 92% among those 75 and older and increased 205% in those age 45 to 54. Unlike traumatic native femoroacetabular disloca-tions, these inherently less stable joints require minimal and trivial forces such as crossing one's leg, arising from a seated position, or even just rolling over in bed. They are reported in 3% of THA procedures. In accordance, recurrent prosthetic hip dislocations may require a revision of the prosthesis to prevent future recurrences. Unfortunately, 8.1% of these revisions tend to dislocate with 70% becoming recurrent. Posterior displacement occurs 80% of the time and is likely to occur in the first 3 to 4 months following THA, although patients may present up to 10 years after THA with a nontraumatic hip dislocation.

Consultation with the orthopedic surgeon who performed the hip prosthesis should be considered prior to attempting reduction in patients who are 3 to 4 months postoperative THA. Please review Table 45.1 for risk factors for instability following THA.

TABLE 45.1 Risk Factors for Instability Following Total Hip Arthroplasty

Patient Factors	Surgical Factors
Female	Surgical approach
Age > 80	Capsular repair
Neuromuscular disorders	Soft tissue tension
Cognitive disorders	Component malpositioning
Alcoholism	Femoral head size
Abductor weakness	Impingement
Prior hip surgery	Surgeon experience

Anterior Hip Dislocations

Anterior dislocation of the hip (10%) occurs from a direct blow to the posterior aspect of the hip, typically from a force applied to an abducted leg that levers the hip anteriorly out of the acetabulum. The hip is forced into abduction and the force pushes the femur medially while the abduction causes the femoral neck or greater trochanter to lock against the superior segment of the acetabulum. The greater trochanter or femoral neck then acts like a lever, propelling the femoral head out of the acetabulum. A medially directed force then pushes the femoral head through the anterior acetabular capsule.

ANATOMY

The femur head is deeply seated in the acetabulum. This ball-and-socket joint, along with ligamentous and numerous strong muscles of the upper thigh and gluteal region, provides joint stability; therefore, a high-energy force is required to destabilize the hip joint. The sciatic nerve rests just behind the hip joint and therefore is at risk for injury following PHD (Figure 45.5)

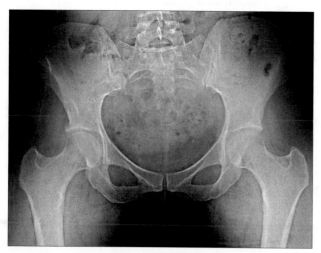

FIGURE 45.5 Normal anterior–posterior pelvis x-ray.

PATIENT PRESENTATION

Patients with native hip dislocations are in severe pain. A theme worth overemphasizing is that because of this, coupled with the extreme energy required to induce such dislocations, a thorough and detailed physical exam must be carried out in order not to miss coexisting and potentially life-threatening coexisting injuries.

Posterior Hip Dislocations

Leg is shortened, adducted, and internally rotated, with the hip and knee held in slight flexion (Figure 45.6).

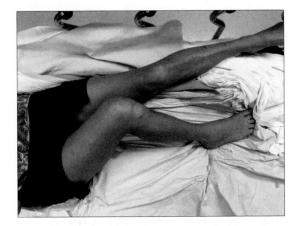

FIGURE 45.6 Posterior hip dislocation—shortening with internal rotation and adduction of the hip.

- Acronym "PID"
  - PHD
  - Internal rotation
  - Adduction
- Inability to walk or adduct the leg
- Signs of a sciatic nerve injury may be present

Anterior Hip Dislocation

Leg is externally rotated, abducted, and extended at the hip (Figure 45.7).

FIGURE 45.7 Anterior hip dislocation. External rotation, abduction, and extension of the hip.

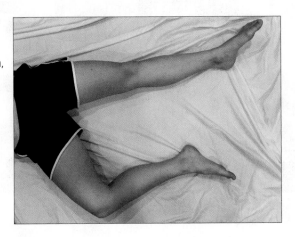

- The femoral head may be palpated anterior to the pelvis.
- Signs of injury to the femoral nerve or artery may be present.

CONTRAINDICATIONS
- Large associated femoral neck, shaft, or pelvic fracture(s)

RELATIVE CONTRAINDICATIONS
- Recent THA within 3 to 4 months

SPECIAL CONSIDERATION
The prosthetic hip can be reduced using any of the previously described methods but warrants special attention. In all hip dislocations, forceful, abrupt reductions should be frowned on, but especially when it pertains to prosthetic hips, as the hip prosthesis may dislodge the acetabular cup, fracture underlying osteoporotic bone, or even loosen or cause subluxation of the prosthesis.

- Neurovascular compromise is cause for a prompt reduction.
- The provider should be comfortable with multiple reduction techniques as no specific technique carries a 100% success rate.

PROCEDURE PREPARATION
- Administer intravenous/intramuscular analgesics early in the course prior to radiographs.

Generally a standard pelvis x-ray is sufficient for the diagnosis (Figures 45.8A, 45.8B, and 45.8C).

- Lateral view helps delineate anterior versus posterior displacement of the femoral head and allows more subtle fracture detection
- CT scan is required for increased fracture detection, especially regarding the acetabulum
  - Less important for THA dislocation
  - Specialty CT required to minimize image degradation from implant

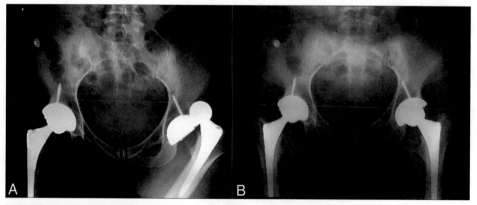

FIGURE 45.8A and 45.B A. Pelvis x-ray demonstrating a posterior hip dislocation in a prosthetic hip pre-reduction and **B.** post-reduction.

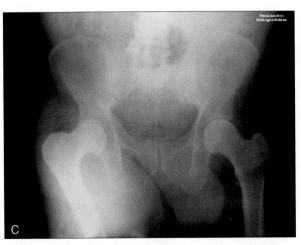

FIGURE 45.8C Pelvis x-ray showing a subtle right native hip dislocation. Note on this anterior–posterior view the right femoral head is smaller in comparison to the left as it is closer to the x-ray plate.

- Prepare for conscious sedation
  - Proper sedation and muscle relaxation cannot be overemphasized in reducing this large ball-and-socket joint with robust ligamentous and muscular support
    - Cardiac monitor
    - Pulse oximeter
    - NCO_2
    - Assistant
    - Potent and short-acting sedative
      - Propofol
      - Ketamine
      - Etomidate

PROCEDURE
Allis Technique (Figure 45.9 and Video 45.1)

- Patient is placed in the supine position.
- An assistant, while facing the clinician, provides stabilization to pelvis by pushing straight down toward the floor on the bilateral anterior superior iliac spines (ASIS) with the goal of not allowing the pelvis "socket" to move during femoral head "ball" positioning.
- The clinician stands on the bed, facing the patient, and places both hands behind the ipsilateral knee/calf, lifting the femur up.
  - In essence, the knee and hip will be in 90 degrees of flexion.
- Steady, constant, and intense traction is applied in an upward force with simultaneous gentle internal and external rotation of the femur.
  - Lateral traction on the proximal femur may help.
- After reduction is successful, hip is brought to the extended position while traction is maintained.

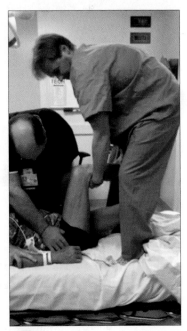

FIGURE 45.9 Allis technique.

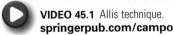

VIDEO 45.1 Allis technique.
springerpub.com/campo

Whistler Technique (Figure 45.10 and Video 45.2)

- Patient is placed in the supine position.
- An assistant, while facing the clinician, provides stabilization to pelvis by pushing straight down toward the floor on the bilateral ASISs with the goal of not allowing the pelvis "socket" to move during femoral head "ball" positioning.
- The clinician stands on the affected side, facing the long axis of the stretcher, and places his or her forearm under the 120-degree flexed ipsilateral knee while the same hand grasps the less flexed contralateral knee.
- Using the other hand, the clinician grasps the ipsilateral ankle and firmly plants it on the bed, stabilizing the ipsilateral leg.
- The clinician, using constant and firm force, raises his or her arm, which subsequently applies an anterior force to the ipsilateral knee, jimmying and raising the femur in the air.
  - The grasping and affixing of the ipsilateral ankle cannot be overemphasized.
- Slight internal and external rotation of the ipsilateral hip using the forearm as a fulcrum under the ipsilateral knee may facilitate.

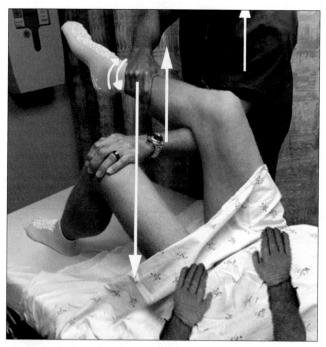

FIGURE 45.10 Whistler technique.

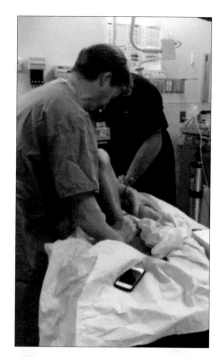

 VIDEO 45.2 Whistler technique. Note the contralateral leg should be in more flexion than shown. **springerpub.com/campo**

Captain Morgan Technique (Figure 45.11)

- Patient is placed in the supine position.
- An assistant, while facing the clinician, provides stabilization to pelvis by pushing straight down toward the floor on the bilateral ASISs with the goal of not allowing the pelvis "socket" to move during femoral head "ball" positioning.

- The clinician faces the patient from the side in a perpendicular manner and places his or her flexed knee on the stretcher under the patient's ipsilateral knee (analogous to the illustration of the infamous rum icon) and places one hand under the same knee for further support.
- Flex the patient's knee and hip to 90 egrees.
- Grasp the ipsilateral ankle and while applying upward force of the femur via the clinician's knee, internally and externally rotate the hip using the patient's ankle.
  - The patient's knee must remain in 90-degree flexion; applying a slight downward pressure on the patient's ankle may facilitate.

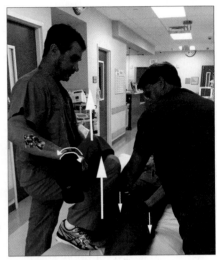

FIGURE 45.11 Captain Morgan technique.

POST-PROCEDURE CONSIDERATIONS

- Neurovascular reassessment is paramount and should always be verified following relocation.
  - Test for sciatic nerve integrity
    - Specifically, the sensory and motor portions of the peroneal nerve
      - Sensation to the anterior foot and lateral legs and to the top of the feet
      - Dorsiflexion

In order to prevent immediate and remote recurrence, immobilize the leg with an abduction pillow or a knee immobilizer (Figure 45.12).
- Postreduction x-rays should be done to verify successful reduction.
- Consultation with the orthopedic surgeon who preformed the THA to ensure a long-term treatment plan following reduction.

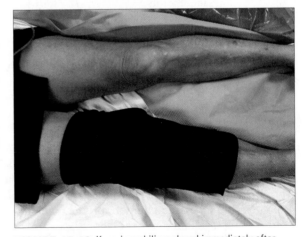

FIGURE 45.12 Knee immobilizer placed immediately after successful reduction to prevent redislocation.

COMPLICATIONS

- AVN of the hip in 15% of cases
- Increased with:
  - Delayed reduction
  - Multiple reduction attempts
  - Open reduction
- Sciatic nerve injury
  - PHD
    - 10%
- Osteoarthritis
- Heterotopic calcification
- Recurrent dislocations

- Complications of immobilization
  - Deep vein thrombosis
  - Pulmonary embolism
  - Decubiti
  - Pneumonia
  - Femoral nerve

EDUCATIONAL POINTS

- Consultation with the orthopedic surgeon who performed the hip prosthesis should be considered prior to attempting reduction in patients who are 3 to 4 months post-operative THA.
- Anterior versus posterior surgical approach gives clues as to the direction of the dislocation.
- Evaluate the surgical site, as invection may also contribute to THA dislocation especially in the early post-operative period.
- Never apply sudden forceful jerking movements on reduction of hip luxations as this increases the chance of iatrogenic fracture.
- Rehabilitation of patients with sciatic nerve injury must begin as early as possible and should focus on the prevention of an equinus foot deformity, which is a chronic foot drop from peroneal nerve injury.
- In all instances, neurovascular examination is imperative before any reduction is attempted.
- The secondary trauma survey should include an assessment of the hips and other large joints.
- Because associated fractures are common (88%) in traumatic hip luxations, minor fractures are not a contraindication for emergent reduction.

PEARLS

- PID can be used as an acronym to describe hip positioning in PHDs; "**P**HD— **I**nternal rotation—a**D**duction."
- The provider should be comfortable with multiple techniques for hip dislocation as no one specific technique is 100% successful.
- Adequate sedation and muscle relaxation are key to a successful hip reduction and attempts without it, in general, are futile.
- Documentation of the patient's neurovascular status pre/postreduction is paramount.
- Admit traumatic hip dislocation and discharge prosthetic dislocation.
- Traumatic native hip dislocations should be evaluated as a trauma due to the high likelihood of multiple injuries and fractures, including but not limited to head, neck, and intra-abdominal traumatic pathologies.
- In a multi-injured patient, on the secondary survey always put the joints through a full range of motion to ascertain a subclinical luxation/subluxation.
- After successful reduction of a prosthetic hip, the patient can be discharged home as trivial trauma is the etiology—this is not the case for traumatic native hip dislocations.
- Resist sudden, jerky, and abrupt forceful movement at all times.
- Always use an assistant.

RESOURCES

Bossart, P. (2013). Hip and femur injuries. In J. G. Adams (Ed.), *Emergency medicine: Clinical essentials* (2nd ed., pp 726–730). Philadelphia, PA: Saunders Elsevier.

Cornwall, R., & Radomisli, T. E. (2000). Nerve injury in traumatic dislocation of the hip. *Clinical Orthopedics and Related Research, 377,* 84–91.

Fillingham, Y. A., Erickson, B. J., Cvetanovich, G. L., & Della Vella, C. J. (2014). Dislocation of a total hip arthroplasty: Acute management in the ED. *American Journal of Emergency Medicine, 32*(12), 1554–1554.

Hendey, G. W., & Avilia, A. (2011). The Captain Morgan technique for the reduction of the dislocated hip. *Annals of Emergency Medicine, 58*(6), 536–540.

Horn, A. E., & Ufberg, J. W. (2014). Management of common dislocations. In J. R. Roberts & J. R. Hedges (Eds.), *Clinical procedures in emergency medicine* (6th ed., pp. 954–998). Philadelphia, PA: Saunders Elsevier.

Murray, B. L. (2014). Femur and hip. In J. Marx, R. Hockberger, & R. Walls (Eds.), *Rosen's emergency medicine: Concepts and clinical practice* (pp. 672–697). Philadelphia, PA: Saunders Elsevier.

Newton, E. J., & Love, J. (2007). Emergency department management of selected orthopedic injuries. *Emergency Medicine Clinics of North America, 25*(3), 763–793.

Stein, M. J., Kang, C., & Ball, V. (2015). Emergency department evaluation and treatment of acute hip and thigh pain. *Emergency Medicine Clinics of North America, 33*(2), 327–343.

Tornetta, P. (2014). Hip dislocations and fractures of the femoral head. In R. W. Bucholz, J. D. Heckman, & C. M. Court-Brown (Eds.), *Rockwood and Green's fractures in adults* (6th ed., p. 1715). Philadelphia, PA: Lippincott Williams & Wilkins.

Werner, B. C. (2012). Instability after total hip arthroplasty. *World Journal of Orthopedics, 3*(8), 122–130.

CHAPTER **46**

Procedures for Patella Dislocation

Keith A. Lafferty

BACKGROUND

The mechanism of injury for knee dislocation usually involves twisting the leg with an externally rotated knee. Most often the patella is displaced laterally over the lateral condyle of the femur. Medial and superior dislocations are rare and may require surgical repair. In order for the patella to be displaced laterally, there must be a tear of the medial patella retinaculum. The typical case involves an adolescent playing a sport that requires a sudden knee extension, external rotation, and valgus maneuver, which is essentially a cutting maneuver of the athlete such as in hockey and gymnastics. Although less common, dislocation can result via a direct blow to the anterior medial patella. Fifteen percent of patients have recurrent dislocations.

Do not confuse a patella dislocation with a femur–tibia (knee) dislocation. Interestingly enough, this is more common in females and up to 24% display a family history of this injury. A true knee dislocation is an absolute emergency and presents spontaneously reduced half of the time. There is a high morbidity, as up to 30% of cases have an associated popliteal arterial injury.

PATIENT PRESENTATION

- Obvious laterally displaced patella (Figure 46.1)
- Sometimes tenting of the skin with the knee in mild flexion
- Inability to ambulate

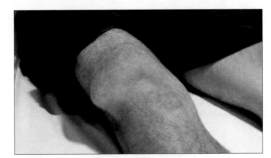

FIGURE 46.1 Patella dislocation.

TREATMENT

Closed reduction can occur spontaneously. X-rays are not routinely required for prereduction but may be done at postreduction to detect osteochondral fractures, which are reported to be as high as 50%, although most are identified by arthroscopy. Sedation is rarely required.

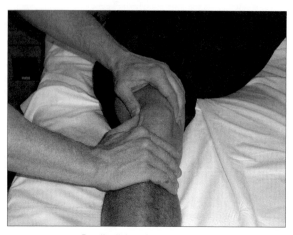

FIGURE 46.2 Patella dislocation—closed reduction.

PROCEDURE

- Patient should be lying in the supine position.
- Apply active knee extension while applying anterior–medial pressure to the lateral edge of the patella (Figure 46.2; watch this video https://www.facebook.com/jerseydemic/videos/10153892933550681).

POST-PROCEDURE CONSIDERATIONS

- A knee immobilizer should be used for 3 to 6 weeks in order for the medial patella retinaculum to heal.
- Patients with recurrent dislocations may require an arthroscopic release of the lateral retinaculum to blunt its pulling force on the patella laterally.

PEARLS

- Reduction can often be done while the patient is on the emergency medical services stretcher.
- If the reduction is unsuccessful, the medial facet of the patella may be locked on the lateral femoral condyle, which will require downward pressure on the lateral edge of the patella.
- Patients presenting with complete ligamentous disruption of the knee with or without a deformity should be suspected of having a spontaneous knee (femoral–tibial) dislocation and should be treated as such (Figure 46.3).

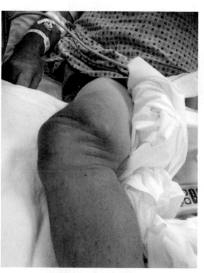

FIGURE 46.3 Femoral–tibial dislocation is a true limb threatening injury secondary to the high incidence of popliteal artery violation and is not to be confused with a patella dislocation.

RESOURCES

Andrish, J. (2008). The management of recurrent patellar dislocation. *Orthopedic Clinics of North America, 39*(3), 313–327.

Arendt, E. A. (2002). Current concepts of lateral patella dislocation. *Clinics of Sports Medicine, 21*(3), 499–519.

Dlabach, J. A. (2007). Acute dislocations of the patella. In T. S. Canale (Ed.), *Campbell's operative orthopedics*. Retrieved from http://www.mdconsult.com/das/book/body/192201420-10/976162489/1584/422.html#4-u1.0-B978-0-323-03329-9..50060-X–cesec4_3265

Geiderman, J. M. (2006). General principles of orthopedic injuries. In J. Marx, R. Hockberger, & R. Walls (Eds.), *Rosen's emergency medicine concepts and clinical practice* (Vol. X, pp. 564–565, 784–786). Philadelphia, PA: Mosby Elsevier.

CHAPTER **47**

Procedures for Managing Nursemaid's Elbow

Keith A. Lafferty

BACKGROUND

The typical presenting age of nursemaid's elbow is usually 1 to 3 years, with the most common being just older than 2 years of age. There are cases in the literature of children from 6 months of age and up to 7 years of age with this condition, although this is rare. The typical mechanism is that of a sudden longitudinal traction of the arm with the elbow extended and slight pronation in the forearm. It typically occurs in the left arm as most caregivers are right handed. Physiologically, the annular ligament stretches and tears at its attachment on the radial neck and slips between capetellum and the head of the radius. Note that 22% of patients report a fall and the recurrence rate is 20%.

PATIENT PRESENTATION

- Patient cannot supinate the arm
- Arm is noted to be in pronation of the wrist and slight flexion of the elbow (Figures 47.1 and 47.2)
- The child is in no distress
- Swelling, ecchymosis, and deformity are absent (unlike a fracture)
- There may or may not be mild nonpoint tenderness
- There is resistance to supination

TREATMENT

For the most part, the treatment of nursemaid's elbow does not require a radiographic examination. Even when the history is vague, if the classic clinical presentation is presented with an absence of point tenderness or swelling and a nondistressed child, a reduction may be done.

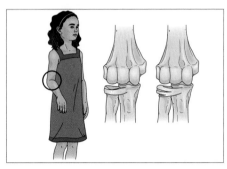

FIGURE 47.1 Note the arm is in slight flexion and the wrist is in pronation. Also note that the underlying pathology is not an "elbow dislocation" but rather a proximal displacement and entrapment of the annular ligament between the radial head and the capitulum.

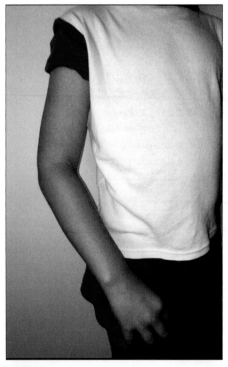

FIGURE 47.2 As stated previously, note slight flexion of elbow and pronation of wrist. Also there is an absence of swelling and distress as would be found typically in fractures.

CONTRAINDICATIONS

- Suspicion of a fracture, septic arthritis, tumor, or osteomyelitis

PROCEDURE PREPARATION

- Have the child sit on the parent's lap.
- Parent holds the ipsilateral humerus in adduction.

PROCEDURE

Two techniques will be described, both of which do not require sedatives. Both methods have equal success rates. If one method fails, the other may be attempted. Regardless of which technique is used, a "click" ensures successful reduction although it is not required. However, it has been shown that the sound has a positive predictive value of 90% and negative predictive value of 76%. Typically, the child is seen using the arm within 5 to 10 minutes and definitely within 30 minutes following the reduction. The practitioner may attempt a second reduction if there is no use of the extremity after the given time is allotted.

Supination Method

- Place pressure on the radial head with the thumb of one hand and then grasp the wrist with the other hand (Figure 47.3A).
- Fully supinate the wrist while maintaining pressure on the radial head (Figure 47.3B).
- Immediately flex the elbow completely to the ipsilateral shoulder while maintaining radial-head pressure (Figure 47.3C).

Pronation Method

- Place pressure on the radial head with the thumb of one hand and then grasp the wrist with the other hand.
- Hyperpronate the wrist.
- Immediately flex the elbow completely to the ipsilateral shoulder.

DIFFERENTIAL DIAGNOSIS

- Fracture
- Septic arthritis
- Tumors
- Osteomyelitis

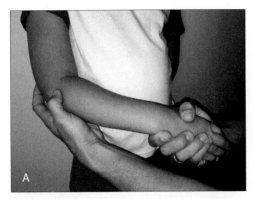

FIGURE 47.3A Place pressure on the radial head with the thumb of one hand and then grasp the wrist with the other hand.

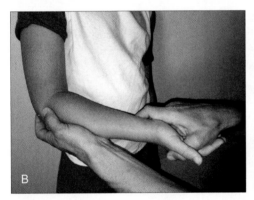

FIGURE 47.3B Fully supinate the wrist while maintaining pressure on the radial head.

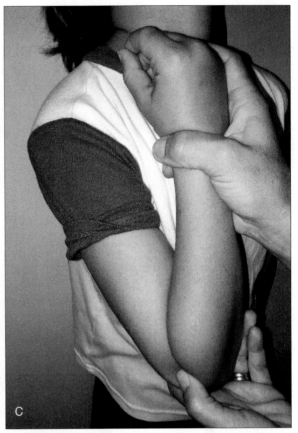

FIGURE 47.3C Flex the elbow completely to the ipsilateral shoulder while maintaining radial-head pressure.

PEARLS

- If the first method fails, the second method can be attempted.
- If all attempts are unsuccessful, place the patient in a posterior splint or sling, and arrange orthopedic follow-up.
- Demonstration of the reduction on the contralateral arm may aid in decreasing anxiety for the patient and the parent.

RESOURCES

Johnson, F. C., & Okada, P. J. (2008). Reduction of common joint dislocations and subluxations. In C. King & F. Henretig (Eds.), *Textbook of pediatric emergency procedures* (pp. 962–963). Philadelphia, PA: Lippincott Williams & Wilkins.

Meiner, E. M., Sama, A. E., Lee, D. C., Nelson, M., Katz, D. S., & Trope, A. (2004). Bilateral nursemaid's elbow. *American Journal of Emergency Medicine, 22*(6), 502–503.

Schunk, J. E. (1990). Radial head subluxation: Epidemiology and treatment of 87 episodes. *Annals of Emergency Medicine, 19*(9), 1019–1023.

Wolfram, W., & Boss, D. N. (2009). *Pediatrics, nursemaid elbow.* Retrieved from http://emedicine.medscape.com/article/803026-overview

CHAPTER 48

Procedures for Splinting of Extremities

Keith A. Lafferty

BACKGROUND

Splints accomplish the following: mechanical stabilization of fractures and dislocations, protection of soft tissue injury, pain control, and protection of the injured area from further trauma. Unlike formal casting, splints accomodate swelling without the risk of external compression while giving similar short-term immobilization. Also, the patient can remove this device to perform wound care, allow range of motion, and allow continued hygiene.

PATIENT PRESENTATION

Although the mainstay of splinting is for the treatment of bone fracture/injury, its use is also amenable to the following:

- Tendon pathology (laceration, tenosynovitis)
- Joint pathology (arthropathies, overlying lacerations)
- Sprains

TREATMENT

Basically, splints can be made from plaster or fiberglass with concurrent use of a stockinette, Webril, and gauze or an elastic roll. However, this is time consuming and, for the sake of discussion, we will limit description to prefabricated splints. These contain essentially all of the aforementioned components in one apparatus. Fiberglass offers an advantage over plaster in that it is stronger, lighter, easier to apply, cures more rapidly, and does not require specific drain traps in the sink.

Proper measurement can be performed on the contraindicated extremity using an Ace wrap to approximate the length. Because most splint material releases heat as it cures, one should use cold water for application.

After proper measurement, the splint is applied and wrapped with an Ace bandage. The splint is thus contoured into the proper position and held until fully hardened. When applying the splint, care should be taken to avoid the following:

- Bunching the Ace wrap
- Circumferential application of the splint around the extremity

- Tight wrapping of the Ace wrap (Figure 48.1)
- Application over a nonaddressed soft tissue wound (note that these must have appropriate wound care and dressing first)
- Creation of sharp edges
- Excessive pressure points that could lead to skin ulcerations
- Burns secondary to heat production during the curing process

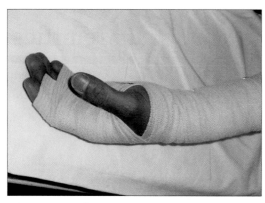

FIGURE 48.1 Inappropriately tight elastic bandage wrap.

The potential of a splint to induce ischemia is much less likely than that of a cylindrical cast, although it can still occur. It is imperative not to apply an Ace wrap too tightly. Also, pain out of proportion to the injury or an increase in pain should alert the provider to consider the diagnosis of compartment syndrome.

PROCEDURE PREPARATION

Unless stated otherwise, extremity position is a constant regardless of the splint used. In general, if a splint crosses over one of the following joints, the position of that joint should be as follows (see Table 48.1):

- Ace wrap
- Commercial splint roll
- Prefabricated splint

TABLE 48.1 Positioning of Joint for Splint Application

Joint	Position
Elbow	90-degree flexion with forearm in neutral position, "thumbs up"
Wrist	Slight extension of 20 degrees*
Thumb	Abducted*
MCP joints	Flexed at 60 degrees*
PIP joints	Slightly flexed at 10–20 degrees*
DIP joints	Slightly flexed at 5 degrees*
Ankle	90 degrees of dorsiflexion
Knee	Minimal flexion

DIP, distal interphalangeal; MCP, metacarpophalangeal; PIP, proximal interphalangeal.

*As if the patient is holding a bottle of beer, also known as the position of function.

PROCEDURE

Upper Extremity Splints (Table 48.2)

TABLE 48.2 Type of Splints

Type and Indication	Length	Width	Note
Volar (Figure 48.2) Forearm, wrist, metacarpal fractures/ injuries	Proximal fingers to just below the elbow on anterior surface	Fully covers the forearm	Allows supination and pronation of the forearm

FIGURE 48.2
Volar splint

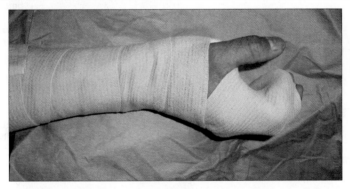

Type and Indication	Length	Width	Note
Sugar tong (Figure 48.3) Distal radius and ulna fractures/injuries	Metacarpal heads on dorsal hand and around the elbow extending over anterior forearm to just distal to the MCP joints	Forearm width without overlap of volar and dorsal surfaces	Treatment of choice because it diminishes supination/pronation of the forearm

FIGURE 48.3
Sugar tong splint

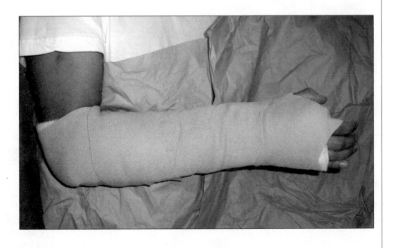

(*continued*)

TABLE 48.2 Type of Splints (*continued*)

Type and Indication	Length	Width	Note
Double sugar tong Elbow and forearm fractures/injuries	Lateral proximal humerus around elbow to the medial humerus up to the inferior axilla	Fully covers the dorsal and volar upper arm without overlap	The forearm component is applied exactly as for the single sugar tong, This device prevents pronation/supination of the forearm more so than does single sugar tong and posterior splint.
			Apply forearm portion before upper arm portion.
Long arm posterior Stable elbow and forearm fractures/injuries	Dorsal aspect of mid-upper arm under elbow along the ulna area of the forearm to the distal palmar flexor crease	Half the arm circumference	Allows some supination/pronation of forearm
Ulnar gutter Fourth/fifth metacarpal and proximal phalangeal fractures/injuries	Just beyond the fifth DIP joint to mid-forearm along the ulna surface	Midline of hand on the dorsal and volar surface incorporating both the little and ring fingers	Gauze should be placed between the fourth and fifth fingers.
Thumb spica First metacarpal, proximal first thumb phalangeal and scaphoid fracture/injuries De Quervain tenosynovitis	Just distal to the interphalangeal joint of the thumb to the mid-forearm along the radial surface	The width of the wrist	Splint all suspected scaphoid injuries as up to 10% of these fractures are missed on initial presentation.
Finger Phalanx fractures, tendon repairs/infections, and arthropathies	No further than the joint below or above the injury	Width of finger	DIP dislocations—the joint should be splinted in slight extension or no more than 5 degrees of flexion PIP dislocations—the joint should be at 20 degrees of flexion.
			Mallet finger is a distal extensor tendon rupture. Immobilization of only the DIP joint is required.
			Apply splint to dorsal surface because this maintains tactile function and is in closer proximity to the bone on the surface.
			Commercially available padded aluminum splints can easily be cut to length.

DIP, distal interphalangeal; MCP, metacarpophalangeal; PIP, proximal interphalangeal.

Lower Extremity Splints (Table 48.3)

TABLE 48.3 Type of Splints

Type and Indication	Length	Width	Note
Short posterior leg (Figure 48.4) Distal tibia, fibula, ankle, and foot fractures/injuries	Posteriorly from the level of the fibula neck, around the heal to the base of the toes	Covers half the leg circumference	When this is combined with the stirrup splint, it gives increased lateral ankle support.

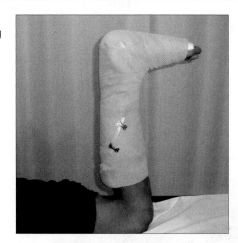

FIGURE 48.4 Short posterior leg splint.

Type and Indication	Length	Width	Note
Ankle stirrup Ankle sprains and minor chip fractures	From just below the fibula head running under the heal and to just below the knee on the medial surface	Half the circumference of the lower extremity	Should be able to place in a shoe for possible partial weight bearing. Commercially available air casts provide similar lateral stability with improved patient comfort (Figure 48.5).
Long posterior leg Knee fractures	Posteriorly just below the buttock crease to 3 cm above the heel	Half the circumference of the leg	

Miscellaneous Immobilization Devices (Table 48.4)

TABLE 48.4 Commercially Manufactured Immobilization Devices

Miscellaneous Immobilization Devices	Indication	Length	Notes
Shoulder immobilizer	Proximal humerus fractures Dislocated glenohumeral joints Sprains of the shoulder	NA	Sling supports the weight of the arm, whereas the swathe immobilizes the arm against the chest wall to maximally minimize shoulder movement.

(*continued*)

TABLE 48.4 Commercially Manufactured Immobilization Devices (*continued*)

Miscellaneous Immobilization Devices	Indication	Length	Notes
Knee immobilizer	Ligamentous injuries to the knee and arthropathies	Posteriorly just below the buttock crease to 3 cm above the heel	Knee should be in almost full extension. Easily removable, comfortable, and can go directly over clothing.
Post-op shoe	Toe fractures/injuries and minor foot injuries	NA	Usually combined with buddy taping of toe fractures. Can be used over a splint for partial weight bearing.
Buddy taping (Figure 48.6)	Finger and toe sprains, dislocations, and arthropathies	NA	Entails taping injured digit to uninjured adjacent digit. Use gauze between digits to prevent maceration and/or pressure ulcers. For treatment of toe fractures but not finger fractures.

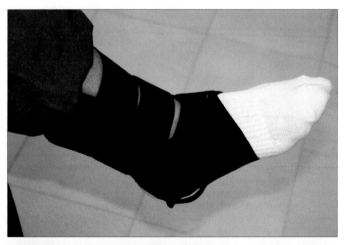

FIGURE 48.5 Ankle air cast splint.

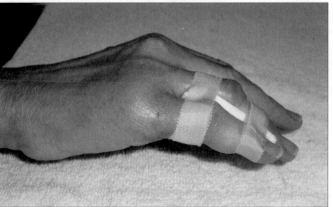

FIGURE 48.6 Buddy tape using adjacent finger as a splint. Note gauze between the fingers, placed in an effort to avoid pressure necrosis of the skin.

POST-PROCEDURAL CARE

- The importance of proper home splint care cannot be overemphasized.
- Apply ice packs no more than 30 minutes at a time.
- Elevation
- Instruct patients to return if pain increases or numbness or parethesia develops

---

PEARLS

- Because occult fractures are occasionally diagnosed as contusions or sprains, splint all injured extremities: "When in doubt, splint."
- Increasing pain in a patient with a splint should alert the provider to consider the diagnosis of compartment syndrome or deep vein thrombosis.
- Volar splints do not eliminate pronation/supination of the forearm as do sugar tongs. They should not be used for the treatment of ulnar or radial fractures.
- When applying a short posterior lower extremity splint, the patient can help keep the ankle at a 90-degree dorsiflexion by pulling up on the foot with an ace wrap (Figure 48.7).
- Application of lower extremity splints is made easier with the patient in the prone position.
- Avoid prolonged periods of splint use of nonfractures in order to prevent the development of joint stiffness, which can be disabling.
- Buddy taping of the fingers is not indicated for finger fractures.
- When applying the ACE wrap, do so in a rolling matter as opposed to stretching the wrap circumferentially around the splint and extremity.
- One must always be cognitive of the notion that, in the acute extremity injury, swelling will increase over the ensuing 24 hours.

FIGURE 48.7 Short posterior leg splint with patient assistance.

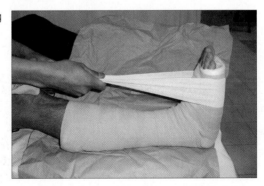

RESOURCES

Boyd, A. S. (2009). Splints and casts: Indications and methods. *American Family Physician, 80*(5), 491–499.

Chudnofsky, C. R., & Byers, S. E. (2004). Splinting techniques. In J. Roberts & J. Hedges (Eds.), *Clinical procedures in emergency medicine* (pp. 995–1007). Philadelphia, PA: Saunders Elsevier.

Gravlee, J. R. (2007). Braces and splints for musculoskeletal conditions. *American Family Physicians, 75*(3), 342–348.

Klig, J. L. (2008). Splinting procedures. In C. King & F. Henretig (Eds.), *Textbook of pediatric emergency procedures* (pp. 919–931). Philadelphia, PA: Lippincott Williams & Wilkins.

Paras, R. D. (2000). Upper extremity fractures. *Clinics in Family Practice, 2*(3), 637–659.

UNIT **XIV**

Procedures for Managing Common Gastrointestinal and Genitourinary Conditions

CHAPTER 49

Procedures for Managing a Thrombosed Hemorrhoid

Keith A. Lafferty

BACKGROUND

Five percent of the population is afflicted with hemorrhoids. Their symptoms run the spectrum from a minor annoyance with intermittent slow bleeding to extreme, excessive, and near-debilitating pain.

The superior hemorrhoidal veins make up internal hemorrhoids and drain into the portal system. The inferior hemorrhoidal veins make up external hemorrhoids and drain into the inferior vena cava. Anatomically, internal hemorrhoids lie above the dentate line (embryologically based, a hemorrhoid is the delineation of anal tissue with mucus-like columnar epithelium and rectal tissue, which has more skin-like squamous epithelium) (Figure 49.1). Also, tissue above the dentate line (anal tissue) receives visceral innervation, whereas tissue below it (rectum) receives a rich supply of somatic innervation. Note that there is communication between these two venous systems, which form a plexus-like pattern.

FIGURE 49.1 Hemorrhoid anatomy.

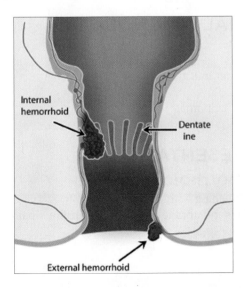

Internal hemorrhoid

Dentate ine

External hemorrhoid

Hemorrhoidal veins are very superficial; internal hemorrhoids are submucosal and external hemorrhoids are subcutaneous. Because of this, symptomatic internal hemorrhoids are beefy red, whereas external hemorrhoids are skin colored.

Internal hemorrhoids form three cushion-like protrusions at the right anterior, right posterior, and left lateral position. These normal anatomic protrusions may aid in the defecation process. External hemorrhoids form a ring-like pattern. Finally, the hemorrhoidal plexus is also composed of muscle fibers, subcutaneous tissue, and a generous arterial blood supply, which contributes to the bright red color of hemorrhoid bleeding.

Only when the hemorrhoidal plexus gets enlarged, prolapsed, or thrombosed are they referred to as hemorrhoids. Mechanistically, contributing to the development of hemorrhoids is the fact that the hemorrhoidal veins are devoid of valves and, as one ages, a loss of the surrounding support of connective tissue occurs. Further causes seem to stem from increased pressure caused from the increased venous drainage of the anal-rectum with pregnancy, portal hypertension, and conditions of increased straining (which also weaken the support of connective tissue). Symptoms are exacerbated by frequent bowel movements, prolonged sitting, heavy lifting, and any condition that leads to increased draining.

External hemorrhoids are symptomatic with either bleeding or acute pain when they are thrombosed. Internal hemorrhoids are classified according to the degree of their prolapse (Table 49.1).

TABLE 49.1 Classification of Internal Hemorrhoids

Type	Prolapse	Reduction
First degree	None	NA
Second degree	Only with defecation	Spontaneous
Third degree	Spontaneous	With digital maneuvers
Fourth degree	Constant	Irreducible

DIFFERENTIAL DIAGNOSIS

- Fissures
- Fistulas
- Abscesses and other infections
- Rectal prolapse
- Gastrointestinal carcinomas

PATIENT PRESENTATION

Internal Hemorrhoids

- Painless, bright bleeding with defecation
- Prolapsed mucous membrane tissue (plus or minus pain depending on whether gangrenous; Figure 49.2)
- Pruritus ani

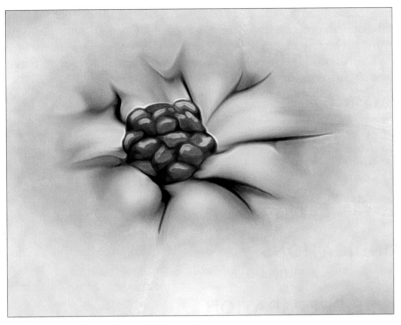

FIGURE 49.2 Internal hemorrhoid.

External Hemorrhoids

- Pain (can be severe with the patient being unable to sit)
- Swelling (skin overlying firm tissue; Figure 49.3A and 49.3B)
- Bleeding
- Pruritus ani

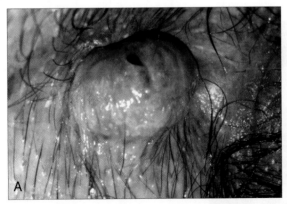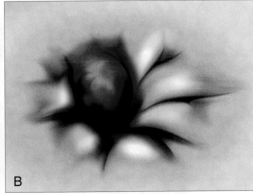

FIGURE 49.3A and 49.3B External thrombosed hemorrhoid.

TREATMENT

First- to third-degree internal hemorrhoids are treated conservatively with surgical follow-up for definitive treatment, which could include banding, sclerotherapy, or hemorrhoidectomy. Fourth-degree hemorrhoids require parenteral antibiotic and emergent hemorrhoidectomy.

External hemorrhoids that are bleeding can be treated conservatively and the patient reassured. Acute thrombosis needs to be excised—not incised. Simply incising the tissue leads to incomplete clot evacuation, reaccumulation, and persistent skin tags. It is imperative that all clots are removed after excision and unroofing of tissue. Conservative therapy consists of the acronym WASH (Table 49.2).

TABLE 49.2 WASH

W	Water—increase oral intake, sitz baths
A	Analgesics—use temporarily to avoid inducing constipation. Topical anesthetic/steroid creams may be a better alternative
S	Stool softeners
H	High-fiber diets

CONTRAINDICATIONS
- Fourth-degree gangrenous internal hemorrhoids

PROCEDURE PREPARATION
- Patient should be placed in the left lateral decubitus position.
- The knee-to-chest position with the buttocks taped to the side rails is an alternative (Figure 49.4)
- Skin antiseptic solution
- Local anesthetic with epinephrine
- No. 11 blade scalpel
- Forceps
- Hemostats
- Gel foam
- Gauze pad

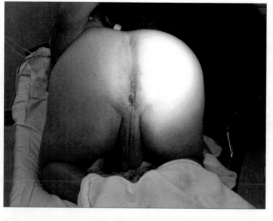

FIGURE 49.4 Knee-to-chest position.

PROCEDURE (Video 49.1)
- Skin cleansing technique as described in Chapter 14
- Sterile technique
- Local infiltrated anesthesia is applied with one stick between the skin overlying the thrombosed hemorrhoid and the hemorrhoidal wall, inducing blanching that covers the entire hemorrhoid.

- An elliptical excision is made in a radial manner, extending from an area just distal to the anal verge outward.
- Unroof the elliptical excision and meticulously remove all clots with manual pressure and forceps (Figure 49.5).
- Place a piece of Gel foam in the wound and cover with a gauze pad, or place a cotton-tipped stick dipped in Monsel's solution in the wound.

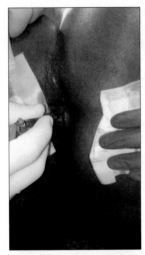

 VIDEO 49.1 Elliptical excision of thrombosed external hemorrhoid.
springerpub.com/campo

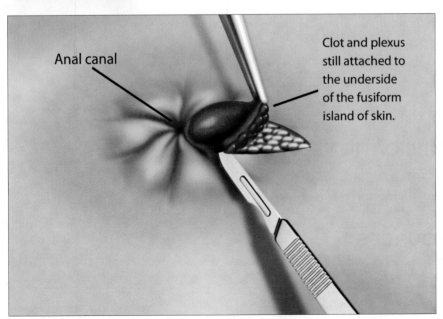

Anal canal

Clot and plexus still attached to the underside of the fusiform island of skin.

FIGURE 49.5 Elliptical excision with clot removed.

POST-PROCEDURE CONSIDERATIONS

- Conservative therapy, implementing WASH for all symptomatic discharged hemorrhoid patients
- Note that the Gel foam packing usually spontaneously dislodges within 24 to 36 hours.

PEARLS

- Patients get almost immediate relief of excision with thrombosed external hemorrhoids.
- Do not incise external hemorrhoids; always excise them.
- All that bleeds rectally are not hemorrhoids. Although hemorrhoids might be seen, the source of bleeding could be secondary to other serious gastrointestinal disorders, especially carcinomas.
- A painful rectal lump needs to be examined and inspected closely because the differential diagnosis is broad.
- The prone knee-to-chest position with buttocks taped to side rails provides the best perianal exposure.
- Bupivacaine lasts longer than lidocaine.
- Inspection of the proximal anus and distal rectum is best done via anoscopy (Figure 49.6).

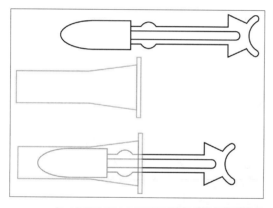

FIGURE 49.6 Anal scope.

COMPLICATIONS

- Bleeding
- Infection
- Perianal skin tags

RESOURCES

Burgess, B. E., & Bouzoukis, J. K. (2004). Anorectal disorders. In J. Tintinalli, G. D. Kelen, J. S. Stapczynski, O. J. Ma, & D. M. Cline (Eds.), *Emergency medicine: A comprehensive study guide* (pp. 539–542). New York, NY: McGraw-Hill.

Coates, W. C. (2006). Anorectum. In J. Marx, R. Hockberger, & R. Walls (Eds.), *Rosen's emergency medicine concepts and clinical practice* (pp. 1507–1514). Philadelphia, PA: Mosby Elsevier.

Kaider-Person, O. (2007). Hemorrhoidal disease: A comprehensive review. *Journal of the American College of Surgeons, 204*(1), 102–117.

Nelson, H., & Cima, R. R. (2008). Common benign anal disorders. In C. M. Townsend, R. D. Beauchamp, B. M. Evers, & K. L. Mattox (Eds.), *Sabiston textbook of surgery* (18th ed.). Philadelphia, PA: Elsevier. Retrieved from http://www.mdconsult.com/das/book/body/192424659-4/0/1565/494.html#4-u1.0-B978-1-4160-3675-3..50055-1-cesec26

Sneider, E. B. (2010). Diagnosis and management of symptomatic hemorrhoids. *Surgical Clinics of North America, 90*(1), 17–32.

CHAPTER 50

Procedures for Treating a Hair Tourniquet

Lee Ann Boyd and M. Bess Raulerson

BACKGROUND

A hair tourniquet occurs when a hair or thread entraps an appendage; it can lead to pain, injury, and possible loss of function or loss of the appendage (Figure 50.1). Epithelialization may occur at the site of the hair or thread, impairing the ability to visualize the tourniquet. Hair has the ability to stretch when wet and contract as it dries. Hair's tensile strength causes ischemic compression as well as a direct cutting action of the appendage. A hair tourniquet is typically accidental; however, incidences of intentional cases consistent with child abuse have been cited in the literature.

Hair tourniquet syndrome may involve fingers, toes, earlobes, nipples, tongue, scrotum, and penis. Most cases involve the fingers and toes, followed by external genitalia (33% of cases). Infants younger than 4 months of age may be at increased risk for development of a hair tourniquet as many mothers experience postpartum hair loss several months after delivery. Our discussion regarding treatment focuses on penile hair tourniquet removal.

FIGURE 50.1 Hair tourniquet: Multiple strands of hair wrapped around mid shaft of the penis.

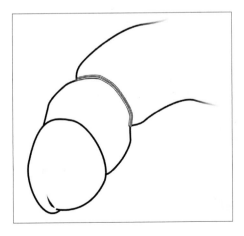

PATIENT PRESENTATION

- Inconsolable crying in the infant
- Painful, edematous appendage
- Presence of sharp circumferential demarcation
- Cyanosis of the appendage distal to the hair tourniquet may occur

TREATMENT

Treatment of a hair tourniquet consists of removal of the hair/thread. The simplest treatment is the use of depilatory creams or the unwrapping technique. Depilatory creams are thioglycolate based, the mechanism of action of which is to break the bonds of keratin in hair. They are not effective for thread tourniquets and should not be used on open skin.

If mild to moderate edema is present, the blunt probe cutting technique may be used. The hair or thread must be visible and not too deeply constrictive in the soft tissues. If the preceding treatments are unsuccessful, or severe edema or epithelialization has occurred, the incisional approach may be necessary.

CONTRAINDICATIONS AND RELATIVE CONTRAINDICATIONS

- A history of an allergic reaction to depilatory creams
- Use caution with the incisional approach in patients with bleeding diathesis

SPECIAL CONSIDERATIONS

- All patients treated for penile hair tourniquet should follow up with an urologist within 24 to 48 hours after the tourniquet has been removed.

PROCEDURE PREPARATION

Prior to initiating treatment to remove the hair tourniquet, you will need to discuss the procedure, potential complications, risks, and benefits with the patient's parents. Instruct the parents on the importance of follow-up and the expected time to return to the treatment center or primary care provider.

Unwrapping Method

- Gloves
- Hemostat or fine-tipped forceps

Depilatory Method

- Gloves
- Depilatory cream

Cutting Method

- Gloves
- Topical or infiltrative anesthetics

- Chlorhexidine or povidone iodine skin cleanser
- Fine-tipped scissors
- Fine-tipped hemostat
- Blunt probe
- No. 11 scalpel blade with handle

PROCEDURE

Unwrapping Method

- Position the patient for maximum visualization of the genitals.
- Most effective when only minimal edema is present, and hair/thread is readily identifiable.
- Put on clean gloves.
- Identify the free end of the hair/thread. If unable to isolate a free end, but a knot is present, break one end of the knot and proceed as follows.
- Grasp the free end of the hair with fine-tipped forceps or a hemostat, and unwind the hair from the appendage.

Depilatory Method

- No anesthesia is required.
- Apply depilatory cream directly to the hair being careful to avoid the urethral meatus, and allow it to sit according to the manufacturer's instructions, typically 3 to 10 minutes.
- After breakage of the hair has occurred, wash off the area with soap and water.

Blunt Cutting Technique

- Gently insert a blunt probe underneath the hair/thread, separating the tourniquet from the skin (Figure 50.2).
- Once the thread is isolated, cut the hair/thread with fine-tipped scissors or a No. 11 scalpel blade, cutting against the surface of the probe to protect the skin.
- Proceed with removal of the remaining tourniquet material using the unwrapping method described previously.

FIGURE 50.2 Use of blunt probe to lift hair or thread tourniquet from shaft of penis prior to cutting.

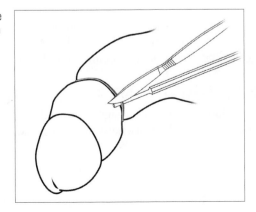

Incisional Approach

- Universal precautions should be used at all times.
- Cleanse the skin with chlorhexidine solution or povidone iodine in a circular motion to remove debris and bacteria.
- Apply a fenestrated drape over the external genitalia.
- A dorsal nerve block is recommended. Topical anesthetics, such as Emla cream, may be used in addition to the nerve block. For a penile nerve block, please see Chapter 10.
- Once the area is anesthetized, make a small longitudinal incision with a No. 11 scalpel blade in the inferolateral surface of the phallus at the 4 or 8 o'clock position (Figure 50.3).
- Care should be taken to stay within the deep penile fascia located between the corpora cavernosum and spongiosum, thus preventing injury to the neurovascular bundle.
- Ensure the removal of all thread/hair tourniquet.

FIGURE 50.3 Cross-cut view of penis just distal to tourniquet demonstrating appropriate depth and position of incision.

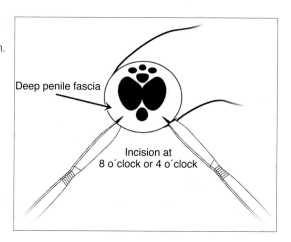

Deep penile fascia

Incision at
8 o´clock or 4 o´clock

POST-PROCEDURE CONSIDERATIONS

- Assess neurovascular status following the procedure.
- Tetanus prophylaxis if indicated.
- Antibiotic therapy should be reserved for those patients who present with localized signs of infection, or those who are diabetic and immunocompromised.
- Pediatric patients should be assessed for child neglect or abuse.
- Urology consultation should be obtained for all tourniquets involving the penis.

EDUCATIONAL POINTS

- Instruct the patient/parents on signs of infection, such as redness or increased warmth of tissue, purulent discharge, or fever, and to report to his or her health care provider.

- Instruct the patient/parents on signs of neurovascular compromise, such as loss of sensation, coolness to the tissue, bleeding, or dusky color to the skin distal to the sight of the injury, and to report to his or her health care provider.
- Report any difficulty eliminating urine or hematuria to the health care provider.
- Instruct on the importance of following up with their health care provider.

COMPLICATIONS

- Skin irritation or contact dermatitis can occur with the use of depilatory creams.
- With incisional method, bleeding, infection, or damage to surrounding structures can occur (i.e., urethra, corpus callosum, corpus spongiosum).
- Ischemic changes can lead to necrosis of tissue distal from the tourniquet site.

PEARLS

- The unwrapping techniques and depilatory creams are commonly ineffective in the clinical setting.
- In the case of symptomatic hair tourniquet syndrome, typically the blunt cutting technique or the incisional approach is necessary.
- Always check for hair tourniquet syndrome in an infant with inconsolable crying (Figure 50.4A and 50.4B).

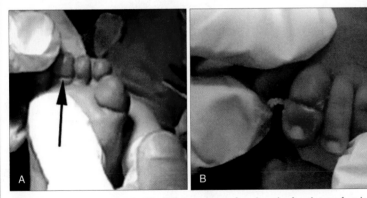

FIGURES 50.4A and 50.4B: Hair tourniquets found on the fourth toe of an inconsolable crying infant.

RESOURCES

Baskin, L. S., & Kogan, B. A. (2005). *Handbook of pediatric urology* (2nd ed., pp. 2–3, 59). Philadelphia, PA: Lippincott, Williams, & Wilkins.

Candriche, D., & Doty, C. I. (2009). *Hair tourniquet removal.* Retrieved from http://emedicine.medscape.com/article/1348969-overview

CHAPTER 51

Procedures for Treating Phimosis and Paraphimosis

Lee Ann Boyd and M. Bess Raulerson

PHIMOSIS
Background

Phimosis is a narrowing of the opening of the prepuce in uncircumcised patients, which prevents the prepuce from being retracted back over the glans penis (Figure 51.1). This condition may be pathologic or may be a normal physiologic finding. When evaluating a pediatric patient with a phimosis, take into account the age of the child. Phimosis is normal in newborns; by 6 months of age, 20% are retractable; and by 3 years of age, 90% are retractable. Inability to retract the foreskin in a pediatric patient requires no treatment in the absence of symptoms.

Pathologic phimosis can occur as a result of poor hygiene, diabetes mellitus, and chronic balanoposthitis. Patients may complain of edema, erythema, and pain of the prepuce with inability to retract the foreskin. Ballooning of the foreskin during voiding may occur, which can increase the risk of a urinary tract infection. Penile discharge may be present, which is often white to yellow in color, and is termed smegma, which is exfoliated skin cells. In severe cases of tight phimosis, urinary retention may occur.

Patient Presentation

- Edema and erythema of the prepuce
- Tenderness with possible induration of the prepuce
- Penile discharge—white to yellow
- Inability to retract foreskin
- Difficulty voiding in some patients with a pin-point opening on the foreskin

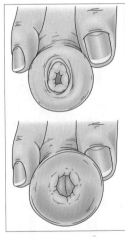

FIGURE 51.1 Phimosis. Note that this can only occur in uncircumcised males.

Image reprinted with permission from *Medscape Drugs & Diseases* (http://emedicine. medscape.com), 2015, available at http://emedicine.medscape. com/article/777539-overview.

Treatment

No treatment is necessary for pediatric patients with asymptomatic phimosis. Treatment of mild cases of pathologic phimosis is local treatment with topical steroids as the first line of treatment. Betamesthasone 0.05% ointment applied at the tip of the penis at the area of the phimosis twice daily for 6 to 8 weeks has a 90% to 95% success rate. After 1 week of treatment, the foreskin should be gently retracted to aid in the release of the phimosis.

Acute or severe cases may require a dorsal slit procedure. The foreskin is pulled taut distally and a hemostat clamp is placed at the 12 o'clock position and held in place for approximately 2 minutes, providing crushing of the tissue with resulting hemostasis; local nerve destruction in the crushed tissue is then incised. The wound edges are approximated horizontally with loose transverse absorbable sutures (Figure 51.2). The cosmetic effects of this procedure may not be aesthetically pleasing. Definitive treatment with a circumcision may be done at a later date. The dorsal slit procedure is a viable option for patients who may be at risk for general anesthesia, because it may be performed with local anesthesia.

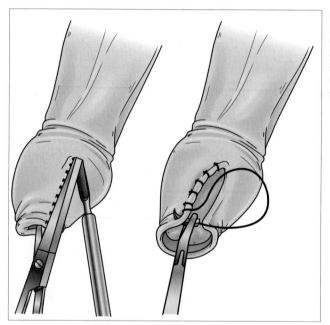

FIGURE 51.2 Dorsal slit.

Image reprinted with permission from *Medscape Drugs & Diseases* (http://emedicine.medscape.com), 2015, available at http://emedicine.medscape.com/article/777539-overview.

Contraindications and Relative Contraindications

- Allergic reaction to betamethasone ointment
- Bleeding diathesis

Special Considerations

Use caution in the use of betamethasone in pediatric patients younger than 3 years—use of topical steroids has not been studied extensively in this age group.

Procedure Preparation

- Skin cleansing solution
- Sterile 4 × 4 gauze
- Sterile drape
- Local anesthetic (LA; see Chapter 9)
- 5-mL syringe
- 27-gauge needle
- Sterile gloves
- Straight hemostat
- No. 15 scalpel blade or iris scissors
- 4-0 absorbable suture
- Topical antibiotic ointment
- Petroleum gauze
- Sterile gauze
- Paper tape

Procedure

- Place the patient in a supine position.
- Using aseptic technique, prepare the perineal area from the suprapubic area to the scrotum using skin cleanser.
- Place a sterile drape over the genital area exposing only the phallus.
- Fill 5-mL syringe with LA and attach a 27-gauge needle.
- Anesthetize the area using local infiltration or penile block (see Chapter 10).
  - Using a hemostat, gently separate any adhesions under the foreskin.
  - Pulling the dorsal foreskin taut, apply a straight hemostat at the 12 o'clock position crushing the tissue of the foreskin. The hemostat should be placed perpendicular to the corona.
  - Leave hemostat in place for 2 minutes.
  - Sharply incise the band of crushed tissue in between the hemostats at the 12 o'clock position using a scalpel or iris scissors.
  - The wound edges should be approximated in a horizontal manner with absorbable suture using running sutures.
  - Reduce foreskin to its natural position.
  - Apply topical antibiotic ointment to the suture line.
  - Apply petroleum gauze and cover with sterile gauze.
  - Adhere with paper tape.

Post-Procedure Considerations

- Observe for bleeding at incision sites for 30 minutes following the procedure.
- Apply bacitracin ointment to the suture line to decrease the risk of developing adhesions during the healing process.
- Ensure that an analgesic prescription is given to the patient for postoperative pain.

Educational Points

Physiologic

- Encourage good local hygiene.
- Instruct on the removal of smegma.
- Instruct parents on gentle and gradual retraction of foreskin in the newborn.

Pathologic

- Encourage good local hygiene.
- Instruct the patient/parents on the importance of completing the course of topical treatment to prevent recurrence.
- Instruct the patient/parents on the application of bacitracin to the glans penis twice daily for 2 weeks to prevent formation of new adhesions following dorsal slit procedure.
- For diabetic patients, encourage tight control of serum blood sugar to prevent recurrence.
- No sexual intercourse for 4 to 6 weeks postoperatively.
- Definitive treatment with circumcision may be done after acute inflammation resolves.

Complications

- If phimosis is not treated, there is an increased risk of persistent balanoposthitis, future phimosis, and development of squamous cell penile carcinoma.
- Bleeding
- Hematoma
- Wound infection
- Glanular adhesions
- Tissue sloughing
- Urinary retention

PEARLS

- Consider the serum glucose level and HGB A1C to rule out underlying diabetes mellitus.
- If the chosen technique for anesthesia is not successful, use a different technique, being cautious not to exceed the usual dosage of lidocaine.
- The tip of the hemostat should be palpable under the foreskin at the coronal sulcus; use care to avoid placing the hemostat within the urethra.

PARAPHIMOSIS

Paraphimosis is a tightening or constriction of the glans penis by the foreskin, which has been retracted behind the corona of the glans penis (Figure 51.3). Prolonged retraction can lead to obstruction of the lymphatics and subsequent lymphedema, which impairs the ability to replace the foreskin to its normal position over the glans penis.

Paraphimosis can occur in children, but is most often seen in uncircumcised adult or elderly men. It is often associated with poor hygiene, chronic balanoposthitis, diabetes, phimosis, chronic indwelling Foley catheter, or patients who perform intermittent self-catheterization. Patients often experience penile pain and edema of the penile shaft proximal to the glans and corona, where a tight phimotic ring is present. If the constriction is severe, venous congestion of the glans is present, which can cause necrosis of the glans penis or distal urethra.

Patient Presentation

- Penile pain
- Edema of the penile shaft proximal to the glans and corona
- Presence of a tight phimotic ring proximal to the corona
- Late finding of venous congestion of the glans with necrosis at the phimotic ring, which may extend to the glans penis.

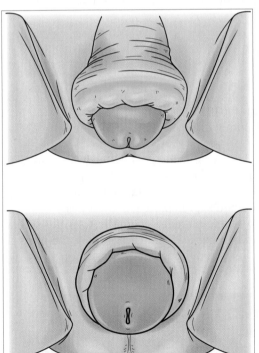

FIGURE 51.3 Paraphimosis. This is a true urologic emergency and must be recognized and treated promptly as the glans is at risk for necrosis in just a few hours and subsequently gangrene; possible amputation may ensue days to weeks later. This can only occur in uncircumcised males and is less common than a phimosis.

Image reprinted with permission from *Medscape Drugs & Diseases* (http://emedicine.medscape.com), 2015, available at http://emedicine.medscape.com/article/777539-overview.

Treatment

Treatment of paraphimosis is closed manual reduction of the edematous glans penis. If manual compression does not resolve the paraphimosis, then a dorsal slit must be performed. Consider circumcision after the inflammation has resolved. Refer to a urologist.

Contraindications and Relative Contraindications

- There are no contraindications to manual reduction of the paraphimosis.
- Use caution with the dorsal slit procedure in patients with a bleeding diatheses.
- Reversal of bleeding disorders, if possible, may be indicated if impending vascular compromise is evident.

Special Considerations

Careful examination should be done to rule out any area of necrosis on the phallus, which would need to be debrided.

Procedure Preparation

- Gloves
- Skin cleanser
- Ice
- 1% lidocaine gel or Emla cream (2.5% prilocaine and 2.5% lidocaine)
- Elastic wrap or Kerlix bandage
- 25-gauge needle (optional)
- 4 × 4 gauze

Procedure

- Apply an ice pack to the distal phallus for 10 to 15 minutes.
- Apply topical anesthetic to the tight phimotic ring, using 1% lidocaine gel or EMLA cream.
- Manually compress the edematous glans penis using gentle, steady pressure with both thumbs on the glans for 5 minutes (Figure 51.4).
- Alternatively, an elastic wrap or Kerlix bandage can be wrapped distal to proximal, from the glans to the base of the penis and kept in place for 5 minutes.
- Adjunctive therapy for moderate to severe glanular edema is to make several superficial (2–3 mm) puncture wounds using a 25-gauge needle in the glans to promote drainage of edema fluid and/or blood from venous congestion.

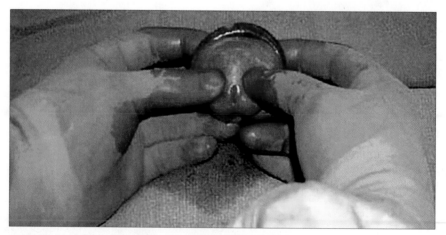

FIGURE 51.4 Manually compress the edematous glans penis.

- Holding the penis with one hand on either side, place both thumbs on the glans for stabilization. Using the fingers of both hands, draw the foreskin down over the glans.
- If the aforementioned procedure does not resolve the paraphimosis, then an emergency dorsal slit or circumcision procedure is required (see Treatment of phimosis section for dorsal slit procedure).

Post-Procedure Considerations
- If there is no definitive treatment, paraphimosis is likely to occur.
- Debridement of necrotic tissue is rarely indicated.
- Observe for bleeding for 30 minutes following a dorsal slit procedure.

Educational Points
Patients and health care providers need to be instructed to replace the foreskin to its normal position over the glans penis after placement of a urinary catheter. Those patients who have a chronic indwelling Foley catheter should be taught routine catheter care with gentle soap and water, stressing the importance of returning the foreskin over the glans.

Complications
- Arterial occlusion with necrosis of the glans penis
- Necrosis of the distal urethra

PEARLS

- If an indwelling Foley catheter is present, remove the catheter to aid in reduction of paraphimosis.
- A successfully reduced paraphimosis needs definitive treatment to prevent a future phimosis.

RESOURCES
Choe, J. M. (2000). Paraphimosis: Current treatment options. *American Family Physician, 62,* 2623–2626, 2628.

Ginsberg, P. C., & Harkaway, R. C. (2000). Phimosis. In L. G. Gomella (Ed.), *The 5-minute urology consult* (pp. 376–377, 388–389). Philadelphia, PA: Lippincott, Williams, & Wilkins.

Paynter, M. (2006). Practice makes perfect: Paraphimosis. *Emergency Nurse, 14*(4), 18–20.

Pulsifer, A. (2005). *Pediatric genitourinary examination: A clinician's reference.* Retrieved from http://www.medscape.com/viewarticle/507161_7

Shlamovitz, G. Z., & Snyder, E. W. (2009, November 10). *Dorsal slit of the foreskin: Treatment & medication.* Retrieved from http://emedicine.medscape.com/article/80697-treatment

Steadman, B., & Ellsworth, P. (2006). To circ or not to circ: Indications, risks, and alternatives to circumcision in the pediatric population with phimosis. *Urologic Nursing, 26*(3), 181–194.

Tanagho, E. A., & McAnich, J. W. (2008). *Smith's general urology.* New York, NY: McGraw Hill.

CHAPTER **52**

Suprapubic Catheter Care and Troubleshooting

Lee Ann Boyd and M. Bess Raulerson

BACKGROUND

A suprapubic catheter is inserted into the bladder via a small incision in the abdominal wall to allow urinary drainage (Figure 52.1). A suprapubic catheter may be used for management of urinary incontinence, urinary retention, and neurogenic bladder. It may also be used temporarily after genitourinary trauma; severe pelvid, perineal, or decubitus ulcers and infections; or surgery.

The benefits of a suprapubic catheter versus a urethral catheter in patients requiring chronic indwelling urinary catheters include decreases in urethral discomfort, urinary tract infections (UTIs), urethral strictures, and urethral trauma. The suprapubic catheter is the indwelling catheter of choice for those patients who remain sexually active.

Suprapubic catheter sizes may vary, but most common sizes used in adult patients are either an 18- or 20-French two-way Foley catheter. Although there is no standard of care as to how often a suprapubic catheter should be changed, it is widely held that these catheters be changed every 4 to 6 weeks. More frequent intervals of suprapubic catheter changes may be necessary in the event of a UTI or an obstructed catheter that cannot be cleared with irrigation.

PATIENT PRESENTATION

Patients may present with a variety of complaints regarding their suprapubic catheter:

- Symptomatic UTI (i.e., fever, hematuria, suprapubic pain, new onset of leakage at the stoma site)
- Bleeding from suprapubic stoma site
- Nondraining suprapubic catheter with suprapubic distention and bladder spasms with possible leakage around the catheter

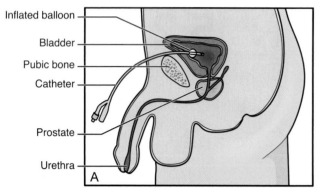
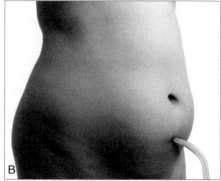

Inflated balloon
Bladder
Pubic bone
Catheter
Prostate
Urethra
A
B

FIGURE 52.1A and 52.1B A. Suprapubic catheter in place; B. Suprapubic catheter in place in lower abdomen.

TREATMENT
Urinary Tract Infection

Patients with chronic suprapubic catheters are likely to have chronic colonization of bacteria in the urine. The bacteria may consist of gram-negative organisms, gram-positive organisms, or yeast. It is recommended that patients with chronic urinary catheters not be treated with antibiotics for asymptomatic bacteriuria. However, a patient who presents with fever, chills, gross hematuria, suprapubic discomfort, or new onset of leakage from the stoma site may have an acute UTI. Leukocytosis may be present. Urinalysis (UA) often reveals white blood cells (WBCs), red blood cells (RBCs), bacteria, positive nitrate, and positive leukocyte esterace.

Obtain the patient's history regarding symptoms of fever, chills, nausea, vomiting, hematuria, suprapubic pain, or flank pain. Perform a physical examination paying special attention to the abdominal, flank, and genitourinary areas. The presence of flank pain may indicate pyelonephritis or an obstructive ureteral calculus. Besides the typical findings on UA with UTI, the patient presenting with pyelonephritis may have proteinuria, WBC casts, and granular casts are found in patients with costovertebral angle tenderness (CVAT) on examination. Consider a renal sonogram or spiral CT scan, to rule out ureteral obstruction from urinary calculi. The suprapubic catheter should be exchanged, urine culture and sensitivity should be obtained, and the patient should be empirically treated with antibiotic therapy. In this situation, this would be considered a complicated UTI and should be treated for 7 to 10 days of antibiotic therapy. Common microorganisms associated with complicated UTIs include gram-negative organisms such as *Escherichia coli, Klebsiella, Enterococcus*, and *Pseudomonas*, with the most common gram-positive organism being *Staphylococcus aureus*. Treatment consists of oral or parenteral antibiotic therapy. Consider hospital admission for those patients with pyelonephritis or urosepsis.

Bleeding From Suprapubic Stoma Site

Minor bright red bleeding at the suprapubic catheter site is normal for 24 to 48 hours after the initial placement of the catheter. If this is noted, do not place traction on the catheter. With well-established suprapubic catheters, the most common cause of new onset of bleeding from the stoma site is excessive growth of granulation tissue. To treat granulation tissue and bleeding at the stoma, use silver nitrate sticks to cauterize the stoma edges and the granulation tissue, being careful to avoid contact with the catheter.

Obstructed Suprapubic Catheter

Patients may present with an obstructed urinary catheter from debris, blood clots, or calcification within the catheter. Assess the patency of the drainage tubing initially to rule out kinks causing obstruction. Irrigate the catheter with sterile water until drainage is reestablished. If obstruction persists, remove the catheter and replace with the same-size catheter.

CONTRAINDICATIONS AND RELATIVE CONTRAINDICATIONS

- For patients with latex allergy, use latex-free or silicone catheters when replacing urinary catheters.

SPECIAL CONSIDERATIONS

If a suprapubic catheter must be changed, always question the patient regarding the date of the last catheter change. If the current catheter has been in place for more than 2 months, use caution when removing the catheter as it may be calcified. A flat plate x-ray of the abdomen may be done to assess for calcification of the catheter prior to removal.

PROCEDURE PREPARATION

Urinary Tract Infection

- Clean gloves
- Sterile gloves
- Skin cleanser
- Foley catheter (use the same size catheter that is currently in place)
- Sterile water-soluble lubricant
- 12-mL Luer Lock syringe
- Sterile water
- Sterile urine specimen container

Bleeding From Suprapubic Site

- Clean gloves
- Silver nitrate sticks or electrocautery

Obstructed Suprapubic Catheter

- Clean gloves
- Sterile gloves
- 500- or 1,000-mL bottle of sterile water
- Irrigation tray with Toomey syringe
- Catheter supplies listed previously as needed

PROCEDURE
Urinary Tract Infection
- Assess the suprapubic catheter for size and patency.
- A Foley catheter of the same size as the catheter presently in place (to prevent difficulty in replacing the catheter in the suprapubic tract) should be readily available for immediate replacement.
- Remove the suprapubic catheter by deflating the balloon, and discard in biohazard container. A corkscrew technique may be necessary to remove the suprapubic catheter.
- Using aseptic technique, clean the suprapubic site with skin cleanser in a circular motion from the stoma outward.
- Lubricate the catheter with sterile, water-soluble lubricant.
- Place the catheter in the stoma and insert a little farther than the catheter that was just removed.
- Wait for urine return. Obtain sterile urine specimen for culture and sensitivity.
- Fill the 5-mL catheter balloon with 10-mL sterile water (to accommodate the fluid contained in the lumen of the catheter).
- Attach the suprapubic catheter to a closed urinary drainage system.
- Antibiotic choice depends on regional antibiograms and local resistance patterns; however, fluoroquinolones, second- or third-generation cephalosporins, or broad spectrum carbapenems may be indicated. In case of systemic symptoms, aggressive antibiotic and sepsis prevention measures should begin immediately.
  - Ciprofloxacin 500 mg orally twice a day for 7 to 10 days.
  - Levofloxacin 500 mg orally once a day for 7 to 10 days.
- Patient should be admitted for urosepsis.

Bleeding From Stoma Site
- Cleanse the stoma site with normal saline.
- Using silver nitrate sticks or elctrocautery, cauterize the stoma granulation tissue until bleeding ceases. The tissue will appear blackened in color.
- Apply triple antibiotic ointment to the site and apply a light sterile gauze dressing.
- Dressing should be removed after 24 hours.

Obstructed Suprapubic Catheter
- Aseptic technique should be used throughout the procedure.
- Ensure that there are no kinks in the tubing.
- Disconnect the Foley catheter from the urinary drainage bag tubing.
- Using an irrigation set with a 60-mL catheter tip syringe, instill 60 mL of sterile water to irrigate the catheter.
- Reassess for catheter patency. If patent, clean the distal tip of the urinary drainage bag tubing with alcohol and reconnect to gravity drainage.
- If the catheter remains obstructed, replace the suprapubic catheter using the aforementioned steps.

POST-PROCEDURE CONSIDERATIONS

- Observe for hematuria following a suprapubic catheter change, irrigation, or manipulation.
- Secure the catheter with tape or a catheter-securing device so that there is no tension placed on the catheter.

EDUCATIONAL POINTS

- Instruct the patient on keeping the catheter drainage tube from becoming kinked, and on positioning the drainage bag below the level of the bladder to promote adequate drainage.
- Explain that minimal bleeding from the catheter is normal and may be intermittent in nature.
- The drainage bag should be emptied when one-half to two-thirds full.
- No urine output in the drainage bag and an urge to void may indicate obstruction of the catheter, and the patient should return for irrigation if needed.
- Notify the provider if a fever develops.
- Instruct the patient to follow up with an urologist in a specified amount of time.

COMPLICATIONS

- Peritoneal placement of suprapubic catheter
- Development of urinary calculi
- Stomal stenosis
- Gross hematuria
- Increased risk of development of squamous cell carcinoma of the bladder

PEARLS

- Odor and discoloration may occur within the urinary drainage bag. The drainage bag may be cleaned with a solution of one part vinegar and three parts water.
- Patients with recurrent gross, painless hematuria should be encouraged to follow up with a urologist for a cystoscopic examination to rule out bladder calculi or bladder tumors.
- Always use gentle, constant pressure; never force the catheter into the stoma.
- If resistance persists, use a smaller sized catheter or call the urologist.

RESOURCES

Anderson, P. J., Walsh, P. M., Louey, M. A., Meade, C., & Fairbrother, G. (2002). Comparing first and subsequent suprapubic catheter change: Complications and costs. *Urologic Nursing, 22*(5), 324–330.

Gotelli, J. M., Merryman, P., Carr, C., McElveen, L., Epperson, C., & Bynum, D. (2008). A quality improvement project to reduce the complications associated with indwelling urinary catheters. *Urologic Nursing, 28*(6), 465–467.

Gray, M., & Moore, K. N. (2009). Urinary tract infections. In *Urologic disorders: Adult and pediatric care* (pp. 92–118). St. Louis, MO: Mosby.

Shabandi, M., & Parulkar, B. G. (2001). Foley catheter problems. In L. G. Gomella (Ed.), *The 5-minute urology consult* (pp. 50–51). Philadelphia, PA: Lippincott, Williams, & Wilkins.

Sinese, V., Hendricks, M. B., Morrison, M., & Harris, J. (2006). Clinical practice guidelines: Care of the patient with an indwelling catheter. *Urologic Nursing, 26*(1), 80–81.

Society of Urologic Nurses and Associates. (2005). Clinical practice guidelines: Suprapubic catheter replacement. *Urologic Nursing, 26*(3), 225–226.

CHAPTER 53

Procedures for Removal of Vaginal Foreign Body

Lee Ann Boyd

BACKGROUND

Vaginal foreign bodies are commonly seen in children and may consist of pieces of toilet tissue, fibrous material from clothing, or small toys. In adolescents and adults, broken condom remnants, pessaries, or tampons may be noted. Vaginal foreign bodies may occur as accidental, intentional during a sexual encounter, or related to sexual abuse. A child who repeatedly and purposely inserts objects into the vagina raises the concern of sexual abuse, and a sexual abuse assessment is required. Vaginal foreign bodies may also be inserted by patients as a result of a psychiatric disorder.

Vaginal foreign bodies may cause symptoms or may be asymptomatic for long periods of time. Patients presenting with symptoms may complain of vaginal discharge, vaginal bleeding, vaginal itching, odor, and, less commonly, vaginal pain or urinary discomfort. If pain is present, it may be caused by vaginal distention or objects with sharp edges.

In the pediatric patient, a vaginal foreign object may not be visible on external genitalia examination. If necessary, a vaginal speculum examination will most often identify the foreign object. Further diagnostics may be indicated if observation of the object is not possible, or if extravaginal penetration of the object is suspected. A flat plate abdominal x-ray, pelvic ultrasound, CT scan, or MRI may be ordered if necessary.

PATIENT PRESENTATION
- Vaginal itching, erythema, rash, and/or edema
- Foul smelling vaginal discharge
- Bloody, brown or yellow vaginal discharge, often malodorous
- Vaginal pain
- Urinary discomfort

TREATMENT

To remove smaller objects, warm-water vaginal lavage may be effective. Objects visible under vaginal speculum examination may be removed with ring forceps. In pediatric patients, a nasal speculum may be used. The foreign body may be expelled from the vagina by placing an examining finger in the rectum and applying gentle pressure on the posterior vaginal wall. Large objects may require removal under anesthesia.

SPECIAL CONSIDERATIONS

Report to child protective services if sexual abuse is suspected. A sexual abuse assessment may be necessary, which includes a forensic interview and anogenital examination by a skilled child abuse health care provider.

PROCEDURE PREPARATION

- Ring forceps (Figure 53.1)
- Nasal speculum for the pediatric patient
- Vaginal or nasal speculum
    - A weighted vaginal speculum can be used for enhanced viewing (Figure 53.2).
- Culturette swab
- No. 8 French infant feeding tube
- 60-mL syringe
- Warm sterile water
- Skin cleanser

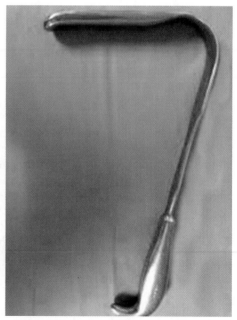

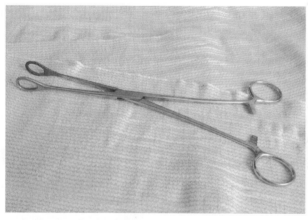

FIGURE 53.1 Ring forceps.

FIGURE 53.2 Weighted vaginal speculum.

PROCEDURE

- Universal precautions should be followed at all times.
- Have the patient positioned in the dorsal lithotomy position for adults and adolescents, and frog-leg position for infants and small children.
- Ensure adequate lighting.
- Examine external genitalia by holding labial traction and separation to open the hymen.
- Perform vaginal speculum examination.
- Small debris may be removed using a no. 8 French infant feeding tube placed vaginally. Fill a 60-mL syringe with warm sterile water and perform gentle lavage.
- Small objects may be removed using ring forceps.
- Larger objects can be removed by hand with added viewing area provided by a weighted speculum (Figure 53.3).
- In pediatric patients, gentle compression of the vaginal wall during a rectal examination may aid in expulsion of the foreign object.
- Perform vaginal culture of drainage, wet prep, and DNA probe for gonorrhea and chlamydia if secondary infection is suspected.
- Swab the vagina with a Betadine solution.

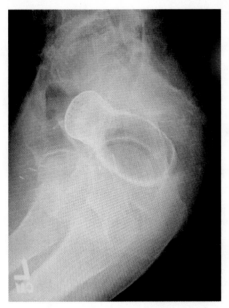

FIGURE 53.3 Large vaginal foreign body (salt shaker) seen on x-ray and easily removed with the aid of a weighted vaginal speculum.

POST-PROCEDURE CONSIDERATIONS

- Question the patient regarding whether the vaginal object was placed by herself or by someone else, and whether it was purposeful or accidental.
- Typically no antibiotics are necessary following the removal of the foreign body.

EDUCATIONAL POINTS

- Advise the patient to return to the clinic if pain, bleeding, or fever develops.
- Discourage the use of douching.
- Instruct the patient to follow up with her pediatrician/primary care provider in a specified amount of time.

COMPLICATIONS

- Urinary tract infection
- Vaginal infection
- Toxic shock syndrome
- Vaginal fistula
- Abdominal or pelvic abscess

PEARLS

- A Foley catheter may be inserted vaginally alongside a foreign object to break the suction, allowing for easier and less traumatic removal of the object.
- To reduce the odor from a retained tampon, pierce the finger of a vinyl glove with the vaginal forceps and immediately pull the glove over the tampon once extracted.
- A weighted speculum can be used to enhance the view.
- Active or passive increases in the intra-abdominal/pelvic pressure may aid in the removal of the foreign object.

RESOURCES

Carey, R., Healy, C., & Elder, D. E. (2010). Foreign body sexual assault complicated by rectovaginal fistula. *Journal of Forensic and Legal Medicine, 17*(3), 161–163.

Dhawan, V.K. (2015). Pediatric toxic shock syndrome overview of pediatric TSS. Retrieved from http://emedicine.medscape.com/article/969239-overview

Kihara, M., Sato, N., Kimura, H., Kamiyama, M., Sekiya, S., & Takano, H. (2001). Magnetic resonance imaging in the evaluation of vaginal foreign bodies in a young girl. *Journal of Gynecology and Obstetrics, 265*(4), 221–222.

Neulander, E. Z., Tiktinsky, A., Romanowsky, I., & Kaneti, J. (2010). Urinary tract infection as a single presenting sign of multiple foreign bodies: Case report and review of the literature. *Journal of Pediatric and Adolescent Gynecology, 23*, e31–e33.

Stricker, T., Navratil, F., & Sennhauser, F. H. (2004). Vaginal foreign bodies. *Journal of Paediatrics and Child Health, 40*(4), 205–207.

UNIT **XV**

Miscellaneous Procedures

CHAPTER 54

Procedures for Performing Skin Biopsy

Joseph Hong

BACKGROUND

A biopsy is performed to ascertain the pathology of the skin. Often it is done to confirm a clinical diagnosis or to help guide appropriate treatment. An old axiom in dermatology is that there are only two times when a biopsy should be obtained: (a) when you believe a biopsy is needed and (b) when you believe a biopsy is not needed. In other words, the information gained from a biopsy is almost always useful, and therefore, a biopsy is usually warranted.

To get the most information from a biopsy, certain factors should be taken into account: duration of lesion, location, healing, and interpretation. The location is important in choosing a site for a biopsy of a rash or another expanding/diffuse lesion. If there is an expanding edge, this area will generally be selected, because a biopsy of the inner aspect of such a lesion will often only show necrotic cells or otherwise give an inaccurate reflection of the true pathology (Figure 54.1).

FIGURE 54.1
Lesion for biopsy.

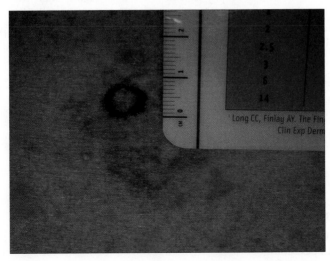

With inflammatory skin lesions, a new or recent lesion is almost always preferred. If the patient's rash is long-standing, with no lesions less than 2 weeks old, a biopsy would be of dubious benefit. A better plan would be to have the patient return when new lesions occur. A biopsy of a lesion within 48 hours of onset will give the best representative pathology and best clues for diagnosis. Evolving processes can be biopsied as long as there are newer lesions present. Of course, if malignancy is suspected, a biopsy can be done at any time.

Location is important in the context of the first rule of medicine: "First do no harm." If the patient is a diabetic, a biopsy of the lower ankle will probably produce a nonhealing ulcer, which could be a more serious problem than the condition you are attempting to diagnose. Other sensitive areas are the genitalia, face, and hands. One must ask the question: Is the information to be gained worth biopsying this site? Can another site provide similar information?

Interpretation of the biopsy cannot be underrated. In this day of managed care and cost cutting, the specimen will often be sent to a predesignated laboratory, which was chosen as a cost-cutting measure. The economic realities will often be of little benefit if the specimen is read incorrectly. There are many subtleties of reading a biopsy that can be easily overlooked by someone without sufficient expertise. For dermatologic biopsies, it is best to have a dermatopathologist review the slide.

SHAVE BIOPSY

The most commonly used technique in biopsying the skin is the shave biopsy. This is performed with a straight edge razor hence the name shave biopsy. Either a sterile scalpel blade or a dermablade can be used. I tend to do most of my biopsies as shaves, which include epidermis and a portion of dermis. If the suspected diagnosis is likely to include deep dermis or subcutaneous tissue, then I would rather do a punch biopsy to obtain a deeper specimen. The scar left from such a biopsy can be more problematic, so location and depth of the biopsy need to be evaluated.

A small pedunculated lesion is ideal for a shave biopsy, whereas a lesion flatter or deeper in the skin would require more depth and lead to more scarring. One of the advantages of a shave biopsy is that it is easier to maintain hemostasis. This is especially helpful in patients who are anticoagulated. Areas which are more prone to keloid and scarring need to be closely monitored for keloid formation. These areas include the bony prominences such as the sternum or elbows and shoulders.

Contraindications and Relative Contraindications
- Location (central face, shin, sternum, or bony prominence)

Special Considerations
- Diabetes
- Immunosuppression

Procedure Preparation
- Electrocautery
- Sterile scalpel blade
- Skin cleanser prep
- Lidocaine 1% or 2% without epinephrine

- Syringe
- Small-gauge needle (30 gauge)
- Formaldehyde with specimen cup
- Bandage

Procedure

- Prepare the area using a skin cleanser—either alcohol or Betadine.
- Then the designated area is anesthetized using lidocaine.
- Lidocaine with epinephrine is generally avoided for these smaller biopsies.
- Using a sterile scalpel blade and scooping, a layer of the skin is taken. Care must be used to not go too deep or remain too shallow.
- Approximately 1-mm depth is usually sufficient.
- Cauterize using electrocautery, chemical cautery (aluminum chloride or ferrous sulfate), or heat cautery.
- Apply a bandage and review wound care.

Post-Procedure Considerations

- Bleeding
- Pain
- Infection

Educational Points

- Cautery should be determined prior to procedure. If the patient is anticoagulated there will be more bleeding. Generally, if a patient has a pacemaker or a defibrillator I will not use electrocautery and substitute chemical or heat cautery.
- Cautery using ferous sulfate: Caution must also be used if using chemical cautery with ferous sulfate. The iron element in the cautery will commonly "stain" or tattoo the biopsy site, even after healing. Therefore, it should only be used as needed and avoided entirely on the face or other cosmetically sensitive area.
- Heat cautery: Caution also needs to be used when using heat. Unlike electrocautery, heat cautery can easily burn through a glove, injuring the caregiver or destroying tissue deeper in the skin.

Complications

- Bleeding
- Scarring, which may lead to keloid formation

PUNCH BIOPSY

Treatment

Generally, the standard biopsy technique used for diagnostic information is the 4-mm punch biopsy. The instrument is a premanufactured cylindrical tube of stated diameter, which is used to create a hole much like an office hole puncher (hence the name). Choosing a smaller biopsy size would be appropriate for the face or other sensitive areas, although 4 mm is the general size as this is enough to provide the pathologist with a good specimen for diagnosis. Another standard biopsy is the shave biopsy, performed with a straight edge razor, or if a larger lesion or deeper biopsy is needed, then an incisional or a "wedge" biopsy is done.

Contraindications and Relative Contraindications
- Immunosuppression
- Anticoagulants (i.e., warfarin, clopidogrel)

Special Considerations
- Diabetes
- Immunosuppression

Procedure Preparation
- 4-mm punch
- Electrocautery
- Skin cleanser prep
- Lidocaine 1% or 2% without epinephrine
- Syringe
- Small-gauge needle (30 gauge)
- Forceps
- Formaldehyde with specimen cup
- Pressure dressing material
- Nonabsorbable suture material
- Suture kit

Suture material used is usually 4-0 for trunk and extremities, 5-0 for neck and other more delicate areas, and 6-0 for the face. A standard tray would consist of the punch, anesthetic, suture, needle driver, pick-ups, and bandage.

Procedure
Hemostasis is normally not needed for a 4-mm punch.

- Prepare the area using a skin cleanser—either alcohol or Betadine.
- Then the designated area is anesthetized using lidocaine.
  - Lidocaine with epinephrine is generally avoided for these smaller biopsies.
- The punch is then applied to the skin with a single, clockwise twisting motion of the punch (Figure 54.2).
  - It is important not to reverse direction in a washing-machine motion, but to keep the motion in one direction.
  - This one motion will help to prevent shearing forces that can separate the layers of the skin, creating artifacts that will make analysis by the pathologist much more difficult.
  - It is also important to obtain a sufficient biopsy. One of the most common mistakes is to puncture only to the dermis. Generally, you have to puncture through the dermis into the subcutaneous fat. This will allow the full thickness of the skin (epidermis, dermis, and the subcutaneous layer) to be evaluated. It is very important to have all these layers, so that a full reading of the pathology of the skin can be obtained.
- After a sufficiently deep biopsy is achieved, the specimen should be maneuvered with a needle to gently elevate the specimen above the skin and then the subcutis attachment is cut (Figure 54.3).

FIGURE 54.2
Performing a
punch biopsy.

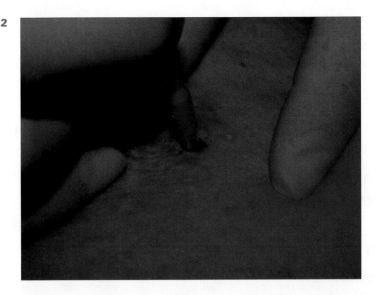

FIGURE 54.3
Maneuvering
a punch biopsy
specimen.

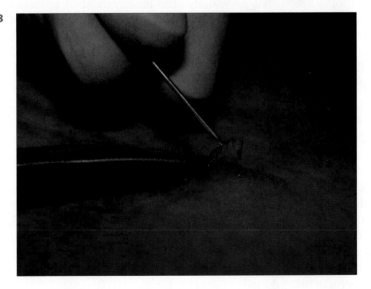

- If forceps or pick-ups are used to grab the tissue, a "crush" artifact can be created, rendering the specimen uninterpretable.
  - If small, single-tooth forceps are used and the tissue is handled gently, this crush artifact is generally avoided. The tissue is easier to handle this way than with a needle.
- The biopsy should be immediately placed in formaldehyde for transfer to the pathology laboratory.
- Once the specimen is removed, the biopsy site can be cauterized if needed, and the defect closed with an appropriately sized nonabsorbent suture.
- Apply a bandage to the wound.

Post-Procedure Considerations

- Bleeding
- Pain

Educational Points

- Depending on the location, the sutures are removed after a suitable time.
  - Face—5 to 7 days; scalp, neck, and arms—8 to 10 days; trunk—10 to 12 days; legs—14 days

Complications

- Bleeding
- Scarring, which may lead to keloid formation

INCISIONAL BIOPSY

Treatment

This type of biopsy is used for a larger lesion, one that is suspicious of metastatic potential, or a lesion that necessitates the procurement of subcutaneous fat. This biopsy can also be called a "wedge" biopsy as it will be used to obtain a full thickness of tissue through the dermis into the subcutaneous tissue, down to muscle.

Special Considerations

- Diabetes
- Immunosuppression

Procedure Preparation

- Lidocaine 1% or 2% (with or without epinephrine)
- Suture material (nonabsorbable and absorbable; 4-0, 5-0, or 6-0)
- Pick-ups
- Scalpel (No. 11 or 15 blade)
- Skin hook
- Hemostat
- Electrocautery
- Gauze
- Duoderm or other dressing
- Sterile drape

Suture material used is usually 4-0 for trunk and extremities, 5-0 for neck and other more delicate areas, and 6-0 for the face.

Procedure

- Prepare and drape the patient.
  - This biopsy should be performed under sterile conditions.
- Anesthetize the surrounding skin with lidocaine alone or lidocaine with epinephrine.
  - If lidocaine with epinephrine is used, wait 15- to 20-minutes before operating to allow the epinephrine to constrict blood vessels.

- Ensure hemostasis by using electrocautery or heat cautery to any bleeding following the excision and then undermining under the dermal layer to allow full closure and healing.
- Incise the area and then remove the necessary tissue.
- Deep sutures are placed using absorbable suture through the papillary dermis. These sutures provide most of the strength and also need to be used to approximate the closure.
- The skin sutures are to approximate the skin, allowing the best cosmetic result.
- Nonabsorbent sutures are used; as a rule, prolene or another synthetic monofilament with good antibacterial properties is used.
- A subcuticular suture may be used, although the long-term cosmetic results may be inferior to other methods of closure.
- Apply a bandage to the wound.
- In these larger excisions that are done under sterile procedure, antibiotics are not needed, but depending on the patient and location, they may be used prophylactically.

As mentioned in the previous section, the need for a proper pathologic diagnosis by a dermatopathologist is essential to provide the best evaluation and diagnosis of the biopsy.

Post-Procedure Considerations
- Pain
- Bleeding
- Infection

Complications
- Bleeding
- Scarring with possible keloid formation

PEARL

- A fine, single-tooth forceps can be used in place of skin hooks to help prevent stick injuries in those not used to handling or assisting with skin hooks.

RESOURCES

Levitt, J., Berbardo, S., & Whang, T. (2013). How to perform a punch biopsy of the skin. *New England Journal of Medicine, 369*, e13. doi: 10.1056/nejmvcm1104849. Retrieved from http://www.nejm.org/doi/full/10.1056/NEJMvcm1105849

Zuber, T. J. (2002). Punch biopsy of the skin. *American Family Physician, 65(6)*, 1155-1158. Retrieved from http://www.aafp.org/afp/2002/0315/p1155.html

Zuber, T. J. (2012). Skin biopsy techniques: When and how to perform punch biopsy. *Consultant, 6*, 712. Retrieved from http://www.consultant360.com/article/skin-biopsy-techniques-when-and-how-perform-punch-biopsy

CHAPTER 55

Procedures for Performing Lumbar Puncture

Keith A. Lafferty

BACKGROUND

As far back as the late 1800s, the subarachnoid space (SAS) was used for spinal anesthesia via cocaine, and shortly after, diagnostic needle sampling of cerebrospinal fluid (CSF) ensued. Current indications for performing a lumbar puncture (LP) in the acute care setting are for the diagnosis of meningitis and possibly subarachnoid hemorrhage (SAH), both of which have time-sensitive treatment-based high morbidities and mortalities. Clinicians must not let their guard down as 4% of all emergency department (ED) chief complaints involve cephalgia. One must always think "worse first" and entertain these two potentially devastating disease states.

Because neuronal tissue itself contains no pain fibers, the suspicion of cephalgia arises from pain in the following structures:

- Scalp (skin, muscle)
- Dura (especially at the base of the brain)
- Venous sinuses
- Meningeal arteries
- CN's V, VII, and IX
- Periosteum

Meningitis

Although it is beyond the scope of this book to go into great detail about the etiology and treatment of meningitis, certain points need to be made. The epidemiology of bacterial meningitis has shifted from a disease of the very young to a disease of adults. For example, the median age for persons with bacterial meningitis was 15 months in 1986, 25 years in 1998, and 39 years of age in the United States in 2007.

Meningitis caused by *H. influenzae* type b (Hib) has been nearly eliminated in the Western world since vaccination against Hib was initiated in the 1980s, which explains why rates of meningitis have decreased in young children. Likewise, the introduction of conjugate vaccines against *Streptococcus pneumoniae* is expected to reduce the burden of childhood pneumococcal meningitis significantly as the vaccine has been shown to have a 97.4% efficacy rate. Although inoculation with a pneumococcal conjugate vaccine is producing herd immunity (increasing immunization is decreasing incidence of the disease and indirectly protecting unimmunized people) among adults, the age distribution of meningitis has now shifted to older age groups who are not routinely immunized until age 65. Rates of neonatal *Streptococcus agalactiae*, also known as Group B *Streptococcus* (GBS), meningitis have also decreased because of routine testing of pregnant women for GBS (25% carrier rate) with prompt treatment via appropriate antibiotics during labor.

Although specific antibiotics for treatment of meningitis are beyond the scope of this book, the clinician needs to administer appropriate antimicrobials pertaining to the patient's age in the most timely manner possible, ideally before the LP is performed.

- Common signs, symptoms, and etiology of meningitis: in a prospective study of 696 patients with proven bacterial meningitis
  - Classic triad of fever, altered sensorium, and neck stiffness occurred only in a minority of patients, 44% overall
  - Two of four had signs/symptoms of headache, fever, neck stiffness, and altered sensorium—95% (4% had one out of four)
  - Altered sensorium—69%
  - Focal neurological deficit—14%
  - Seizure—5%
- Most common organisms causing meningitis include:
  - *S. pneumoniae.*
    - Classic triad—58%
    - Most common cause—60%
      - Most common community-acquired cause in HIV
    - Spread by airborne droplets
    - Incidence of pneumococcal disease is highest in those younger than 2 years and those older than 65 years of age.
    - Fully vaccinated children show an overall 97.4% efficacy in disease prevention.
    - Before introduction in 2000 of a 7-valent pneumococcal conjugate vaccine (PCV7), invasive pneumococcal disease among children less than 5 years old was 80 cases per 100,000 population and after the introduction of PCV7, rates of disease dropped dramatically to less than 1 case per 100,000 by 2007 (PCV13 now exists).
  - *Neisseria meningitides*
    - Classic triad—27%
    - Among adults, 5% to 10% are carriers in the nasopharynx.
    - Crowded living conditions can facilitate respiratory droplet transmission of meningococci (college dormitories).
    - Fifty percent of invasive diseases cause meningitis.
    - Second most common cause—20% (decreasing incidence of *S. pneumoniae* and Hib have been achieved as a result of using conjugate vaccines).
    - Although adolescents and young adults are the highest carriers, few carriers actually develop invasive disease.
    - Petechial rash is absent in 1/3 of patients.
    - 98% of cases are sporadic.
    - Of those who survive invasive disease, 10% to 20% experience sequelae, including limb loss from gangrene, extensive skin scarring, or cerebral infarction.

- Patients with meningococcal meningitis who do not develop septic shock are less likely to die or experience these sequelae, but are at risk of developing neurosensory hearing loss, mild to moderate cognitive defects, or seizure disorders.
- Recent vaccine recipients develop antibodies against the four major strains that are responsible for 82% of disease in the United States.
- Recent vaccine develops antibodies against the four major strains in 82% of those immunized that cause meningococcal disease in the United States.
- *Haemophilus influenzae* type b
  - Hib was the leading cause of bacterial meningitis in the United States among children younger than 5 years of age and a major cause of other life-threatening invasive bacterial diseases in this age group.
  - Meningitis occurred in approximately two thirds of children with invasive Hib disease, resulting in hearing impairment or severe permanent neurologic sequelae, such as mental retardation, seizure disorder, cognitive and developmental delay, and paralysis in 15% to 30% of survivors.
  - Hib vaccine, introduced in the 1980s, has dramatically decreased the overall incidence and has almost eradicated the disease in the United States.
- GBS
  - Two thirds of all cases occur before the first 3 months of life.
  - Thirty-fold reduction of early-onset neonatal GBS disease with the use of intrapartum antibiotics in rectovaginal positive pregnant carriers.
- *Listeria monocytogenes*
  - Two percent of bacterial meningitis.
  - Alcoholics, the elderly, and pregnancy.

Bacterial and viral etiologies have similar presentations (HA, fever, and stiff neck); however, viral meningitis is associated with an extremely low morbidity rate and most recover fully in 7 to 10 days (exception herpes simplex virus [HSV]).

- No treatment is generally the rule.
- Most are treated as if bacterial until cultures are negative; empiric antibiotic therapy is often selected pending cerebral spinal fluid (CSF) studies.
- HSV is an important cause of encephalitis that presents with characteristics similar to viral meningitis, coupled with an altered mental status and is treated with antiviral therapy.

Subarachnoid Hemorrhage

- Eighty-five percent of cases originate in a ruptured cerebral aneurysm within the brain's main arterial supply at its base (Circle of Willis), 10% are from a ruptured arteriovenous malformation (AVM) and 5% is from another etiology.
- Because the etiology is from an aneurysmal (occasionally AVM) rupture, the presentation is abrupt and severe (often describes as "the worst headache of one's life" although, clinical presentations can vary greatly). The leaking blood may act as a chemical irritant to the meninges and, if so, may induce meningeal irritation and accompanying meningeal signs.
- One percent of the population has cerebral aneurysms.
- Current high-resolution CT scans rule out SAH in nearly 100% of patients within the first 24 hours of HA (after this time, the sensitivity decreases as the hyperdense blood-filled SAS catabolizes through myoglobin breakdown and becomes increasingly homogeneous within the CSF) (Figure 55.1).

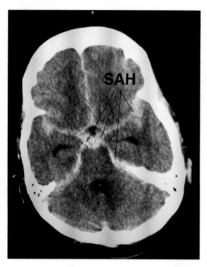

FIGURE 55.1 CT subarachnoid hemorrhage.

- McCormack and Hutson (2010) have shown that the combination of a negative CT and computed tomography angiography (CTA) in later presentations excludes a visible SAH and vascular abnormality in 99.4% of patients (CTA detects cerebral aneurysms as small as 3 mm) (Figure 55.2).

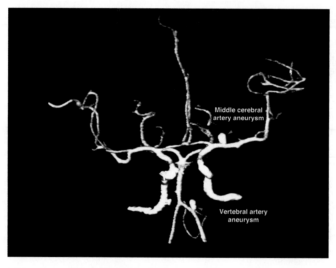

FIGURE 55.2 Brain computed tomography angiography. Notice 7-mm left vertebral artery aneurysm and 8-mm middle cerebral artery aneurysm.

- Through extrapolated data based on the Hiroshima bomb survivors and a few retrospective pediatric cohort studies, the risk of radiation-induced cancer death from a single CT of the head is less than 1/100 in neonates and less than 1/10,000 in patients 15 years and older.
- In similar presenting cases beyond 24 hours, LP has increasingly fallen out of favor in definitively excluding SAH if CTA is available because CTA allows for a quicker diagnosis and avoids an invasive procedure, coupled with the fact that LP lacks the ability to detect:
  - Aneurysmal expansion
  - Thrombosis
  - Dissection

- Dural venous sinus thrombosis
- Vasospasm

Note that LP has a 15% risk of inadvertent puncture of the epidural venous plexus, introducing blood into the CSF (traumatic tap) thereby complicating the diagnosis of SAH.

As red blood cells (RBCs) age in the CSF they lyse and, through myoglobin breakdown, heme molecules are released and enzymatically metabolized to produce bilirubin and xanthrochromia (yellowish colored CSF) ensues. Though this discoloration of the CSF may last for 2 weeks, interpretation via visual inspection carries a low sensitivity, whereas detection via spectrophotometry carries a low to moderate specificity.

ANATOMY
Cerebral Spinal Fluid

The CSF has the following functions:

- Provides buoyancy to the brain and by doing so decreases its functional weight by 75%, effectively decreasing its weight from 1,400 to 50 g
- Buffers neural tissue from trauma
- Because the brain's parenchymal tissue lacks a lymphatic system, the CSF and its circulation takes on this role.
- Contains antibacterial properties

CSF is made in the choroid plexuses, which are finger-like extensions with an ependymal structure that merge into the innermost ventricular lining located in the paired lateral third and fourth ventricles. These epithelial-like microvilli are composed of tight junctions on the CSF side of the ventricles and contain capillaries in their projections that are fenestrated, creating an ultrafiltration of plasma, which comprises the CSF (Figure 55.3). This in turn leads to its composition being 99% water, giving it its clear appearance.

The CSF is propelled along the neuronal axis by cranial–caudal directional pulsatile waves stemming from cerebral artery pulsations. The majority of the CSF is reabsorbed in the arachnoid granulations draining from the SAS into the dura venous sinuses and subsequently into the internal jugular veins. Twenty percent of the CSF is confined to the ventricles, 60% is in the convexities of the brain, and 20% is around the spinal cord.

After its production, the CSF circulates out of the roof of the fourth ventricle through the foramen of Luschka and foramen of Magemdie to the cerebellom-

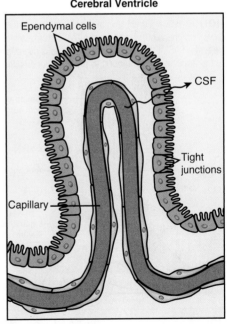

FIGURE 55.3 Choroid plexus lining the cerebral ventricles.

edullary cistern. This is a CSF reservoir secondary to a large space between the arachnoid and pia matter. From there it flows in the SAS throughout the convexities of the cerebral hemispheres and the spinal cord (Figure 55.4). The ependymal lining is freely permeable to the CSF and in this way is in constant chemical communication with the

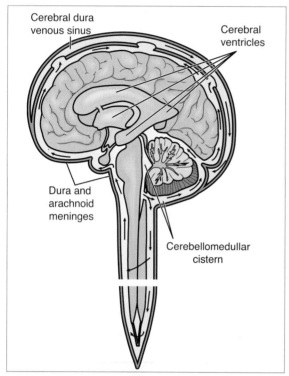

FIGURE 55.4 Cerebrospinal fluid (CSF) flow. Notice the CSF flows from the ventricles to the cerebral cisterns where it than fills the entire SAS of the brain/spinal chord and is eventually reabsorbed by the arachnoid granulations to the dura venous sinuses.

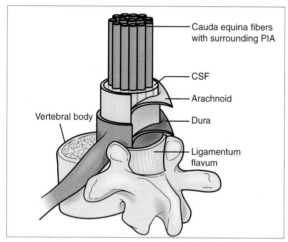

FIGURE 55.5 Meninges. Notice the rich venous plexus in the epidural space as a potential source of traumatic lumbar punctures.

interstitial fluid that surrounds the neurons. Therefore, the CSF is representative of the brain's physiology and/or pathology.

A total volume of 500 mL/day of CSF is made at a rate of 20 mL/hr with an average volume at any one time of 150 mL. The 3 to 4 mL removed in a typical LP is fully replenished within 30 minutes.

Meninges

The brain and spinal cord are surrounded by three meninges that help protect and support the central nervous system (CNS): the dura, arachnoid, and pia maters (Figure 55.5). The outermost dura is a fibrous dense membrane attached to the skull and foramen magnum via the periosteum and hence there is no true epidural space. In the spinal cord, however, the dura is not attached to the vertebral spinal canal but rather separated by a true epidural space, which contains the vascular internal vertebral venous plexus. The arachnoid mater is anatomically deep to the dura and is a delicate membrane closely adhered to the dura.

The potential space between the two is known as the subdural space. The innermost meninge, the pia mater, is an ultrafine membrane that closely adheres to the convexities of the brain and spinal cord. The space between the arachnoid and pia mater is the CSF-filled SAS.

Needle Passage (Figure 55.6)

- Epidermis/dermis/subcutaneous tissue
- Supraspinous ligament
  - Connects the spinous processes
  - May calcify in the elderly and dictate a lateral LP approach
- Interspinous ligament
  - Connects the inferior and superior border of the spinous processes together
- Ligamentum flavum
  - Thick elastic ligament that covers the interlaminar space between the spinal cord and the vertebral canal

- Posterior epidural space
  - Contains the internal vertebral venous plexus
- Dura
- Arachnoid
- SAS
  - Contains the cauda equina nerve roots

During gestation the spinal cord and the vertebral column are both the same length, but normal growth allows the spinal column to grow more rapidly than the spinal cord and, as such, at birth the conus medullaris (the most inferior portion of the spinal cord) is already at the level of L3 while continued growth into adulthood causes the conus to end at L1 (68%), T12 (22%), and occasionally L2 (10%). Though the conus medullaris ends here, the posterior and anterior roots constituting the cauda equina fill the rest of the inferior lumbar and sacral portions of the spinal canal. The lumbar cistern, which is filled with CSF, is an enlargement of the SAS between the conus medullaris, the inferior end of SAS (large area of separated pia and arachnoid membranes) and the dura mater about vertebral level S2 (Figure 55.7). This area is most amendable to CSF sampling.

PATIENT PRESENTATION

LP is used primarily as a diagnostic modality with the majority of indications entertaining the diagnosis of meningitis. There are approximately 3,000 to 6,000 cases per year of bacterial meningitis in the adult population with the mortality being 5% to 25%. An expedient diagnosis decreases the morbidity and mortality. Challenges hindering timely diagnosis and subsequent treatment include:

- Very young age (because of lack of nuchal rigidity)
- Elderly (comorbidities)
- Comatose state
- Immunocompromised (decreased inflammation) patient

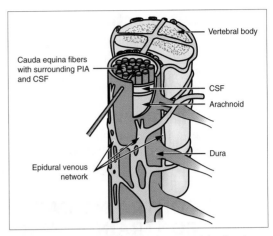

FIGURE 55.6 Needle passage. In sequential order, the needle penetrates skin, supraspinous and interspinous ligaments, ligamentum flavum, posterior epidural space, dura, arachnoid, and finally rests in the subarachnoid space containing the cerebrospinal fluid.

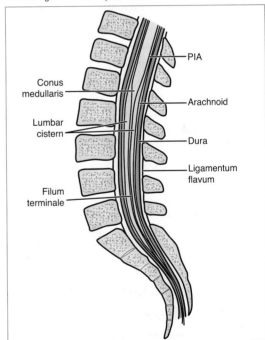

FIGURE 55.7 Lumbar cistern. This reservoir is most amendable to cerebrospinal fluid sampling, is below the conus medullaris, and contains the cauda equina fibers.

LPs are indicated in patients presenting with signs and symptoms of meningitis. Historically, it has been used in those patients with thunderclap, or the worst headache of their lives, in which a CT scan of the brain is normal; LP is used less often for diagnostic and therapeutic reasons in other disease states.

Diagnostic

- Infectious—meningitis, encephalitis, myelitis
- SAH
- Inflammatory—multiple sclerosis, Guillain–Barré
- Oncologic—leukemia

Therapeutic

- Decompression of fluid in pseudotumor cerebri
- Introduction of chemotherapeutic agents and antibiotics
- Spinal and epidural anesthesia

CONTRAINDICATIONS AND RELATIVE CONTRAINDICATIONS

- Signs of elevated intracranial pressure (ICP) are an absolute contraindication to performing an LP to avoid unchal herniation and is ruled out by the following:
  - CT head
  - Fundoscopic exam for evaluation of papilledema
  - Bedside ocular ultrasound for detection of papilledema (higher sensitivity than previous two)

Elevated ICP is transmitted to the contiguous optic nerve sheath and may be detected via bedside ultrasound, which will show an increased optic nerve sheath diameter (ONSD). This allows a quick and simple indirect assessment of a patient's ICP as the optic sheath is a continuum of the brain, contains meningeal covering (SAS), and its size directly correlates with an increasing ICP.

- Place patient in a supine position with eyes closed and apply ultrasound gel covering outer lid. Use the high-frequency linear probe over the eye to visualize the optic nerve and the posterior retina and freeze the image. Measure the ONSD 3 mm posterior to the globe and, if the ONSD is greater than 5 mm, an elevated ICP should be entertained (Figure 55.8).
- Cardio respiratory compromise (positioning may worsen especially in children)
- Focal neurological exam
- Bleeding diathesis (coagulopathy/anticoagulation therapy)

SPECIAL CONSIDERATIONS
Ultrasound-Guided Landmark Identification

Though this modality for landmark identification has been described since the 1970s, its use has not been mainstream until recently. With ultrasound machines becoming more ubiquitous in clinical arenas and familiarity gained by such common procedures as central venous catheter (CVC) placement and diagnostic abdominal sonography (FAST, AAA), its use in other areas, including its static use in identifying the midline spinous processes in anatomically challenging patients, is warranted and literature supported.

Landmarks that are normally palpated by the clinician may not be appreciated or may be altered in some patients.

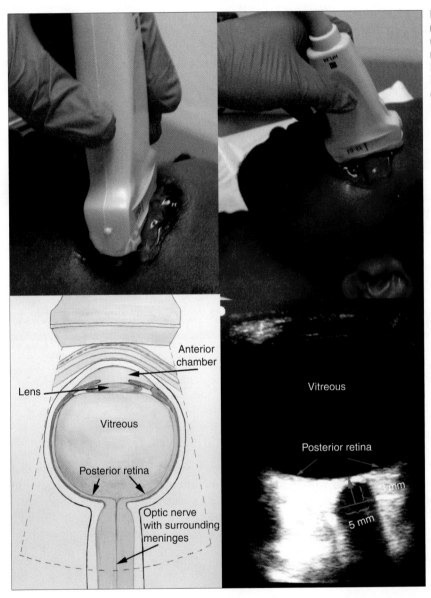

FIGURE 55.8 Optic nerve sheath diameter ultrasound. Consider this modality before every lumbar puncture, as it is highly sensitive for detecting an elevated intracranial pressure.

- Obesity (ultrasound-guided landmark identification [USGLMI] is successful in the majority of patients with a body mass index [BMI] greater than 30)
- Osteoarthritis
- Ankylosing spondylitis
- Kyphoscoliosis
- Previous lumbar surgery altering landmarks
  - In cases involving lumbar fusions, if a laminectomy was done at the same time, one may pass the needle in this area void of bone

- A lumbar x-ray or CT may identify lateral fusions in which case a medial approach still may be obtainable.
- May need to perform the procedure at a level above or below the previous surgery.
- In patients with spinal stenosis, one may need to use the L2/L3 interspace.

The use of bedside ultrasound in a static manner may act as the "hands" of the provider in identifying landmarks used for needle insertion. The inability to identify landmarks may lead to the clinician's reluctance to perform the procedure, higher rates of complication, and increasing patient discomfort. Furthermore, USGLMI prevents treatment without a CSF sample and may avoid fluoroscopy (transport, radiation, availability).

Ferre and Sweeney (2007) found that nonradiology clinicians can identify five structures (spinous processes, ligamentum flavum, dura, epidural space, and SAS) in patients with an average BMI of 31 with 88% doing so in less than 1 minute and 100% in less than 5 minutes. Stiffler et al. (2007) have shown that as a patient's BMI increases, so does the difficulty in palpating landmarks and the needle depth.

TABLE 55.1 Needle Depth Based on BMI

BMI	Difficulty Palpating Landmarks	Needle Depth
< 25	5%	4.4 cm
> 25	33%	5.1 cm
> 30	68%	6.4 cm

A meta-analysis has shown that there is an inherent 15% traumatic LP rate that is higher as BMI increases when greater than one attempt is required. This may add confusion to the diagnosis and possibly the administration of unnecessary antibiotics. USGLMI has been found to reduce the risk of failed attempts and needle insertions.

Transverse View

- Exact position of a spinous process

Sagital View

- Interspinous process area
- Depth to the SAS
- Needle angle

PROCEDURE PREPARATION

Most supplies listed are available in commercially packaged kits (Figure 55.9).

- Sterile gloves
- Skin cleanser (chlorhexidine or betadine)
- Sterile drapes
- Topical anesthetic

- Spinal needle with stylet
  - Infant 1.5"/3.8 cm
  - Child 2.5"/6.3 cm
  - Adult 3.5"/8.9 cm
- Manometer
- Collection tubes

Needle Type

Though noncutting needles (Whitacre, Sprotte, etc.) have been in use since the 1920s, their use has been recently validated in multiple studies in decreasing the incidence of post-dural puncture headaches (PDPHs). Regular cutting needles that are still supplied in most LP trays cut the dura (the larger the needle, the larger the defect) allowing a subsequent leak, giving rise to a 30% rate of PDPH. Noncutting or pencil-tipped needles are blunter at the tip area: they spread the dura fibers and have an incidence of PDPH as low as 2%. Holst et al. (1998) have shown that in an in vivo human cadaver model, less CSF leaks through the dural hole were made by the pencil-point noncutting needles as opposed to the traditional cutting ones (Figure 55.10).

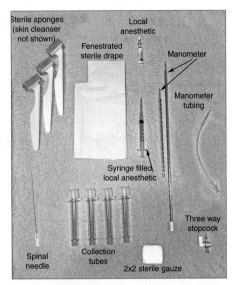

FIGURE 55.9 Open LP kit.

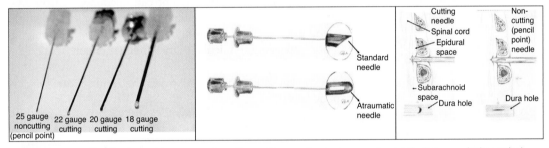

FIGURE 55.10 Needle size and type comparison. Non-cutting needles have a pencil point tip that spreads the vertical dura fibers instead of cutting them as beveled needles do. This creates less dura trauma and subsequently minimal if any post-procedure cerebrospinal fluid leak.

In a meta-analysis of 38 trials including 8,184 patients, Demaerschalk and Wingerchuk (2002) found that pencil-point noncutting needle use significantly decreased the odds of a PDPH to the point that for every six LPs done by the pencil-point needle, one PDPH will be prevented. The distinction is so convincing that the American Academy of Neurology and the American Society of Anesthesiology have published statements as class-one evidence for the use of noncutting needles. Though the noncutting needle may require minimal familiarity for first use (loss of the resistance or "popping" feeling through the dura/ligamentum flavum may be lessened), a meta-analysis by Halpern and Preston (1994) further found that procedure difficulty is greater and failure rates higher with the use of cutting needles.

PROCEDURE

- Place patient in either the sitting or the lateral recumbent position.

Patient Positioning

The goal of positioning the patient is to maximally flex the lumbar vertebrae and widen the interspinous distance by means of stretching the supraspinous/interspinous ligaments and ligamentum flavum. It helps to ask the patient to arch the lumbar region out, mimicking the arch of a cat. The sitting position makes this procedure somewhat easier for clinicians to perform, but if one needs a CSF pressure reading the lateral recumbent position must be used.

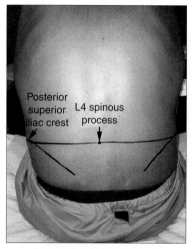

FIGURE 55.11 Sitting position. The L4 spinous process can be found by drawing a line connecting both posterior superior iliac crests and marking its midpoint.

Sitting Position (Figure 55.11)

- Have the patient lean over a bedside table with their spine perpendicular to the stretcher, hugging a pillow.
- Ensure the shoulders are even.
- Studies have shown that maximal hip flexion increases the interspinous space the most. This can be accomplished by placing a stool under the patient's feet or towels under his or her thighs.

Lateral Recumbent Position

- Have the patient lie on his or her left lateral side with the lumbar spine parallel to the stretcher and the hips and shoulders flexed so they're perpendicular to the stretcher.
- An assistant facing the patient can encourage an optimal position by placing one arm behind the patient's flexed knees and the other behind the shoulders to ensure the shoulders are equally perpendicular to the stretcher (Figure 55.12).

- Avoid flexing the neck because this does not widen the lumbar interspinous space and may impede breathing.
- Using sterile gloves, apply the skin cleanser using a concentric motion from the needlepoint entry site outward.
- Place the fenestrated sterile drape on the patient.
- Inject the local anesthetic over the needle site entry point subdermally.
    - One can apply local anesthetic in a long-track manner using a long 27-gauge 1.5" needle and anesthetize the interspinous ligament up to the point of

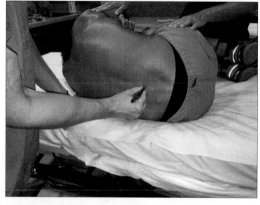

FIGURE 55.12 Lateral recumbent position.

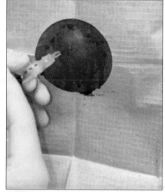

VIDEO 55.1 Long-track local anesthesia.
springerpub.com/campo

the ligamentum flavum in the same direction of the LP needle placement (Video 55.1).
- In pediatric patients, randomized trials have shown that both infiltrative and topical anesthesia can reduce pain associated with performing an LP, even in a neonatal patient.

Needle Positioning

Palpate the posterior superior iliac crests and note the midpoint as it intersects the L4 spinous process. Mark this area by using a skin marker or pressure divot (Figure 55.13). USGLMI should be used if the tactile appreciation of pertinent anatomy is challenging in either the lateral decubitus or the sitting position (Figure 55.14).

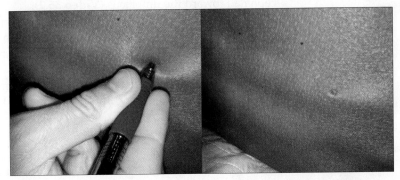

FIGURE 55.13 Skin divot. Because the skin cleansing occasionally removes marker ink, depression of the skin may serve as better guidance on commencement of needle placement.

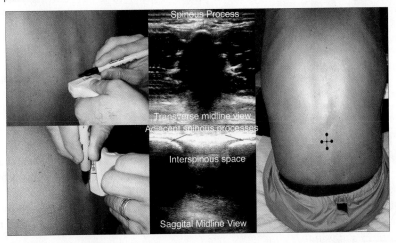

FIGURE 55.14 USGLMI.

- Using the transverse view with the high-frequency linear probe, find the center of the L3 or L4 spinous process (hyperechoic crescent shape with acoustic shadowing) and mark a point above and below in the midprobe area.
- Place the probe in the sagittal plane and place over adjacent spinous processes in the already identified midline (already marked by the two vertical points) and mark a point in between two adjacent spinous processes on either side of the midprobe area.

- Connect the horizontal and vertical points.
- This dot represents the exact midline coordinate and the interspinous space between the two adjacent spinous processes and the needle insertion point.
- The curvilinear probe may be required for the obese patient (lower frequency/greater depth) and for identification of the ligamentum flavum/dura, SAS, and needle depth.

Because the spinal cord usually ends at the level of L1 in adults, insert the needle at the L3/L4 or the L4/L5 interspace, whereas in younger pediatric patients the spinal cord ends at L3, so the L4/L5 level is recommended.

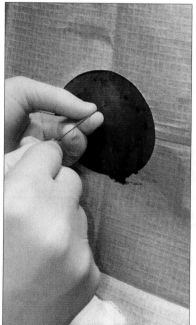

FIGURE 55.15 Holding the needle.

- Insert the needle with a stylet at the superior aspect of the inferior spinous process and angulate 15-degree cephalad toward the umbilicus (**Video 55.2**).
- In the classic way of holding the needle, both thumbs are placed on either side of the proximal needle hub while both index fingers are used to support the distal needle close to the skin to advance forward.
- Another technique has the hub between the dominant thumb and index finger and the nondominant thumb and index finger support the distal needle close to the skin to advance forward (Figure 55.15).
  - In pediatric patients, the needle should be inserted with less of an angle and possibly with no angle as their spinous processes are flatter.
  - If using a cutting needle, ensure the bevel is in the sagittal plane in order to lessen cutting the vertical dura fibers.
  - As the needle passes through the ligamentum flavum and/or dura, one may appreciate a decrease in resistance and a "popping" sensation.
    - In the very young pediatric patient, this popping sensation may be absent.

NOTE *Because of this decreased tactile sensation when the needle pierces the dura/ligamentum flavum ligaments the "Cincinnati" method includes continuing to advance the needle and stylet past the dermis. The stylet is then removed (avoids dislodging a plug of skin that could be transported into the SAS), and the needle is slowly advanced until CSF is seen flowing. In this technique, one avoids inserting the needle too far into the anterior epidural space and its venous plexus contents. Studies have shown this method decreases traumatic LPs in pediatric patients.*

- At this point, stop, withdraw the stylet, and, if no fluid returns, reinsert the stylet and repeat at 2-mm increments.
  - If fluid is not acquired and/or bone is encountered, withdraw the needle to the level of the subcutaneous tissue without exiting the skin and redirect the needle (typically more cephalad)
  - If CSF flow is poor, a cauda equina nerve route may be obstructing the needle and one should rotate the needle 90 degrees.

If one encounters blood and it clears, the needle is in the SAS and tube collection can follow after a few drops are discarded and sequential cell counts are obtained on tube 1 and tube 3 or 4.

If the blood does not clear, the needle has most likely been advanced into the venous plexus within the ventral epidural space and must be removed completely.

- If obtaining an opening pressure, the patient must be in a lateral recumbent position.
  - Attach a stopcock to a flexible connector or to the spinal needle itself while pointing the lever away from the patient.
  - Record the CSF column level at the highest point of respiratory and cardiac variations (an abnormal reading is anything above 25 cm of water).
  - Now turn the lever of the stopcock toward the patient so fluid in the manometer may be collected.
- Collect fluid by allowing it to drip into the collection tubes.
  - **Never aspirate the CSF, as even a small amount of negative pressure can precipitate a hemorrhage.**
  - The amount of CSF collected should be limited to the smallest amount needed for testing, typically 3 to 4 mL with approximately 1 mL placed in each tube.
- After adequate CSF fluid collection, replace the stylet and remove the needle.
- In older patients, the supraspinous and possibly the interspinous ligaments may calcify, requiring a lateral approach.
  - In this technique, the needle entry point is lateral to the calcified ligaments mentioned and it is vectored toward the midline to bypass all extramedullary ligaments, piercing the ligamentum flavum after passing through various paraspinal muscles (Figure 55.16).
  - Place the needle just above the transverse process of L3 or L4 and direct it medially and cephalad.

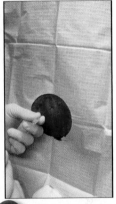

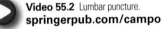

Video 55.2 Lumbar puncture.
springerpub.com/campo

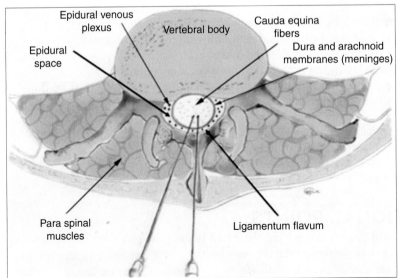

FIGURE 55.16 Medial and lateral approach. In cases in which the supraspinous/ interspinous ligaments are calcified, one may enter lateral to the spinous process (all the while vectoring toward the midline) while bypassing these ligaments and piercing the ligamentum flavum via the paraspinous muscles.

POST-PROCEDURE CONSIDERATIONS
CSF Analysis in Bacterial Meningitis

- CSF culture (CSF exam and clinical picture is only 70% sensitive).
- Regardless of the causative organism of bacterial meningitis, CSF findings in acute bacterial meningitis are often similar.
- Expedient transport to the laboratory is mandatory as cells begin to lyse within an hour and this process is slowed by refrigeration (especially meningococcal organisms).
- The white blood cell (WBC) count of CSF is almost always between 1,000 to 10,000 WBC and rarely is less than 100.
  - In 90% to 95% of patients, polymorphonuclear (PMN) cells account for the total WBC count of the CSF and in less than one quarter of cases do PMN cells comprise less than 80% of the total leukocyte count.
- Gram stain is only 80% sensitive.
  - Streptococcus/Staphylococcus—gram-positive cocci
  - Neisseria—gram-negative intra/extracellular diplococcic
  - Haemophilus—gram-negative bacilli
- The polymerase chain reaction (PCR) has a sensitivity over 90% and 100% specificity for *S. pneumoniae, Neisseria meningitides,* and *Haemophilus influenzae*
  - In some centers, *N. meningitides* is being solely diagnosed via PCR without cultures
  - Also detects HSV and enteroviruses
- The opening pressure is typically increased in almost all patients, with 90% of cases having an opening pressure of over 200 mmHg
  - Pressure will increase parallel with the progression of the disease and it returns to normal with recovery.
- The CSF glucose is usually moderately to severely reduced; in 75% of patients it is less than 50 mg/dL and in 25% of cases it is less than 10 mg/dL
  - The normal range for CSF/serum glucose ratio is greater than 0.6 (two thirds the serum glucose)
  - Usually normal in viral meningitis but may be slightly low
  - Higher sensitivity than protein
- The CSF protein concentration is almost always increased and in more than 80% of patients the absolute value is more than 80 mg (usually greater than 500)
  - Viral infections with lymphocytic pleocytosis have a lesser (sometimes normal) elevation of protein, usually between 50 and 100 mg/dL
- Other studies that may be obtained depending on the clinical scenario:
  - India ink—Cryptococcal surface antigen
  - Viral specific IgG/IgM for mosquito borne viral encephalitis
  - Acid-fast smear—bacilli (culture for *Mycobacterium tuberculosis* to be done in countries with high incidence of TB)
    - Most commonly seen in the United States in cancer and/or immune-compromised patients
    - Induces very high CSF protein levels
  - *Borrelia burgdorferi* antibodies—Lyme disease
  - HSV analysis

EDUCATIONAL POINTS

- Though clinical dogma states lying flat 2 to 3 hours post-procedure decreases CSF leakage and risk of post-procedural headache, there is no evidence to support this.
- Never aspirate CSF as even a small amount of negative pressure can precipitate a subdural/epidural hemorrhage.

- CT of the brain does not rule out meningitis nor does any imaging modality; only an LP does.
- If the blood clots, suspect a traumatic tap (SAH blood has already been defibrinated and therefore will not clot).
- When obtaining an opening CSF pressure, the patient must be in the lateral decubitus position, as changes in CSF pressure are seen in varying body positions.
  - This is due to changes in venous pressure that are related to cerebral perfusion pressure and, therefore, CSF pressure.
- Although the detection of bacterial antigens, the gram stain (less commonly done anymore) and/or an affirmative culture ensure the diagnosis, the following have a high correlation with the diagnosis of an bacterial etiology:
  - CSF glucose/blood glucose < 0.4
  - CSF WBC > 500/uL
  - CSF lactate > 30 mg/dL (not routinely tested)
- Although recent antibiotics may decrease the sensitivity of the Gram stain and culture, they have no adverse effect on the WBC, glucose, or protein measurement.
- Nuchal musculature is poorly developed until 8 weeks of age, and therefore fever in infants usually warrants an LP.
- If a noncutting needle is not available, use the smallest needle gauge possible and assure the bevel is oriented in the sagittal plane of the spinal column in order to spread vertical dura fibers.
- One third of ED patients will experience difficulty with LPs without USGLMI.
- Have a high suspicion of HAs that are abrupt in onset or "worst of life" as Vermeulen and Schull (2007) have shown that 5% of SAHs are missed on initial ED presentation.
- Besides significantly decreasing the incidence of PDPH, Engedal et al. (2015) have shown in 501 patients that switching from a 22-gauge to a 25-gauge noncutting needle decreased hospitalization rates from 17 to 2, missed workdays from 175 to 55, and the number of blood patches needed went from 10 to 2.
- Engedal et al. (2015) found in a prospective study that switching to a 25-gauge noncutting needle (more expensive needles) decreased cost by reducing PDPH treatment modalities by 76%.
- An epidural blood patch is effective in the treatment of PDPH in at least 85% of patients treated, usually within 30 minutes.
- One small clinical trial in postpartum women who had received spinal anesthesia found that infusing 500 mg of caffeine had an absolute risk reduction of 61% in patients with PDPH, although a 30% recurrence rate was reported. However, its efficacy in emergency settings is unknown.

COMPLICATIONS

Most complications can be avoided by careful assessment and physical exam prior to the procedure, including a thorough neurological exam and fundoscopic or ocular ultrasound for detection of papilledema.

- Cerebellar herniation
  - In cases in which there is a potential brain-space-occupying mass and hence a pressure gradient, performing an LP may precipitate this devastating complication.
  - In cases, such as pseudotumor cerebri, in which the elevated ICP is uniform throughout, an LP is not only safe but also therapeutic.
- Epidural/subdural hematoma
  - Bleeding diathesis
  - Thrombocytopenia (correct platelets > 50,000)

- ITP
- Leukemia
- PDPH
  - Occipital or cervical HA that arises within 5 days after a dura puncture associated with either nausea, neck stiffness, tinnitus, hypoacusia, or photophobia that is aggravated within 15 minutes of assuming an erect posture and improves within 15 minutes after laying flat
  - Besides cutting needles and larger sizes, other factors that increase the risk:
    - Young age
    - Female gender
    - History of chronic HAs
    - Lower BMI
  - A persistent CSF leak can lead to intracranial hypotension (bouyancy of the brain as it sits in the cranial vault is decreased) and subsequent traction on the pain sensitive dura at the base of the brain
  - The Monro–Kellie doctrine states that the sum of volumes of the brain, CSF, and blood must remain the same and, as such, vasodilation of cerebral arteries may be an accompanying culprit secondary to compensation for intracranial hypotension (migraine like)
  - Exacerbated by an erect position
  - Greatly avoided by using a smaller needle size, especially pencil-point needles
  - PDPH occurs in 80% of patients on whom 16-gauge needle was used
  - Associated symptoms may include vertigo, tinnitus, and hypoacusia from a decrease in the endolymph volume in the semicircular canals as well as diplopia and blurry vision from stretching of cranial nerve VI.
- Subarachnoid epidermal cyst formation
  - Occurs when a skin plug is introduced and embedded in the SAS upon needle placement
  - The standard use of a stylet prevents this
- Infection
  - Meningitis
  - Discitis
  - Osteomyelitis
- Paresthesia
  - Needle may irritate the cauda equina nerve route in which case the needle should be repositioned

PEARLS

- The most feared complication is cerebellar herniation, therefore it is paramount that a detailed a thorough neurological and fundoscopic exam precedes the procedure.
- Patients will usually not have an adverse outcome if an LP is omitted but may indeed have an adverse outcome if definitive treatment such as antibiotics are delayed.
- Ultrasound-guided landmarks double the success rate in the obese patient.
- Meticulous patient positioning is critical to procedure success.

- Accurate landmark identification can occur via the use of a pen-induced skin indentation.
- Collect no more CSF fluid than needed for testing (3–4 mL).
- Always remove the needle with a stylet in place.
- Bed rest, number of needle attempts (assuming unsuccessful dura penetration), IVF, supine position, and clinical experience of the clinician have not shown in any studies to decrease the rate of PDPH.
- Only smaller needle size and noncutting type have shown to decrease the rate of PDPH.
- Flow rate does not change with needle type or size.
- Apply sterile drapes to the patient while the skin cleanser is still wet in order to facilitate added drape adherence.
- Ensure collection tubes are in sequential order at procedure setup.
- Re-identify landmarks just before insertion of the needle, as subtle movements may change the overlying skin and spinous process relationship.
- If the CSF flow is poor, a cauda equina nerve route may be obstructing the needle and one should rotate 90 degrees.
- Dehydrated patients may require the sitting method to collect CSF.
- Bacterial meningitis usually causes some alterations of the sensorium, whereas a viral etiology does not (inflammation limited to the meninges) except HSV.
- In a traumatic tap, using an RBC threshold of 100 can rule out a SAH, whereas RBCs greater than 10,000 increase the likelihood of an SAH by a factor of 6.
- The best treatment for bacterial meningitis is prevention via vaccination against the common pathogens.
- CSF glucose less than 50% of the serum glucose should raise the suspicion of bacterial meningitis.
- Blood culture has a 50% to 80% sensitivity in bacterial meningitis.
- Crul et al. describe a patient with a persistent PDPH refractory to three epidural blood patches who was treated with 3 mL of fibrin glue with success.

RESOURCES

Abo, A., Chen, L., Johnston, P., & Santucci, K. (2010). Positioning for lumbar puncture in children evaluated by bedside ultrasound. *Pediatrics, 125*, 1149–1153.

Arendt, K., Demaerschalk, B. M., Wingerchuck, D. M., & Camann, M. D. (2009). Atraumatic lumbar puncture needles after all these years, are we still missing the point? *Neurologist, 15*(1), 17–20.

Blaivas, M. (2012). *Emergency medicine: An international perspective.* Medicine Public Health.

Bonadio, W. (2014). Pediatric lumbar puncture and cerebrospinal fluid analysis. *Journal of Emergency Medicine, 46*(1), 141–150.

Brouwer, M. C., Tunkel, A. R., & Van de Beek, D. (2010). Epidemiology, diagnosis, and antimicrobial treatment of acute bacterial meningitis. *Clinical Microbiology Reviews, 23*(3), 467–492.

Chong, S. Y., Chong, L. A. & Ariffin, H. (2010). Accurate prediction of the needle depth required for successful lumbar puncture. *American Journal of Emergency Medicine, 28*, 603–606.

Cronan, K., & Wiley, J. (2008). Lumbar puncture. In F. M. Henretig & C. King (Eds.), *Textbook of pediatric emergency procedures* (2nd ed., p. 507). Philadelphia, PA: Lippincott, Williams, & Wilkins.

Crul, B. J., Gerritse, B. M., van Dongen, R. T., & Schoonderwaldt, H. C. (1999). Epidural fibrin glue injection stops persistent postdural puncture headache. *Anesthesiology, 91*(2), 576–577.

Czuczman, A. D., Thomas, L. E., Boulanger, A. B., Peak, D. A., Senecal, E. L., Brown, D. F., & Marill, K. A. (2013). Interpreting red blood cells in lumbar puncture: Distinguishing true subarachnoid hemorrhage from traumatic tap. *Academy of Emergency Medicine, 20*(3), 247–256.

Demaerschalk, B. M., & Wingerchuk, D. M. (2002). A traumatic dural puncture needles for preventing post-dural puncture headache: Meta-anaylsis of randomized controlled trials. *Neurology, 58*(3), A285–A286.

Dery, M. A., & Hasbun, R. (2007). Changing epidemiology of bacterial meningitis. *Current Infectious Disease Reports, 9*(4), 301–307.

Engedal, T. S., Ording, H., & Vilholm, O. J. (2015). Changing the needle for lumbar punctures results from a prospective study. *Clinical Neuro and Neurosurgery, 130*, 74–79.

Euerle, B. D. (2014). Spinal puncture and cerebrospinal fluid examination. In J. R. Roberts, & J. R. Hedges (Eds.), *Roberts and Hedges' clinical procedures in emergency medicine* (6th ed., pp. 1218–1242). Philadelphia, PA: Saunders.

Farzad, A., Radin, B., Oh, J. S., Teaque, H. M., Euerle, B. D., Nable, A. T., … Witting, M. D. (2013). Emergency diagnosis of subarachnoid hemorrhage: An evidence-based debate. *Journal of Emergency Medicine, 44*(5), 1045–1053.

Ferre, R. M., & Sweeney, T. W. (2007). Emergency physicians can easily obtain ultrasound images of anatomical landmarks relevant to lumbar puncture. *American Journal of Emergency Medicine, 25*, 291–296.

Glatstein, M., Zucker-Toledano, M., Arik, A., Scolnik, D., Oren, A., & Reif, S. (2011). Incidence of traumatic lumbar puncture experience of a large, tertiary care pediatric hospital. *Clinical Pediatric, 50*, 1005–1009.

Gupta, M., Barrett, T. W., & Schriger, D. L. (2013). Every peddler praises his own needle: Have clinical rules in the diagnosis of subarachnoid hemorrhage supplanted lumbar punctures yet? *Annals of Emergency Medicine, 62*(6), 633–640.

Halpern, S., & Preston, R. (1994). Postdural puncture headache and spinal needle design meta-analysis. *Anesthesiology, 81*, 1376–1383.

Hassen, G. W., Nazeer, O., Manizate, F., Patel, N., & Kalantari, H. (2014). The role of bedside ultrasound in pretherapeutic and posttherapeutic lumbar puncture in patient with idiopathic intracranial hypertension. *American Journal of Emergency Medicine, 32*, 1298.e3–e4.

Holst, D., Mollmann, M., Ebel, C., Hausman, R., & Wendt, M. (1998). In vitro investigation of cerebrospinal fluid leakage after dural puncture with various spinal needles. *Anesthesia and Analgesia, 87*, 1331–1335.

Hunter, B. R., & Seupaul, R. A. (2013). Are there pharmacologic agents that safely and effectively treat post-lumbar puncture headache? *Annals of Emergency Medicine, 61*(1), 84–85.

Kim, S., & Adler, D. K. (2014). Ultrasound-assisted lumbar puncture in pediatric emergency medicine. *Journal of Emergency Medicine, 47*(1), 59–64.

Lam, S. H. F., & Lambert, M. J. (2015). To the editor, in reply: Ultrasound-assisted lumbar puncture in pediatric patients. *Journal of Emergency Medicine, 48*(5), 611–612.

Liu, W. H., Lin, J. H., Lin, J. C., & Ma, H. I. (2008). Severe intracranial and intraspinal subarachnoid hemorrhage after lumbar puncture: A rare case report. *American Journal of Emergency Medicine, 26*, 633.e1–633.e3.

Lo, B. M., & Quinn, S. M. (2009). Gross xanthocromia on lumbar puncture may not represent an acute subarachnoid hemorrhage. *American Journal of Emergency Medicine, 27*, 621–623.

McCormack, R. F., & Hutson, A. (2010). Can computed tomography angiography of the brain replace lumbar puncture in the evaluation of acute-onset headache after a negative noncontrast cranial computed tomography scan? *Academy of Emergency Medicine, 7*, 444–415.

Moghtaderi, A., Alavi-Naini, R., & Sanatinia, S., (2012). Lumbar puncture: Techniques, complications and CSF analyses. In M. Blaivas (Ed.), *Emergency medicine: An international perspective* (pp. 43–62). Iran: InTech. Retrieved from http://www.intechopen.com/books/emergency-medicine-an-international-perspective/lumbar-puncture-techniques-complications-and-csf-analyses

Nomura, J. T., Leech, S. J., Shenbagamurthi, S., Sierzenski, P. R., O'Connor, R. E., Bollinger, M., … Gukhool, J. A. (2007). A randomized control trial of ultrasound-assisted lumbar puncture. *Journal of Ultrasound Medicine, 26,* 1341–1348.

Seupaul, R. A. (2007). How do I perform a lumbar puncture and analyze the results to diagnose bacterial meningitis? *Annals of Emergency Medicine, 50*(1), 85–87.

Shlamovitz, G. Z., & Lutsep, H. L. (2014). Lumbar puncture medication. *Medscape Drugs, Diseases & Procedures.* Retrieved from http://emedicine.medscape.com/article/80773-medication

Stiffler, K. A., Sharhabeel, J., Wilber, S. T., & Robinson, A. (2007). The use of ultrasound to identify pertinent landmarks for lumbar puncture. *American Journal of Emergency Medicine, 25,* 331–334.

Swaminathan, A., & Hom, J. (2014). Does ultrasonographic imaging reduce the risk of failed lumbar puncture? *Annals of Emergency Medicine, 63*(1), 33–34.

Turnbull, D. K., & Shepherd, D. B. (2003). Post-dural puncture headache: pathogenesis, prevention and treatment. *British Journal of Anaesthesia, 91*(5), 718–729.

Vermeulen, M. J., & Schull, M. J. (2007). Missed diagnosis of subarachnoid hemorrhage in the emergency department. *Stroke, 38,* 1216–1221.

Vettivel, S. (1991). Vertebral level of the termination of the spinal cord in human fetuses. *Journal of Anatomy, 179,* 149–161.

Younggren, B. N. (2008). Lumbar puncture and post-dural puncture headaches-letter to the editor. *Journal of Emergency Medicine.* doi:10.1016/j.jemermed.2008.12.018 http://www.cdc.gov/vaccines/schedules/hcp/imz/adult.html

Index

Note: Page numbers followed by "*f*" and "*t*" denote figures and tables, respectively